Culture, Religion and Childbearing
in a Multiracial Society

To the babies, of every culture, colour and creed. Each one of them deserves to be cherished and to be fully and joyfully welcomed into the world.

*   *   *

Nothing has changed except our attitudes, so everything has changed.

Anthony de Mello (1983) *Wellsprings*

Culture, Religion and Childbearing in a Multiracial Society

A handbook for health professionals

Judith Schott and **Alix Henley**

Foreword by Dora Opoku

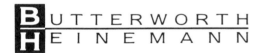
BUTTERWORTH
HEINEMANN

Butterworth-Heinemann
Linacre House, Jordan Hill, Oxford OX2 8DP
225 Wildwood Avenue, Woburn, MA 01801-2041
A division of Reed Educational and Professional Publishing Ltd

℞ A member of the Reed Elsevier plc group

OXFORD   AUCKLAND   BOSTON
JOHANNESBURG   MELBOURNE   NEW DELHI

First published 1996
Reprinted 1997, 2000, 2001

© Judith Schott and Alix Henley 1996

All rights reserved. No part of this publication
may be reproduced in any material form (including
photocopying or storing in any medium by electronic
means and whether or not transiently or incidentally
to some other use of this publication) without the
written permission of the copyright holder except in
accordance with the provisions of the Copyright,
Designs and Patents Act 1988 or under the terms of a
licence issued by the Copyright Licensing Agency Ltd,
90 Tottenham Court Road, London, England W1P 0LP.
Applications for the copyright holder's written permission
to reproduce any part of this publication should be addressed
to the publishers

British Library Cataloguing in Publication Data
Schott, Judith
    Culture, Religion and Childbearing in a
    Multiracial Society: Handbook for Health
    Professionals
    I. Title II. Henley, Alix
    362.198200941

ISBN 0 7506 2050 1

Composition by Genesis Typesetting, Laser Quay, Rochester, Kent
Printed and bound in Great Britain by
Athenæum Press Ltd, Gateshead, Tyne & Wear

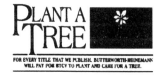

FOR EVERY TITLE THAT WE PUBLISH, BUTTERWORTH-HEINEMANN
WILL PAY FOR BTCV TO PLANT AND CARE FOR A TREE.

Contents

Foreword

Over the past ten years or so I have often found myself very frustrated, and indeed overwhelmed, when confronted with evidence which appears to support the view that certain maternity clients continue to experience cultural and religious insensitivity and hurt.

As this period coincides with a dramatic change in the thinking and practice of many people concerned with the provision of maternity care, perhaps some of you will understand why I have privately wondered whether the challenge that health professionals have set themselves – to identify and meet the needs of all the different cultural and religious groups – is attainable. Laudable though this goal is, how does such a huge organisation as the National Health Service equip all its staff to respect and value the cultural and religious needs of all clients?

I suspect that one response to this seemingly unassailable hurdle is for health professionals to make assumptions and generalisations which, on the face of it, can sometimes seem like useful short cuts. In their analysis, however, the authors of this book remind us of the drawbacks of stereotyping and the potential effects on relationships with clients/patients.

For me personally some of the most fascinating insights in *Culture, Religion and Childbearing in a Multiracial Society* come from hearing clients speak for themselves. For example, the Sikh mother who said '.... don't judge me by the way I look or dress. Talk to me and try to understand who I am not what I am' (page 11). I intend to keep reminding myself of these words. I had no difficulty in visualising the situations that clients spoke about and in some I could share the hurt and obvious disappointment.

My initial crisis of faith has therefore been lessened somewhat by knowing that this book is available and provides a systematic approach to the study of providing care in a multicultural society.

No one can reasonably expect any educational programme to completely prepare students for the many facets of this complex area. I believe, however, that everyone is responsible for identifying their own learning needs and for filling the gaps. The material contained in the five parts of this book provides a robust framework for study in an area which is arguably going to be one of the most challenging hurdles. I can only admire the impressive number of written sources which, together with interviews and discussions with professional people, clients and people of different religious and cultural groups, have been critically used to present a useful, analytical and worthwhile book.

Culture Religion and Childbearing in a Multiracial Society recognises and draws on the reader's knowledge and experience and invites health professionals to reflect on particular situations in their own sphere of work. A further strength of this inter-active approach is the ability of the authors to sustain the reader's interest.

Of course what this book cannot do is to claim that, as a result of its publication, all cultural and religious insensitivity in childbirth will disappear. It can, however, rightly claim that it contains up-to-date, extensive and well-sourced material on a wide variety of relevant issues which should prove invaluable to anyone who makes 'a personal effort and commitment to let go of old assumptions and practices and open themselves to new ways of thinking and doing things'.

I feel honoured to have been given this opportunity and offer the authors my wholehearted congratulations for the skill, sensitivity and breadth of vision they have brought to the task of writing this book. It fulfils a real need.

Dora Opoku, RGN, RM, MTD, BEd(Hons), MA
Head of Midwifery Education
St Bartholomews School of Nursing and Midwifery

The authors

Judith Schott is a freelance writer and trainer with PROSPECT. She has worked in and around the health service, as a health professional, an antenatal teacher, a consumer representative and researcher. Her particular interest is in devising and running experiential training for health professionals in order to support them in their work of providing optimal care. She runs workshops throughout the UK on various topics including: parent education; communication skills; loss and grief; team building, stress management, and culture, religion and childbearing. She is co-author with Judy Priest of *Leading Antenatal Classes: a Practical Guide*, published by Butterworth-Heinemann and, with AVERT, of *AIDS and Childbirth*. She lives in London.

Alix Henley is a freelance writer, researcher and consultant. She specializes in matters to do with health and health care and has a particular interest in communication between professionals and consumers and in equal opportunity issues. Her most recent books include *Equality in Action: Introducing Equal Opportunities in Voluntary Organisations*, written with Mee-Yan Cheung-Judge and published by NCVO Publications; *When a Baby Dies: the Experience of Late Miscarriage, Stillbirth and Neonatal Death*, published by Pandora, and *Miscarriage, Stillbirth and Neonatal Death: Guidelines for Professionals* for the UK Stillbirth and Neonatal Death Society, both written with Nancy Kohner. At present she is living in Switzerland.

They have previously worked together on *Breaking the Barriers: A Training Package on Equal Access to Maternity Services*, available from the Obstetric Hospital, University College London Hospitals, NHS Trust.

Note to readers

Writing anything about people's needs, beliefs and lifestyles is like walking a tightrope. So called 'facts' that health professionals might perceive as 'useful information' may in practice be misleading or even cause offence. It is essential to avoid stereotypes and generalisations and to show the subtleties and variety that exist within each culture. It is important to help people think sensitively about providing care for people whose culture they do not share. This is what we have tried to do.

For these reasons permission to reproduce any material in any form from this book must be sought from the authors who will wish to ensure that the context in which the material will be used is consistent with this philosophy and approach.

Judith Schott and Alix Henley

Acknowledgements

This book would not exist without the help we have received from many people. We would like to thank everyone and in particular, the people of different cultures and religions who were willing to be interviewed and to read what we subsequently wrote. Meeting and listening to them was a privilege. We are indebted to everyone who trusted us enough to invite us into their workplace and into their homes and who answered our questions, bore with our ignorance and our occasional inadvertent insensitivity and helped us to discover the questions we did not even know we needed to ask. Each one of them helped us to examine and re-examine our own attitudes and assumptions and taught us a great deal. We are grateful to them for their patience, tolerance and encouragement and for reminding us that although there are cultural and religious variations between people, fundamentally we all share many more similarities than differences.

We should like to thank, in particular, Jyoti Ahluwalia, Aisha Ahmed, Lindsey Ahmet, Shanaz Akhtar, Iman Ali, Esther Amidu, Jill Aston, Bridget Baker, Rajes Bala, Nicky Barnard, Sara Barnett, Carol Bates, Jo Begent, Valerie Betts, Marti Biswas, Alan Brash, Elizabeth Buggins, Auriol Burrows, Mee-Yan Cheung-Judge, Shelly Choudhery, Alice Clifton, Ruth Cochrane, Daphne Crossfield, Lemuel Crossfield, Cherry Cunningham, Champa Desei, Frances Drain, Dr Ian Ellis, Myra Farnworth, Dr Yohannes Fassil, Ann Ferreira, Ros Finlay, Amira Fletcher, Donald Franklin, Jo Garcia, Dr A.R. Gatrad, Carla Gavsey Jacobs, Supinder Ghatora, Jonathan Gibbs, Jagdev Gilbert, Penny Gillinson, Jill Gingell, Gulçin Gökul, Jane Grant, Sheila Gray, Members of the Church of Haile Selassie 1, Rashida Hunzai, Mohamoud Omer Ibrahim, Suryakala Jacob, Lea Jamieson, Naveen Jeevan, Saryu Joshi, Gulshan Karbani, Lila Kibria and the Health Aides at the Royal London Hospital, Nancy Kohner, Estriana Lewin, Louise Long, Alison Macfarlane, Amran Mahmoud and Aisha Ahmed at the Somali Women's Centre, David Malyon, Lesley Marks, Ingred Mariott, Mary McCaffrey, Vicky McIntosh, Kathy McKnight, Sabera Mirza, Dr R.F.M. Mueller, Bill Nathanson, Jo Naylor, Joan Nelson, Nancy Ng, Mary Nolan, Bridget Okereke, Lola Oni, Dora Opoku, Greta Ottway, Pauline Palmer, Regina Parry, Minat Patel, Pushpa Patel, Maria Peppos, Rabbi Alan Plancey, Hansa Patel-Kanwal at the Naz Project, Kem Kit Poon, Jackie Powell, George Priest, Anne Rider, Ruth Rosenfelder, Jacqueline Rothschild, Walter Rothschild, Kai Rudat, Carla Rusconi, Agnes Sampare Kwateng, Caroline Shepherd, Shabnam Sharma, Aliya Sheikh, Rabbi Dr Nissan Shulman, Dr Maurice Sifman, Pastor Paul Sinclair, Joan Small, Sonia Stewart, Richard Taylor, Veronica Taylor, Kirpal Vedwan, Judy

Walder, Gem Wason, Marie Webb, Dee Wheater, Moya de Wet, Allyson Williams, Dianne Williams Trottman, Richard Willis, Kuang Peng Wong, Saulan Yim, Tina Young, and Fawzia Zaidi. We are also grateful for the encouragement and help we received from many health professionals, and particularly from Susan Devlin of Butterworth-Heinemann whose unfailing faith, support and flexibility have been invaluable.

We should also like to express our appreciation of Hansy Josovic who contributed to this book shortly before her untimely death. Her work to ensure that the needs of women in her community were met is a model to us all.

Despite all the help we have received we may have made mistakes or unwittingly caused offence. We take full responsibility for this and apologize.

Our thanks also go to both our families who have lived with this book throughout its long gestation. Fred Adelmann and Geoff Schott have tolerated large telephone bills and have supported us both emotionally, practically and financially. Tana, Sofia and Robbie Adelmann have been more patient than was reasonable. Lotti Henley acted as courier between London and Basel, stepped in from time to time to run the Basel household and gave invaluable practical help. Benjamin Schott bailed us out when our word processors refused to collaborate. Geoff and Jonathan Schott kept an eye on the medical literature for us and tracked down papers and references. Between them Lotti, Fred, Geoff, Jonathan and Benjamin have also read and commented on various drafts and from time to time challenged our thinking and broadened our view.

The logos were designed by Helen Chown, BA (Hons) Fine Art, to whom we offer many thanks.

We are grateful to Camden and Islington Health Authority, London, for permission to reproduce some of the material previously published in *Caring in a Multiracial Society* by Alix Henley. We are also very grateful to Ros Morpeth and the National Extension College (NEC), Cambridge for permission to reproduce some of the material by Alix Henley previously published in their publications *Health Care in Multiracial Britain* (1985) (co-authored with Penny Mares and Carol Baxter), *Asian Names and Records* (1981), *Caring for Muslims and their families* (1982), *Caring for Hindus and their Families* (1983), *Caring for Sikhs and their Families* (1983), and *Caring for Everyone: Ensuring Standards of Care for Black and Ethnic Minority Patients* (1991). For more information about all NEC publications, contact NEC Customer Services, 18 Brooklands Avenue, Cambridge CB2 2HN. Tel. 01223–316644.

Crown copyright material is reproduced with the permission of the Controller of Her Majesty's Stationery Office.

The label 'multi-ethnic Britain' will, to many people, still signify just its ethnic minority communities. This, of course is wrong. Multi-ethnic Britain means **all** of Britain and all of its people. Britain **is** multi-ethnic just as it **is** a parliamentary democracy.

Herman Ouseley, Chairman of Commission for Racial Equality, 1994

Every woman has unique needs. In addition to those arising from her medical history these will derive from her particular ethnic, cultural, social and family background. The services provided should recognise the special characteristics of the population they are designed to serve. They should also be attractive to all women, particularly those who might be less inclined to use them.

Changing Childbirth, 1993

The NHS must address the particular needs of the black and ethnic minorities living in this country, and take positive steps to eliminate discrimination.

Chief Medical Officer, 1991

As a registered nurse, midwife or health visitor, you are personally accountable for your practice and, in the exercise of your professional accountability, must recognise and respect the uniqueness and dignity of each patient and client, and respond to their need for care, irrespective of their ethnic origin, religious beliefs, personal attributes, the nature of their health problem or any other factor.

UKCC Code of Professional Conduct, 1992

Introduction

Britain, like most other countries, is a multiracial, multicultural society. The major period of New Commonwealth immigration that followed the Second World War was part of a process that has gone on for many centuries. The legacies of industrialisation, European imperialism and colonialism, combined with modern mass media and transport, have made the movement and settlement of people a permanent feature of our world. Over 90 per cent of the independent states in the world are now ethnically mixed, containing people of different origins, cultures and religions (Cheung-Judge, 1993).

The needs of parents

Whatever our cultural origins or our religious beliefs and practices, we all need to feel that we are respected, accepted, valued and understood. This is especially important for people embarking on the adventure of parenthood. Pregnancy, birth and the transition to parenthood are major life events, accompanied by heightened sensitivity and vulnerability. They can be positive and life-enhancing, but they can also be traumatic and demoralising. The quality of care and the support that parents receive crucially affect their response to these challenges, how they feel about themselves and their baby, and their ability to care for their family in the future.

Over the past ten years there has been a dramatic change in the thinking and practice of many people concerned with the provision of maternity care. It is now widely accepted that providing the same inflexible services for everyone, of however high a standard, cannot meet the needs of all the different groups that make up our society. Policy documents at all levels, including the government's Patients' Charter, acknowledge the importance of providing care that takes full account of different cultures and language barriers, and that deals with racial discrimination.

But knowing what the goal is does not necessarily mean knowing how to achieve it. Change requires personal effort and commitment, letting go of old assumptions and practices, and opening up to new ways of thinking and doing things. The racial prejudices and attitudes that are the legacy of Britain's imperial and colonial past also make change in this area more difficult. Unconscious as well as conscious resistance and hostility lead some health professionals to oppose changes that would increase equality of access to health care for members of black and minority ethnic groups. There are still people who feel that the issues will go away if they are ignored, that members of minority groups who maintain cultural and other differences are in some way less entitled to appropriate services, or that racism is not a major factor in health and health care.

The needs of a multiracial, multicultural society are a major challenge to everyone involved in providing, managing or purchasing health care. Skill, imagination, knowledge and self-awareness are needed to deliver high-quality care to people of different cultures and religions, and to challenge the discrimination built into so many of our existing systems. Health professionals need to start by reflecting on how services are currently organised and examining the assumptions which underlie them. They need time, information and support, as well as opportunities to examine their own beliefs and ideas so that they can re-assess what they do and work out how to improve care for cultural and religious minorities.

The role of information

Information about many of the cultural and religious issues that surround childbearing has not been readily accessible, and one of the aims of this book is to bring such information together. However, 'facts' about culture or religion are, for many reasons, not the answer. No set of 'facts' applies to any one individual. Culture and religion are only two of many factors that may influence people's needs and wishes, and no culture or religion is static, especially when its members are in a minority. None of us wants to be treated as a stereotyped bundle of facts, however accurate; we are all individuals. Good care is only possible when we find from each client what her own wishes, needs and concerns are. As one mother told us, 'I want someone who thinks **with** me, not **for** me'.

We therefore do not see this book, nor want it to be seen, as providing a set of answers which can simply be applied to people of certain cultural or religious groups. Our primary belief and message is that the answers lie with each individual woman and her family. At the same time, if health professionals are to identify and meet the needs of different religious and cultural groups, they need a framework of knowledge as well as increased self-awareness. In this book we offer both, and hope that the benefits of the information-based sections outweigh their potential disadvantages.

A note to readers in different countries

In this book we look at different cultures and religions primarily from the perspectives of Britain, the British health care system, and traditional English culture. However, the issues we address apply to all multiracial societies. The ideas and principles can be used to reflect on any system of health care in order to meet the needs of women and families of different cultures and religions.

ABOUT THIS BOOK

The book is divided into five sections. Each is followed by a list of references and recommended further reading. Certain ideas and themes are repeated in different sections of the book because we realise that many people will not read straight through from beginning to end and will need to consult different sections at different times.

Part One discusses the concepts of culture, 'race' and difference and looks at inequalities in health and health care and the importance of equal access to care. It also includes opportunities for personal reflection, because our own beliefs and assumptions about people of different origins, cultures or creeds are likely to affect the care we give.

Part Two focuses on communication skills, the foundation of all good health care. It looks at the skills and awareness needed to communicate across cultural and language barriers, including ways of working well with professional interpreters. It also outlines different naming systems and how to address and identify people correctly.

Part Three looks at areas of everyday life and at a range of childbearing issues from the perspective of a number of cultural and religious groups. It includes opportunities for reflection as a basis for understanding and responding to other people's perspectives and needs.

Part Four covers health issues that have specific relevance to certain cultural or religious minorities.

Part Five focuses on five traditional cultures and seven religions in relation to everyday life and maternity care. The content is based on what we have learned from meetings and discussions with people of different cultural and religious groups.

Caution!

Some readers may be tempted to turn to Part Five first, to find out, for example, about Jews, Sikhs or Chinese people. We strongly urge you not to do this but to read and reflect on Parts One to Three first. Only by understanding our own culture-based beliefs and values can we avoid stereotyping and develop a sensitive and intelligent understanding of what the issues **might** be for people of other groups or communities. And only then can we usefully find out from each client what she or he really needs.

LANGUAGE AND SOME DEFINITIONS

The power of language in defining and creating attitudes to individuals and groups is increasingly understood. Each of us is very sensitive to the terms used, particularly by others, to define us or the groups we belong to. Part of respecting people is listening to and respecting the way they define themselves and the labels they use. In this book we have tried to use terms that are acceptable to members of the communities we are talking about, but language and awareness are constantly developing, and in many cases there is no term that is universally accepted by every member of a particular group.

People's views of what is acceptable also changes with time, whereas the words we have used here are necessarily fixed on the printed page and cannot change. Where we have used words and phrases that are offensive or unacceptable to some of our readers we should like to apologize. It is our intention to increase mutual respect and understanding, not in any way to diminish or insult people.

BCE   (Before the Common Era) is used as an alternative to BC which has a specifically Christian reference point. **CE** (Common Era) is used as an alternative to AD.

Black   The term increasingly used by people of African-Caribbean, African and South Asian origin as well as others to underline the unity of their experience of discrimination on grounds of skin colour (Mares, Henley and Baxter, 1985).

Black and minority ethnic groups   Means the same as minority ethnic groups (see below) but may be more acceptable to many people who define themselves as black rather than as members of a minority ethnic group (Runnymede Trust, 1994).

British   Refers to everyone living in Britain, whatever their heritage. A statement of nationality and residence.

Client   Used in this book to refer to women and their partners. We appreciate that this term is not universally accepted and that many health professionals consider the word patient more appropriate. However, patient has connotations of passivity, dependence and potential ill health. People using maternity services are, on the whole, healthy and it is vital for their future role as parents that their autonomy is respected and their self-esteem enhanced.

Equal access   Ensuring that an organization's policies and practices do not result in any group receiving less favourable treatment on grounds that are not material; for example, 'race', colour, ethnic or national origin, creed, gender, marital status, class, disability or sexuality (Cheung-Judge and Henley, 1994).

English   Used in this book for convenience and for lack of comprehensible alternatives when discussing contemporary white British culture, though in full recognition of the limitations of the term, and without any intention of causing offence to white people of Scottish, Welsh or Irish heritage.

Ethnic group   A social group with a distinctive language, values, religion, customs and attitudes (Hillier, 1991). Also used in majority ethnic group (roughly speaking, the white British) and minority ethnic groups.

Health professional   Used in this book to refer to everyone working in health care, whether in hospitals or in the community, who comes into direct contact with clients, or whose work influences the way care is given. This includes hospital doctors, general practitioners, midwives, health visitors, nursery nurses, neonatal nurses, physiotherapists, gynaecology nurses, family planning nurses, receptionists and clerks, hospital and community managers and those purchasing services.

Immigrant   A person who was born in another country and has settled in Britain.

Midwife   In some sections of the book, in particular where the issue of modesty is discussed, we imply that all midwives are women. We have done this for the sake of brevity and apologize to the small and growing number of male midwives who also fulfil the role of being 'with woman'.

Minority ethnic groups or communities   Groups or communities which are distinguished in some way from the majority by, for example, their skin colour, their first language, or their religion.

New Commonwealth   The official term used to indicate Commonwealth countries whose populations are predominantly black, for example, India, Pakistan, Bangladesh, the West Indies, Nigeria, Ghana and Kenya.

Old Commonwealth The official term used to indicate Commonwealth countries whose populations are predominantly white, for example, Australia, New Zealand and Canada.

Racism Conscious or unconscious belief in the superiority of a particular 'race'. Acts of discrimination and unfair treatment, whether intentional or unintentional, based on this belief.

South Asian People born in India, Pakistan, Bangladesh and Sri Lanka – the Indian subcontinent – or descended from people born in those countries.

References

Cheung-Judge, L. M. (1993) *Equal Opportunities in Management Education and Development*, Q & E Consultancy Services, 18–24 Middle Way, Oxford

Cheung-Judge, M. Y. and Henley, A. (1994) *Equality in Action: Introducing Equal Opportunities in Voluntary Organisations*, NCVO Publications, London

Hillier, S. (1991) The health and health care of ethnic minority groups. In *Sociology as Applied to Medicine* (ed. G. Scambler), Bailiere Tindall, London

Mares, P., Henley, A. and Baxter, C. (1985) *Health Care in Multiracial Britain*, National Extension College, Cambridge

Runnymede Trust (1994) *Multi-ethnic Britain: Facts and Trends*, Runnymede Trust, London

Part One Culture, 'Race' and Health Care

1 Culture and difference

None of us is simply a package of culture. We are all affected by a myriad of different influences and, above all, each of us has our own unique personality. But our culture, the culture of the society or community in which we grew up, is one of the key influences on the way each of us sees and reacts to the world, and on the way we behave. In some ways the effects of culture on each of us cannot be overestimated. Almost everything in our behaviour is influenced by our culture. At the same time it is important to bear in mind that culture is a framework, not a straitjacket. Within our own culture there is a wide range of choices and options for each of us, a million ways in which we express our individuality and live our unique lives. When working across cultures, therefore, we need **both** to be aware of the possibilities that may exist within a culture other than our own, **and** to avoid assuming that any individual will conform to a particular cultural pattern.

WHAT IS CULTURE?

Culture is a shared set of norms, values, assumptions and perceptions (both explicit and implicit), and social conventions which enable members of a group, community or nation to function cohesively. Our culture vitally affects every aspect of our daily life, how we live, think and behave and how we view and analyse the world. But because, like the air we breathe, our culture is all around us from the day of our birth, and because we acquire almost all of it unconsciously in early childhood, most of us grow up unaware that we have a culture at all. We often also find it hard to distinguish, even in ourselves, what is cultural from what is individual or personal (Helman, 1986; Hoecklin, 1993; Hofstede, 1991; Keesing, 1981; Reber, 1985; Trompenaars, 1993). We may not realise that what we regard as normal, universal values and ways of behaving are in fact cultural, and may therefore be normal only to us.

Although most aspects of culture are invisible and intangible, some are apparent. Hofstede (1991) compares culture to the layers of an onion; Trompenaars (1993) also uses a model of culture with concentric layers.

- The outer layer, **artefacts and products** (see Figure 1.1) consists of things which can be seen, heard, tasted or otherwise observed fairly easily. These include, for example, the way we dress, the food we eat, our buildings and the way we fill and use them, written and spoken language, and art.

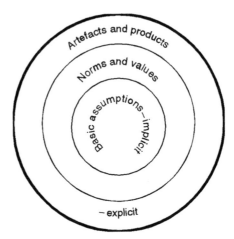

Figure 1.1 A model of culture. (Reproduced from *Riding the Waves of Culture: Understanding Cultural Diversity in Business* by Fons Trompenaars 1993. Nicholas Brealey Publishing Ltd, by permission)

- The middle layer consists of the shared **norms and values** of our group, community or society; shared ideas about how people should behave, about right and wrong, good and bad. These can usually be put into words when necessary, though within any culture most people take them for granted as normal and even universal.
- The inner layer consists of the implicit, **basic assumptions** of our society or community, based on solutions that have been developed over centuries in response to local geography, climate and available resources. These are so fundamental that they are both unconscious and absolutely self-evident to the members of the society that holds them. They underpin the other two layers.

Culture is not genetically inherited. It is acquired during childhood when we absorb the basic values and norms by which our family, our society and community live. Hofstede (1991) sees culture as one layer of our 'mental programming' (see Figure 1.2). He also identifies two other layers of human mental programming:

- Human nature – inherited, universal characteristics, needs and abilities that all human beings share, such as the ability to feel emotions. (How people express their emotions is partly influenced by their culture.)
- Personality – mental programmes, both inherited and learnt, that are unique to each individual.

Within every society there are also 'micro-cultures'; families, social groups, religious groups and occupational groups all have, to some extent, their own cultures. Organisations too have their own micro-cultures which people adapt to, often unconsciously, when they join. Each of us is therefore not only affected by the wider culture of our society or community, but also by several micro-cultures.

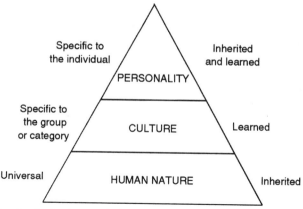

Figure 1.2 Three levels of uniqueness in human mental programming. (Reproduced from *Cultures and Organisations. Software of the Mind* by Geert Hofstede 1991. McGraw-Hill Book Company, by permission)

Cultural differences

The cultural values and norms that individuals learn differ from one society to another. What makes sense and is normal and acceptable to people in one culture may be odd, shocking or even completely abhorrent to people in another. Few values are universal. Every culture makes sense to the people within it (though they may not like every aspect of it). Part of treating individuals with respect involves respecting and trying to understand their culture and values as they see them.

> In German-speaking Switzerland people believe strongly that children should remain almost exclusively with their mothers until they are seven years old and start school. Even then, most children only go to school for two or three hours a day until they are eleven. All children and almost all fathers come home for a cooked lunch every day. It is expected and assumed that mothers will remain at home all day. Mothers who work even part-time are widely disapproved of and are sometimes called 'crow mothers'.

> In traditional South Asian culture marriages are arranged. This is regarded as the best way to ensure a successful life-long marriage and the stability of the whole extended family. Parents and older relatives are involved in the selection of a suitable partner. They know and understand the young people involved and the kind of partner who will be most suitable for them. Parents who do not arrange a marriage for their children are often strongly disapproved of for neglecting one of their most important parental duties.

> In contemporary English culture marriage is regarded as the business of the two young people concerned. Parents, close relatives and friends may give an opinion if asked, but usually do not for fear of being thought to intrude. Increasingly, young English couples live together before marriage or decide to live in a stable partnership without getting married. Some people then decide to marry before they have children or once a baby is on the way. People generally have high emotional expectations of the marital relationship and may decide to end the marriage if these are not fulfilled. The emotional aspects of marriage are generally regarded as the most important.

Take a moment to reflect on your own experience of being in a different culture. You may find the following exercise helpful.

Think back to a time, maybe when you were a child, when you felt out of place. Perhaps you stayed with another family or started a new school.

■ How did the 'culture' in which you found yourself differ from your own?
■ How did you find out what the unwritten and unspoken rules were, what was acceptable or unacceptable?
■ How did you feel?

In this situation it is likely that there were more similarities than differences between your culture and the culture into which you moved. But you probably did not notice the similarities nearly as much as the differences. And the people you were with probably also noticed mainly what was different about the way you behaved.

'People fail to appreciate that our culture and traditions are of equal value and that they were evolved in response to the land and to the situation in which they arose.'   South Asian midwife

Changes and variations within cultures

Culture is not fixed or static. The culture of a nation varies between and within regions. Cultures also change over time in response to new situations and pressures. Frequently the practical adaptations that people have to make in response to external circumstances then seep into and change their culture.

Some societies and communities change faster than others. Since the Industrial Revolution, for example, the pace of cultural change in Western Europe and North America has been unprecedented. Rack wrote of Britain in 1982:

'In the last twenty years the list of conventions that have been challenged, shibboleths abandoned, hierarchies dismantled, and moral restrictions lifted is a very long one indeed. Social inequality, acquisitive materialism, and the subordination of women have all come under fire. The public face of sexual morality has altered entirely, and the institution of marriage is under attack. Innovations in music and the other arts have been bewilderingly rapid. Dress and speech are no longer the insignia of class. Hair can be worn long, short, absent altogether or green and purple. The pace of social change is unparalleled, and appeals to tradition are greeted with derision'. (From Rack, 1991, p.67, by permission)

The speed of change has not diminished since then. Not everyone is happy about some of these changes, especially those that affect people's family and personal lives. But cultural change is a powerful force, and it is difficult for individuals to withstand it.

Some societies are more conservative, either because they are not confronted by the same pressures to change, or because their culture contains strong features that enable it to withstand such pressures. Societies that are more religious may, for example, be slower to change. Communities that are uprooted from their own society may also become more conservative, often as a response to fear of losing their identity in the face of external pressures. British expatriate communities during the period of the Empire and since, for example, have often been more 'old-fashioned' than their contemporaries in Britain. Similar patterns occurred among some South Asian communities in East Africa (Roberts, 1977).

ATTITUDES TOWARDS DIFFERENT CULTURES

Us and them

> However we conceive of our group, whether a class, nation or a race, we define it by those we exclude from it ... However we define them, we perceive them as an undifferentiated mass with no individual variations. (Littlewood and Lipsedge, 1989)

We learn about our own culture from a very early age. Babies and young children are acute observers. We copy the things that adults say and do, and the way that they say and do them. If we behave in ways that do not fit in with the culture of our family or peers, we are left in no doubt about their disapproval. So we are strongly encouraged to conform, to fit in with accepted, though often unspoken, norms of right and wrong, of behaviour, speech, dress, language and manners. A child from a religious family is taught an additional and specific set of values and beliefs and learns what is acceptable to her or his particular religious group. Although many of us may rebel against some of these values, especially in adolescence, they remain a subtle yet powerful influence on us throughout our lives.

As we learn what is acceptable within our own culture and/or religion, the foundations for regarding difference with suspicion are laid. If we are taught that what we do and how we do it are 'correct' and 'right', we can be forgiven for assuming, however unconsciously, that people who do things differently are wrong and less deserving of our respect.

In extreme cases differences may be labelled pathological. In the former Soviet Union dissidents who expressed political views which were different from the ruling group ran the risk of being incarcerated in psychiatric hospitals. In societies where one ethnic group is dominant, the cultural practices and values of groups which differ from the majority 'norm' are all too easily regarded as deviant, wrong or pathological, and there is but a small step from 'cultural' to clinical pathology (Smaje, 1995).

Inaccurate information about other groups

Much of the information we get from the media, our peers and our families about societies or groups other than our own is also inaccurate. It often focuses on differences and on negative characteristics (real or imagined) while ignoring the qualities we all share. In many cases it plays on our fears. Extremes and the bizarre make better entertainment than normal people living ordinary lives. Few of us would want to be judged on the basis of the most extreme or notorious members of our group or society. Few of us would want people in other countries to think that the headlines of our tabloid newspapers accurately represent our values and those of our families.

Stereotyping, misinformation and prejudice are also perpetuated through jokes. The British make jokes about the Irish, the Canadians about New-foundlanders and so on. Jews forestall others by telling jokes against themselves, but can be deeply offended when similar jokes are told by non-Jews. Such 'humour' helps boost the sense of superiority of the teller and his or her group.

Assumptions and stereotyping

'No matter where I go or who I am, as an Asian I am stereotyped. There is an assumption that I don't speak English and that because I am not white and middle class, I am not well educated.'   South Asian midwife teacher

'White people don't see me, they see my colour and they automatically judge me negatively. But when I speak, you can almost see them having to change their minds as I sound very English and cultured.'   African-Caribbean woman

Stereotyping is an intellectually crude and limiting way of understanding (or seeming to understand) individuals (Modood, 1990). We all use stereotypes and assumptions to make sense of the world, and to save time and effort. We make assumptions based on what we know or what we *think* we know. This can be particularly true of health professionals who are traditionally expected (by themselves and by society in general) to have all the answers and always to know what to do and when to do it.

The further people are from our own experience and the less we know about them the more we tend to stereotype them. We do not, for example, usually stereotype members of our family and close friends. We do tend to stereotype people in groups that we do not belong to and that we know little about. The less we know about a person the more we tend to rely on stereotypes in deciding what they are like and what they need, especially if there is also a language barrier (Bowler, 1993). But stereotypes have a life and a quality of their own. They are often negative, belittling or even hostile (Green, *et al.*, 1990). They are useless as a basis for delivering sensitive individual care.

To see how stereotypes can work, cover the box below and try reading the lines one at a time. Think about the assumptions that come to your mind and observe how they change as you read.

- Mrs X is in her thirties,
- she is pregnant,
- she has two school-age children,
- she speaks five languages,
- her husband is a consultant surgeon,
- she is a head teacher,
- she is Bengali.

Which of these statements tells you most about Mrs X? None of them. They all offer you possibilities, but Mrs X is no more defined by the fact that she is Bengali than by the fact that she is pregnant. All these facts about her are true. All of them affect her in some way (only she can tell you how) but she is more than the sum of all of them, and only by asking her will you find out what she needs.

Identity

In reality, all of us have many different identities. Our ethnic or cultural identity is only one of these. Depending on where we are and who we are with, different identities may become more important. When we are with our children, we may be primarily parents and the professional part of us may move out of the foreground. At work, we may become entirely professional and forget that we even have children. With people who know us socially, or within our religious community, other identities may be more important.

Many people also have multiple ethnic or cultural identities. Some are of mixed heritage. Some are the children or grandchildren of immigrants, who have learnt to operate effectively in two or more cultures, taking and adapting what they consider most valuable from each, and moving smoothly between them.

'I was born and brought up in North London. My parents came from the West Indies when they were children. My father is African-Caribbean with one black parent and one white parent. My mother's family are Asian. In my family there has been intermarriage like this for several generations. I suppose I would describe myself as black but I get fed up with people assuming they know where I 'come from'. Some call

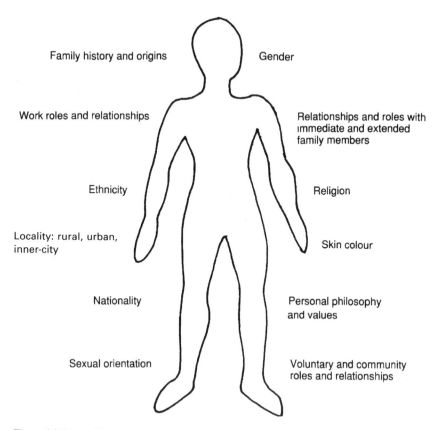

Figure 1.3 Some of the influences that may contribute to an individual's identities

me West Indian and I have also been called a Paki. Just as well my father brought me up to stand up for myself and not to put up with that sort of racist nonsense.'   Young black woman

'I was born and brought up in the UK. My mother is English and my father was a German Jewish refugee, but I'm not sure where I really belong. There are bits of both that I really like and bits I'm uncomfortable with. I do know that in some circumstances I am careful about disclosing my Jewish identity. Orthodox Jews don't consider me to be Jewish at all and that denies an important part of me. With Gentiles I prefer people to know me as an individual first and to judge me on my own merits rather than making assumptions about me based on any pre-conceived ideas or prejudices about Jews. Once I think people know me for who I am, I often say I am partly Jewish, if only to explode the stereotypes! That's a luxury my black friends don't have. They cannot hide or escape people's assumptions and prejudices about who they are and what they are like.'   Mother of two

Our identities are influenced by many factors including the culture(s) in which we grew up, our gender and sexual orientation, our 'race', our position in the family, our occupation(s), our experiences and our personal situation.

Using Figure 1.3 as a starting point, you may like to make a list of your own identities, including the different relationships you have with various members of your family.

■ How do your different identities emerge in different situations.
■ Which are most important to you?
■ How do you feel when other people focus on one aspect of your identity (probably the one most visible to them) and ignore others which are equally or more important to you?

'When people see me they simply see an 'Asian woman'. What I would like is to be seen as a normal human being with normal feelings, wants and needs. I may have different cultural perspectives but I still buy my knickers at Marks and Spencer's. Don't section me off and treat me differently. I don't want to be put in a separate category from white, British people.'   South Asian health worker

First impressions

Many people place great value on first impressions and consider them reliable. Research confirms that judgements made on the basis of first impressions are powerful and difficult to reverse. We are particularly unlikely to change our minds if our first impression is negative (Roberts, 1985).

Obvious physical characteristics, such as skin colour, gender, age and physical ability, form a crucial part of our first impressions. If we have negative stereotypes about people who are, for example, black or male or overweight or physically disabled, these contribute towards our initial judgement. We then tend to behave towards the person on the basis of that judgement, setting up a circle of misunderstanding. Even when it becomes apparent that a stereotype is not true, people find it hard to adjust their assumptions.

'I was at a consultants' dinner at the hospital where my husband worked and I sat next to a senior physician. Halfway through the meal he turned to me and asked in a rather patronising way, "And what do you do, my dear?" I said I also worked in the Health Service. "You are a secretary or a receptionist," he said. I began to answer but he cut me off: "Then you must be a nurse." "Actually no," I said, "I'm a doctor." "In general practice are you?" he said, seeming slightly put out. "Well, not really," I said. "You work in a hospital? You are a registrar in geriatrics or psychiatry", he said condescendingly. "Actually, I'm a consultant thoracic surgeon," I said. You should have seen his face!' Fifty-year-old woman

Gender, age, skin colour and other things that help create a first impression are merely the visible tip of the iceberg. They do not reveal the myriad of qualities and attributes which make up the character of each human being. They convey nothing about an individual's history and background, educational attainments, values, beliefs, experience, knowledge, skills or wishes. But they are often used as a basis for making assumptions about people and a 'reason' for treating them in certain ways.

Think back to a time when someone made an inaccurate assumption or judgement about you.

■ How did you feel?
■ How did you react and behave?
■ How did it affect your attitude to the person who made that assumption?
■ How did you react to them afterwards?

The dangers of stereotyping

'Stereotyping – I find that the hardest thing. Don't judge me by the way I look or dress. Talk to me and try to understand **who** *I am not* **what** *I am.'* Sikh mother

Assumptions and generalisations can sometimes seem like useful short cuts, but they block our ability to understand and communicate and to meet clients' real needs.

Rachel and David were visited by the health visitor soon after Joshua's birth. Rachel was confused and alarmed by the un-asked for, detailed information she was given about the content of various baby milks which, because they contained animal products, were apparently not suitable for her baby. She worried that the health visitor knew that Joshua had some kind of problem with his digestion. She felt that the problem must be serious if the doctors had not told her about it. It later emerged, that because they live in an area where there are a large number of Jews and had names which could be Jewish, the health visitor had assumed that they too were Orthodox Jews and ate only kosher food. Rachel and David are Catholics.

A Health Education Authority survey (HEA, 1994) found that a high percentage of Bangladeshi and Pakistani women had never had a cervical smear test. It is often assumed that a low take-up of smear tests is inevitable among these communities because of religious prohibitions or modesty. In fact, the survey found that the main problem was that women did not know what a smear test was and/or had never been called for one. Embarrassment and fear accounted for only about 5 per cent of those women who had not had a smear test.

People whose needs and behaviour are unfamiliar to health professionals are often treated as if they are strange or abnormal, or are regarded as a nuisance. Nobody should be labelled difficult simply because of their culture, religion or skin colour. Each person should be seen as an individual who deserves respect, and responsive and appropriate care.

Sharon and Geoff were expecting their first baby, They read a lot and attended National Childbirth Trust classes. Like many couples in their area, they wanted to know exactly what would be done and why and were keen to exercise choice and control over the care Sharon received during pregnancy and birth. However, the reactions of their carers were negative and unhelpful. The staff in that district had become used to responding positively to the demands of white middle-class women, but Sharon and Geoff, who are black, were perceived as aggressive, difficult and demanding. They did not receive the information and care that they asked for.

The dangers of ignorance

Equally dangerous and damaging is the failure to recognise that in a plural society the same norms and assumptions cannot be applied to everyone. It may be necessary to re-assess existing practices, or to try to find out more about the needs and wishes of clients of different communities.

'During the 1980s there was a very high incidence of "small for dates babies" amongst the Bengali women we were looking after. As a result many of them were induced or delivered by Caesarean section. This continued until someone realised that the definition of "normal" we were using was based on Caucasians and that measuring Bengalis against this scale was totally inappropriate.'   Community midwife

'A West African woman who spoke no English refused to eat in hospital. Every time she was offered food she would shake her head and chant "ramadan-ramadan-ramadan". The staff didn't understand that she was observing the Muslim fast of Ramadan and could therefore only eat during the hours of darkness. They thought she was mad.'   Nursery nurse

'The midwives observing a Jewish man who stayed with his wife during a long and difficult labour became very concerned about the couple's relationship. They saw the fact that he did not touch her once during the whole time as pathological. After the birth, they sought a psychiatric opinion. Actually the couple were loving and close. The midwives simply did not know about the Orthodox Jewish prohibition against touch between husband and wife whilst the wife has any vaginal blood loss. They assumed that there was something wrong with the couple rather than finding out what was really going on. They then went on to cause unnecessary distress.'   Orthodox Jewish antenatal teacher

LEARNING ABOUT CULTURE

The reason that we operate so effectively and confidently within our own community is that we have a profound and detailed understanding of its culture with all its richness, variety, connections and contradictions. We automatically see people and their behaviour within our shared cultural context and can make appropriate assessments and interventions. We are able to go beyond generalisations and to understand each person as a rounded individual with their own needs and wishes.

Working with people whose culture we do not share can be far harder. They may seem one-dimensional. Their behaviour may appear bizarre, contradictory, off-putting or frustrating. In order to get beyond simplistic and offensive stereotypes, we need to find out much more about the cultural, social, religious and economic frameworks within which people live. Only then can we see the individual properly in their own right and not merely as a member of a stereotyped group. 'Till one can penetrate into the forest one cannot see one tree as being different from another' (Modood, 1990). At the same time it is important to be aware of the possible pitfalls of information. In some cases, believing that they have all the information can lead professionals to take short cuts, avoiding human contact rather than deepening it.

'When I went into hospital I only got vegetarian food. After a few days I realised other people were getting more interesting meals. When I asked I discovered that it was because I had given my religion as Muslim. I was brought up a Muslim but I'm not at all religious. I thought you had to give an answer and I didn't know what else to say.' Iranian woman

Finding out about the context in which a person moves, their cultural heritage, their social and economic circumstances and so on, does not tell you anything reliable or specific about the real person in front of you. What it can do is to give you a framework within which to ask the right questions.

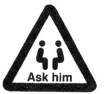
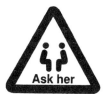

Thinking about our own culture

'We do not see things as they are, but as we are.'

Immanuel Kant (1724–1804)

The culture barrier is a double barrier; our own culture is the first part of the barrier. Only when we become aware of what in ourselves is cultural can we step outside our cultural constraints and care for other people in terms of their own needs. Judging people of other cultures on the basis of what is 'normal' or 'appropriate' to us can lead to misunderstanding, serious misjudgements and failures of care.

We often find it difficult to define our own culture because it is so much part of who we are, how we understand the world and how we lead our lives. We may never think about it unless we see it through the eyes of someone whose culture is different. People who have grown up as members of a minority group, or who have moved to live and work outside their own society, are generally far more aware of culture and how it influences them. Other people may have to work harder at developing such awareness, but in a multicultural society it is crucial.

The problems of finding out about culture

People of minority cultures interact with the culture of the majority. It may be useful, therefore, to reflect on what this is. In Britain, it is clear that there are tremendous national and regional variations. Scotland, Northern Ireland, Wales and England all have their own cultures. To try to simplify the process of defining a culture we have restricted ourselves in the next reflection to English culture.

Consider, whatever your own cultural heritage, how you would answer these questions about traditional English culture:

- What could you say about relationships between English men and women and about the structure of the family?
- How would you define the English diet, and style of dress?
- What are English attitudes to modesty, morality and sex?
- How would you describe English views on codes of behaviour and ways of expressing feelings?
- What are the attitudes of the English to health care and to doctors, midwives and nurses?
- How do the English view pregnancy, birth and child care?
- How would you define English attitudes to death and dying?
- What are the English customs related to funerals and grieving?
- Would you say these are the same throughout England and that they apply to everyone?

You could say that the English are reserved, xenophobic, do not express their feelings openly, eat fish and chips, stop for tea at 4 pm, are concerned about their bowels, worry about catching a chill, are prudish about breast feeding but have photos of topless models in the most popular daily newspapers, and behave badly at football matches and on the Costa del Sol. Some of these statements might be true for some people some of the time, but, if your cultural heritage is English, how would you feel if someone assumed **and then treated you** as if they were all true of you?

Thinking about other people's culture

Other people's culture is generally far more obvious to us than our own. Even if we do not understand why people do things differently it is often abundantly clear that they do. And when we notice cultural differences in others it is common to assume that it is the other culture that is odd or deviant and that what we do is 'normal'. This is particularly dangerous in the context of health care.

Figure 1.4 shows what happens when people of one culture, symbolised by the rectangle, look at a different culture, symbolised by the circle. Although most of the values and assumptions of the two cultures (indicated by the area in the middle) are in fact shared, what the people of each culture tend to notice is what is different in the other. It is easy to focus on cultural and other differences and to miss the large amount of common ground.

Every culture is also inherently logical and makes sense in its own terms. Every culture answers the age-old needs of a society. In an imperfect world,

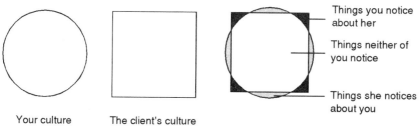

Your culture   The client's culture

Figure 1.4 Working across cultures

every culture contains a balance of advantages and disadvantages. For example, in some cultures there is a high level of social control, in others there is relatively little. One advantage of greater social control is that crime rates are generally lower; one advantage of less social control is that individuals have greater freedom. In a culture where the extended family is extremely important very few people are ever lonely or unsupported, though everyone is expected to conform to certain, often inflexible rules. In a culture where the individual is paramount, many of the weaker members are lonely and unsupported, in many cases no one takes responsibility for them. On the other hand, those people who can cope in such a culture enjoy greater freedom and less restriction.

Our reaction to other people's cultures often tells us more about our own culture than it does about theirs. If something in another culture seems illogical or incomprehensible, this is usually a sign that we do not understand it properly and need to find out more.

A middle-aged South Asian man with three children recently lamented the total lack of family love and morality in Britain. 'English people do not love or protect their daughters,' he said. 'All they think about is money. As soon as their daughters are 16 the parents let them go out and sleep around. Then when the girls get pregnant they are married off to the man so the parents don't have to support them any more.'

It is helpful to think carefully when considering aspects of a culture other than your own and to find out more about the practical or historical reasons behind what people do.

The custom amongst Orthodox Jews of holding a funeral as soon as possible after the death may seem to some people like indecent haste. It makes more sense when one considers the Jewish prohibition against embalming, the absence (until recently) of refrigeration, and the consequent health risk posed by unburied corpses in the heat of the Middle East.

The dangers of cultural and other 'information'

Health professionals often feel under tremendous pressure to have all the answers, to know everything. Not knowing, or needing to ask, may feel like failure or incompetence. But 'information' carries its own dangers. Even if it is accurate it can be crudely and insensitively applied, used to stereotype and to avoid genuine contact (Phoenix, 1990). It can become a barrier to understanding the person in front of us rather than an aid, especially in the complex field of 'race' and culture.

Acquiring cultural understanding that is genuinely respectful, accurate and sufficiently complex to be useful takes time. People who are hard-pressed and concerned about getting through the day's tasks may feel that they cannot afford it. Bowler (1993) describes an incident that occurred during her study of the delivery of maternity care to South Asian women. A midwife, genuinely concerned to give better care to the women in her care, asked her to recommend a source of helpful information. When Bowler suggested a short book the midwife looked surprised. 'I don't have time to read books,' she said, 'What we need is an A4 bit of paper with it all on so we can look things up when we need them'. The midwife assumed that all the 'facts' she needed about South Asian women to help her look after them could be written on one piece of paper.

Information is only useful if it is accurate, up-to-date, acknowledges the complexity and variation of the real world **and** is relevant to the individual concerned. It must also be combined with self-awareness and the skills to ask the right questions, to listen well, and to offer sensitive and effective care.

When trying to understand more about the cultural frameworks in which people operate it is always important to:

- Be aware of your own cultural assumptions and how these may affect your understanding and responses.
- Listen with respect and a genuine wish to learn.
- Find out how people see themselves and their culture, what they value, what they see as important.
- Beware of negative or pejorative 'information'; it usually indicates prejudice or incomplete understanding.
- Understand that in discussing culture we are discussing possibilities, not certainties, a framework, not a straitjacket.
- Be prepared to change your understanding as new information becomes available.
- Sort out what information is useful and helpful to your work with clients and what is merely exotic or personally fascinating.
- Understand the importance of factors such as age, generation, life experience, occupation, education and so on.
- Realise that culture is one factor, but not the only factor in anybody's life.
- Remember that the person you are working with is always the expert on their own life, wishes and needs.

Culture and health care

DIFFERENT BELIEFS AND SYSTEMS

Our beliefs about health and about what makes us ill, where to seek treatment for what, and how to prevent illness are as much influenced by our culture as our views on family patterns, acceptable dress and what constitutes normal behaviour (Mares *et al.*, 1985). For people who have grown up in societies where Western medicine and maternity care are taken for granted as uniquely effective, the existence of other flourishing systems can be a surprise. Many Westerners assume, for example, that when people have access to Western medical care they will gladly abandon the system they grew up with.

But even within Western medicine, which is often considered to be purely scientific and therefore impervious to culture, there are tremendous variations in practice and attitude. For example, French people are more likely to attribute their physical symptoms to the liver, whereas German people are more likely to attribute them to the heart. In much of Europe, low blood pressure is regarded as dangerous and requiring treatment; in Germany drugs for low blood pressure account for the third largest percentage of all drugs prescribed. In contrast, in the UK and the USA people with low blood pressure are regarded as fortunate and may get lower insurance premiums. In the USA the fight against disease is often regarded as justifying any treatment, no matter how 'heroic'. In some countries breast cancer has been treated with radical surgery; in France, where the quality of life has more to do with having an attractive body, breast cancer is usually treated with the minimum possible surgical intervention (Payer, 1989).

There are similar clear variations in patterns of care and belief about best practice in maternity care. Such variations may be due to local culture, tradition and fashion; to the views and preferences of those who control the system; to differences in the availability of staff and physical resources; to differences in the extent to which professionals fear malpractice litigation and in the way they are paid; and to different pressures from drug and equipment manufacturers and others (Enkin *et al.*, 1989). (For more about cultural differences in attitudes towards maternity care see Part Three.)

In Britain allopathic medicine and practitioners have been dominant for some time and have driven other systems into the fringes of society, though they are now making something of a comeback. In most of continental Europe, systems such as homeopathy and herbal medicine have always been important. Many European pharmacists are trained to give homeopathic and herbal advice as well as advice on allopathic preparations. In most parts of the world allopathic and local medical systems exist side by side. People select which system and practitioner to use depending on the condition, its seriousness, and on the costs and accessibility of the different options.

Culture and experience

Both people's culture and their previous experience of health care systems influence the way they relate to health professionals and what they expect of them. When a woman visits the doctor expecting a prescription for her sore throat, she may feel neglected and uncared for if all she receives is information and advice. Another woman with the same symptoms might be dismayed to be given antibiotics when all she wanted was advice and reassurance.

> 'I see a lot of foreign students and they often walk out looking so dejected. They have come to me with something they clearly regard as important and needing treatment, but which means nothing to me. Either I can't see the significance or it just doesn't add up to any disease process I can diagnose or treat.'   GP in South London

Culture influences what people regard as healthy and normal in terms of the way their body functions. For example, the English are said to be preoccupied with their bowels and with having a 'good clear out'. In some cultures menstrual loss and lochia are seen as a means of cleansing the body of impurities, so women may be concerned if their flow is light.

Culture also influences what people see as causing illness. Depending on the condition, most Western Europeans see illness as caused by some combination of bad luck, external factors and individual behaviour. In other societies the causes may be seen as, for example, bad behaviour, spiritual affliction, emotional stress or the ill-will or jealousy of another person. People's view of the cause obviously affects what they regard as sensible methods of diagnosis and treatment. In the Western bio-medical system, biochemical and other physical tests are very important. In other systems practitioners may use, for example, a complex system of pulse taking, or may spend a lot of time finding out about what is happening in the patient's life and relationships. If health problems have a spiritual explanation, or if people see their whole life as having a spiritual dimension, it may be very important to consider moral and spiritual factors in deciding on the right course of action.

Physical methods of treatment also vary. For example, people may be given a combination of chemicals or herbs to take, they may be massaged or injected with needles. In France and Switzerland rectal suppositories are popular; in the UK they are generally regarded as disgusting and most medication is given by mouth. In some countries injections are regarded as more effective. Multinational pharmaceutical companies are careful to market their products in whichever form will be most acceptable in each country and will therefore sell best.

People's confidence in health care often depends to a large extent on whether it fits in with what they have come to expect. We tend to have faith in the system we have grown up with. We assume that practitioners in this system know what they are doing and often mistrust practitioners who do things differently. For some immigrants this can pose a real problem. They may have little faith in the effectiveness of diagnostic methods and treatments in their new country. They may prefer to find a practitioner who understands their culture and assumptions, from whom they can get care that makes sense to them. Where there is a language barrier this can be particularly important.

A research project in central London on the health care needs and expectations of Chinese families found several people who went to a private Chinese doctor to find out what was wrong with them in their own language and in terms that they understood. Since private prescriptions are very expensive they then went to their English-speaking GP for a second diagnosis (which they often could not understand) and a prescription for medication (Bloomsbury Health Authority, 1984).

The client/professional relationship

The kind of relationship people expect with health professionals varies a good deal. In many societies doctors must be treated with great respect. Below an American journalist summarises humorously, but perhaps with some truth, the contrast between the attitudes of the British and American public to the medical profession:

[The American attitude] A doctor is a necessary evil . . . a man in a white coat who gets you when you're down, overmedicates, operates at the drop of a chin-line and uses your misfortunes to pad his annual income. Watch him like a hawk. Ask plenty of questions and don't let him come near you with a wet cotton-swab unless

1. It's a matter of life and death.
2. You've had a second opinion.
3. You've negotiated his fee.

Remember that you can never win in any encounter with the medical profession. The rule is simple, and the odds are on their side. They get the money, but the results are never guaranteed.

[The British attitude] Respect all medical men and women, dedicated servants of the community. Overworked healers with a sense of vocation, bleary-eyed with sleepless hours of service to mankind. Do not ask too many questions. Your case is paltry, and your life one tiny speck of light in the doctor's vast firmament. Anyway – being challenged or called to account or asked what is in a prescription seems to annoy him. (From Walmsley, 1986, by permission)

You may like to take a moment to observe your own reactions to the above paragraphs.

■ Do you find it easier to accept stereotypes about a culture you don't belong to?
■ Most of us find it hard to deal with stereotypes or misunderstandings of our own culture. It is rather like an outsider criticising one's family. We may also feel threatened and offended when our culturally-conditioned values are scrutinised (Seelye, 1993). Cross-cultural discussion always requires sensitivity and tact.

The relationship between professional and client in a Western, bureaucratised health system can appear peculiar to people who are new to it. People from countries where health care is less formalised may sometimes expect a more equal relationship with balanced mutual responsibilities. For example, in many countries, although a midwife is highly respected, she is also a member of the local community and often a close friend.

- Take a few minutes to think about the kind of relationship that you, as a trained professional, expect with your clients and their families:
- What is it suitable for you and your client to discuss? Is it the same in both directions?
- What do you give advice to your client about? What does she give advice to you about?
- Are you equally involved in each other's personal lives?
- Where does your involvement with her stop? Where does her involvement with you stop?
- What are your obligations to your client and her family? What are her obligations to you and your family?
- What kind of demands is it reasonable for you to make on her? What kinds of demands is it reasonable for her to make on you?
- Do you have authority over your client? Does she have authority over you? How far does this authority go?
- Are there certain times when you do not have obligations to your client? When are they?
- How long does your relationship usually last?
- How do you both know all this?

LEARNING ABOUT A NEW HEALTH CULTURE

Every health system has its own culture, its own language and its own accepted, if unspoken, ways of doing things. People who are new to a health care system have to learn what is available, how to get it, and the appropriate behaviour for each situation. They have to adapt to new patterns and styles of care.

The culture of the British National Health Service, for example, can pose real problems even for people born and brought up in Britain, let alone for people who are used to different systems.

When you joined the health service, you entered a new world. What did you need to learn:
- About the way staff communicate with:
    their peers?
    with those more senior or more junior?
    with staff from other disciplines?
- About the way staff relate to:
    patients?
    relatives?

- About language, medical terms, phrases and acronyms?
- About the different ways, different wards and departments did things?
- About what was expected of you?
- How did you need to change?
- How did you feel during this learning process?
- Were there things that shocked or upset you?
    how did you feel?
    how did you react?

Although to an outsider the health service may look like a uniform whole, it contains many micro-cultures. Insiders know that each unit and department functions differently and that each discipline has its own characteristics. The cultures of midwives, doctors, nurses, physiotherapists and so on are very different even though they work side by side. An outsider might wrongly assume, for example, that obstetricians and midwives have identical approaches to pregnancy and birth.

Becoming a client of the National Health Service means learning the skills of a world organised and run largely according to white, middle-class English values. Pregnant women are expected to understand and fit in with the way services are organised and with the routines, procedures and timetables of the people who control the system. This is generally easiest for those who are themselves white, middle-class and English. It can be hard for everyone else and particularly for people of other cultures or who speak little or no English.

THE COSTS OF CULTURAL MISMANAGEMENT

In today's international commercial markets the management of cultural differences is increasingly recognised as essential to a company's competitiveness. Successful multinational companies realise the importance of taking cultural differences into account both in managing international subsidiaries and in marketing to people in different counties. Even the ways in which meetings are run, decisions made, memos written and titles used within a company varies depending on the local culture. Advertising that works brilliantly in one country may flop completely or cause extreme offence in another. The same product often has to be given different names in different countries to avoid unfortunate connotations or the wrong impression. In a world where failure to take cultural differences into account visibly costs money, managers and staff become very culture-conscious (Hoecklin, 1993; Hofstede, 1991; Trompenaars, 1993).

The financial costs of cultural mismanagement in the National Health Service are likely to be just as great; the human costs far greater. The differences are that most of the costs are not visible on the balance sheet and that many of them are borne by clients rather than by the service or by managers.

Likely costs to the service include:

- wasted staff time
- wasted tests, treatment and medication
- staff frustration and loss of job satisfaction.

Likely costs to the clients include:

- untreated conditions or conditions treated only after they have become unnecessarily serious
- increased perinatal morbidity and mortality
- pain, anxiety, fear, hopelessness
- wasted time
- frustration and anger
- alienation (NAHAT, 1988).

To avoid the high human and financial costs of cultural mismanagement in the area of maternity care, all health professionals must take responsibility for ensuring that care is provided in such a way that it is accessible and effective for people of different cultures.

3 Immigration and change

Britain saw a major period of immigration and settlement between the end of the Second World War and 1980. According to the 1991 census, half of all members of black and ethnic minority groups now in Britain were born here (OPCS, 1993). Nevertheless, a large number of people have had to make the major changes required of anyone who moves to another country. For recently arrived refugees, and for dependants joining long-settled heads of families, these changes are still pressing.

Living in another culture

Learning about and adjusting to the spoken and unspoken norms and culture of a new society is always difficult and stressful. Whatever the reasons for the change, and however positive it may be in many ways, there is inevitably loss; loss of family and friends, of home, of emotional and social support, of familiar places and things, of competence, of status and of acceptance.

Everyday practical tasks are handled differently in each society. People have to find out about and manage a huge number of such tasks in creating a home and life in a new country. They have to cope with complicated and often unsympathetic bureaucratic systems in order to gain access to basic provision such as health care and education. Systems whose workings seem natural and obvious to people who are used to them may be frightening and anything but obvious to newcomers.

'Living in a foreign culture is a constant assault on one's self-esteem.' Director, Centre for International Briefing, Farnham, Surrey

Very few immigrants foresee the complex emotional pressures and difficulties of living within another culture and society. For many, life outside the security of the home becomes a series of exhausting compromises and adjustments, many of them touching people's deepest feelings and undermining their confidence. The personal and social skills that worked in their own culture may no longer be effective. And it can be hard to understand those that are effective in the new culture and harder still to adopt them.

'Culture is not like a coat. You cannot take off your own culture when you leave your country and put on someone else's. Culture is woven into each of us as into a piece of cloth. If we pull out and discard the vital threads of culture, the whole cloth falls apart.' Researcher

Culture shock

The difficult and exhausting process of adapting to a new environment is well-documented and has been described as 'culture shock' or 'culture stress' Although everyone experiences culture shock differently, the most common symptoms can include depression, anxiety, irritability, hypersensitivity, a feeling of loss of control, a sense of bereavement, grief, anger and psychological weariness (Furnham and Bochner, 1986; Seelye, 1993). These symptoms can last for many years, possibly, with varying degrees of severity, for a person's whole life. Recognition of culture shock and the toll it can take has prompted some multinational organisations to invest heavily in training and support for employees and their families when they move to live and work in another country.

Changes, even those that are welcomed and chosen, are not easy to deal with. Those imposed by outside pressures are much more difficult to accept and adjust to. Change demands that we let go of the familiar and adjust to the unfamiliar. It can be a long and painful process. Graphic examples of the effects of changes initiated and imposed from outside and of how people respond to them can be found in the National Health Service of the 1980s and 1990s.

Pressure to change

Immigrants often come under great pressure from outsiders to give up important aspects of their culture. Such pressure is ill-conceived and damaging for several reasons. First, although communities and groups may sometimes look as though they are not changing and have not changed, from the inside the picture is completely different. People have made tremendous personal, practical and emotional changes. Second, it is both very difficult and undesirable for people to change the deepest aspects of their culture and identity. For their own emotional stability and mental health it is important that they do not (Furnham and Bochner, 1986; Rack, 1991). Third, nobody has a right to demand that anybody changes any aspect of their personal behaviour unless it is infringing the law. And fourth, however much people change and at whatever cost, some of their critics will never be satisfied. They do not want black people to change but to go away.

> 'They see us as looking inwards and clinging together in an 'unhealthy way' and 'refusing to change'. We see ourselves as having made the most tremendous adaptations and as pulled apart by life in this society. People can only change so much in their lives. If we change any more we shall lose our souls.'   Vietnamese woman

All of us also need to see a good reason for changing before we give up something that is working perfectly well or makes sense to us. New ways are not automatically better. Currer, in a detailed study of the lives of Pathan (Pakistani) mothers in Bradford, found that most of them were keen to learn new ways of doing things provided these seemed a genuine improvement on what they were doing already and made sense to them. But the decision had to be a rational one:

> It was not the women's ignorance but their intelligence that led to their refusal to adapt or abandon certain habits. They sought to understand the reason for such changes in terms that made sense to them. Not all those put forward by health workers did. (From Currer, 1986, by permission)

GROWING UP IN TWO CULTURES

For many British-born black and minority ethnic people the key issues are not cultural change, but living in two cultures, and dealing with racism and stereotyping from the white majority.

For each of us, the most powerful influences on our values and lifestyle are our family and the wider society in which we grew up. For children in minority families the culture of their childhood may have been very different from that of wider society. All children move between the cultures of their home and of the wider world and learn the skills they need for each, choosing to some extent as they grow up what of each culture they wish to maintain. But where the values of the family and of the majority community conflict strongly this is more difficult. Children may feel under pressure from their peers to reject the culture and values of their parents. In some cases, their parents may also become stricter or more conservative in the way they bring up their children, often in response to what are seen as the loose morals and crumbling values of Western society. They may, for example, try to protect children by sending them to religious schools to learn traditional values. Some parents may try to ensure the continuity of their cultural values by arranging or encouraging a marriage within their own community. Others may hope that the values their children learn at home will protect them from damaging outside influences. Occasionally the process is reversed. For example, some younger people have become more traditional and more religiously observant than their parents.

Occasionally the conflicting values of home and of wider society lead to problems between parents and children. Usually these are not very different from the normal inter-generational problems of contemporary Western society and are resolved with time (Ballard, 1979). In a few cases they are more serious and lead to young people leaving their families. Black and minority ethnic young people who leave home may face particular problems since they are unlikely ever to be fully accepted by white society (Coombe and Little, 1986).

> '*When I meet people they often ask me where I come from. So I say Coventry. And you can see they're not happy with that. "No, but where do you really come from?" they often say. "Coventry," I say . "I was born in Coventry." Sometimes I take pity on them and say, "My parents come from Jamaica," and then they look relieved. But it irritates me being asked where I come from all the time. I'm British, as British as they are, and I wish they'd recognise it.*'   Health visitor

Racism is an important factor for black and minority ethnic young people. Research has shown that children distinguish between racial groups from about two or three years old and learn the racial values of the society in which they are growing up within the next four or five years (Milner, 1975). Black children in Britain become aware from an early age, despite their parents' and communities' attempts to protect them, that to many white people they are 'second class citizens', not 'real Britons'. As they grow older, racist abuse and even violence, and patronising references to their culture and colour reinforce the message (Mares *et al.*, 1985; Milner, 1975). Once they enter the job market, the reality of discrimination becomes very clear (see Chapter 4). Alienation, anger and mistrust, especially towards white people in authority, can easily result.

Part of racism is the belief that white British culture is inherently superior and that immigrants, and even more, their descendants should reject the 'inferior' or 'backward' values of their communities and become culturally British (though what this means is never defined). But culture is not a simple issue. None of us chooses our culture, though there are choices involved. Culture is both a sign of the community to which one belongs, and a way of belonging. No culture is better or worse than others, most of us simply understand and prefer our own. For many British-born black and ethnic minority young people, the culture of their family and community is a crucial source of support and identity.

'I find that it is hard for English people to understand that I can be both British and Indian. Because I look Indian and wear a sari they first assume that I speak no English and am very conservative. As soon as I open my mouth I see their eyes light up. I speak with a Yorkshire accent. I must be one of them. I must be culturally English. But I'm not. I still wear a sari, I'm still a vegetarian, I still live with my in-laws. I'm part of both cultures, and both are important to me.'   Teacher

4 Racial discrimination in society

Racism: Conscious or unconscious belief in the superiority of a particular 'race'. Acts of discrimination and unfair treatment, whether intentional or unintentional, based on this belief.

Mares *et al.*, 1985

THE ORIGINS OF RACISM

There is no scientific validity for dividing up humanity into neat groupings on the basis of identifiable physical characteristics. While human variation is obvious for all to see, the existence of definable groups or races is more of a social construction than a scientific reality. (From Sheldon and Parker, 1991, by permission)

The idea that there are several separate and biologically distinct human races and that each has its own unique genetic make-up which is linked to psychological and behavioural characteristics and abilities, is false. It originated in the eighteenth century as part of an attempt to understand evolution and human variation (Godrej, 1994; Senior and Bhopal, 1994). In fact, all people come from a common genetic stock and share most of their genetic inheritance. Most genetic variation occurs at the level of the individual, and there are more genetic differences **within** any so-called racial group than **between** all the different 'racial' or national groups. Geographically, genetic variation is gradual; populations merge into one another. The genes responsible for skin colour and other physical features, the basis for dividing people into so-called racial groups, are few and atypical. They are only one small difference amongst a myriad of genetic differences. There is no rational basis for racism or for regarding one 'race' as biologically superior to another (Godrej, 1994; McKenzie and Crowcroft, 1994; Senior and Bhopal, 1994; Sheldon and Parker, 1992).

Skin colour and other physical features have therefore no meaning in themselves. They only gain importance when societies load them with meaning, or use them to assign people to different groups and then treat those 'groups' differently, allocating them different jobs and so on. Physical differences are not the cause of racism; they are used as an excuse to justify racism.

Colour is the greatest single factor which governs society's attitudes to members of minority groups and influences their own self-image, and it is inescapable. (Rack, 1991).

Although the ideas of race and of superior and inferior races are only social constructs, they are powerful and damaging. In British popular belief they have also been given weight and credibility by the way that successive governments and those in authority have explained and justified British policies towards people in other parts of the world.

> For 400 years the British systematically conquered territories in the four corners of the globe. These lands provided Britain with wealth, power and glory. Commerce and trade flourished as Britain and the other Imperial powers gained access to the natural resources of half the world. Through this accumulation of wealth and materials the momentum was gained for the industrial revolution which transformed agrarian Britain into the modern industrial country in which we now live.
>
> For the peoples of Africa and Asia this process involved a complete disruption of their former ways of life. It was not only coffee and cotton which was extracted from these lands but the people themselves. For 200 years, the trade in black African slaves drained that continent of millions of its most able-bodied men and women. This occupation of other countries and enslavement of their peoples was justified by defining black people as inferior beings to whites. (From Klug and Gordon, 1983, by permission)

RACIAL DISCRIMINATION AND THE LAW

In the UK, the Race Relations Act 1976 covers employment, service provision and racial harassment. It is illegal under this act to discriminate against a person on racial grounds. Racial grounds are defined as grounds of colour, race, nationality (including citizenship) and ethnic or national origins.

The Race Relations Act forbids two kinds of discrimination, direct and indirect:

- **Direct discrimination** means treating someone less favourably on racial grounds than a person of a different racial group would be treated in the same circumstances.
- **Indirect discrimination** means imposing a requirement which applies equally to everyone (so may appear fair) but the proportion of people of a particular racial group that can comply with it is considerably smaller than the proportion of people of other racial groups, and it cannot be objectively justified, and it is to the disadvantage of the person concerned.

It is the **effects** of any action on people that makes an act discriminatory under the law, not the motives of the organisation or of the individual(s) responsible for the action.

Direct, intentional racism in any form in health care is clearly unacceptable and should be treated as a disciplinary offence. However, indirect and unintentional discrimination are also illegal. Once such discrimination has been identified, both organisations and individuals have a legal responsibility to remedy it.

Liability for racial discrimination rests both with the person who does the discriminating and with the person who instructs them, or applies pressure on them, to discriminate. An employer is responsible for any racial discrimination by employees in the course of their work, unless the employer can show that he/she has taken practical steps to prevent discrimination. It is no defence for employers to plead ignorance of their employees' actions. It is also illegal to victimise a person in any way because that person has asserted, or intends to assert, their rights under the Act (CRE, 1994).

Discrimination in the provision of services

Under Section 20 of the Race Relations Act it is illegal to discriminate in the delivery of any services to the public on racial grounds. It is illegal to discriminate, directly or indirectly:

- By refusing or deliberately omitting to provide services.
- In the quality of the services provided.
- In the manner or terms on which the services are provided.

Direct discrimination in the provision of health services includes, for example:

- Making racially prejudiced remarks.
- Refusing to register clients who require an interpreter.
- Only asking black people or people who do not speak English for passports to prove their right to free health care.

Indirect discrimination is more insidious and usually more difficult to identify. It occurs when **exactly the same services** are provided to everybody (so that they appear fair) but when for cultural, religious, linguistic or other reasons it is not possible for members of one or more black and minority ethnic groups to benefit equally from them.

Examples of indirect racial discrimination include:

- Ruling that women having an ultrasound scan can only have a husband or partner with them. Women of some ethnic groups may strongly prefer a female relative or friend (CRE, 1994).
- Running only mixed-sex antenatal classes. This cuts out women who find it offensive to discuss childbirth issues in male company (CRE, 1994). (For more examples of discrimination in the provision of maternity care see Chapter 5.)

Both direct and indirect discrimination can be institutionalised in routines and even in written protocols.

Discrimination in employment

It is illegal to discriminate, directly or indirectly, against a person on racial grounds in recruitment and selection, in the treatment of employees in their terms of employment, in access to opportunities for training, promotion, transfer or other benefits, or in dismissals or other detrimental acts, including racial harassment or abuse (CRE, 1994).

In employment, **direct discrimination** includes, for example:

- Requiring higher qualifications of black applicants for a job than of white applicants.
- Promoting a white person with less experience over a black person with more experience, when the two are equally qualified and suitable for the job.

- Not employing or promoting someone of a particular racial group because of stereotypes or assumptions about their abilities or other qualities, or, for example, because a previous employee of that racial group did not work well.

Indirect discrimination in employment includes, for example:

- Requiring all female nurses and midwives to wear skirts. This may make it impossible for women of some ethnic minorities to enter these fields. Skirts cannot be objectively justified as an essential requirement of the job.
- Using word-of-mouth recruitment. This tends to favour members of those ethnic groups currently employed within the organisation.
- Using culturally biased tests, or subjective selection criteria such as hobbies and outside interests, which cannot be objectively justified in terms of ability to do the job, in selecting people for employment, promotion and training (Open College, 1992).
- Advertising in places where, for example, only white people are likely to see the advertisements, or using agencies based in largely white areas who only recruit locally.
- Requiring minimum selection criteria which are not related to the needs of the job, simply to cut down the number of applicants. People of black and ethnic minorities have historically been disadvantaged in the education system and are more likely to have under-achieved academically or at work. Fewer black and minority ethnic people can therefore meet formal requirements for certain qualifications. If these requirements are not necessary in terms of the needs of the job, they are indirectly discriminatory (CRE, 1989).

Positive action

Under the 1976 Race Relations Act it is permissible in certain cases to take 'positive action' to recruit a suitable person of a particular ethnic group to provide a service for members of his or her own community. An employer can claim a 'genuine occupational qualification' (GOQ) if it can be shown that it is particularly important to recruit someone who will understand the customs, culture, experience and, where appropriate, speak the language of the racial group with which he or she would work.

It is also legal in certain circumstances to take 'positive action' to try to increase the proportion of people in the workforce of a particular ethnic group which is currently under-represented in comparison to their presence in the local population. But the positive action rules are tight: employers are not allowed to recruit suitable people simply because they are members of a particular ethnic group that is currently under-represented. They are only allowed to take special steps to encourage such people to apply for jobs, or, where appropriate, to give them training so that they can compete more equally with other applicants. Employers are not allowed to set employment or other quotas for different racial groups.

RACIAL DISCRIMINATION IN SOCIETY

There is abundant evidence that ethnic minorities in Britain are at a disadvantage in every important socio-economic variable. They experience prejudice and rejection in everyday situations, and the Race Relations Act devised for their protection touches only the tip of the iceberg. Insult is added to injury when they are accused of having caused the problems under which they suffer. Many settled in inner-city areas because housing was cheap, large Victorian houses suited extended-family lifestyles, and in any case they were barred from 'white' suburbia. Now they are accused of causing the decay of those areas – which were actually dilapidated before they arrived. They attend the most ill-equipped schools – and are then derided for failing in academic attainment. They are refused jobs – and then criticised for living on social security. Most of the criticisms are quite unfair. It is not the immigrants who have caused the defects in British society, it is truer to say that they act as a marker, identifying and rendering visible some of the defects that were already present in the structure. (From Rack, 1991, by permission)

Government and other research over the past forty years has repeatedly shown that racial discrimination – discrimination on the basis of skin colour – is a major factor affecting every area of the lives, experiences and opportunities of most black and minority ethnic people in Britain. According to the Joseph Rowntree Foundation (1995) black people are almost twice as likely to be in the poorest fifth of the population as white people. Poverty and poor health are powerfully correlated (Smaje, 1995; Townsend *et al.*, 1988). In the next few pages we summarise the situation in five areas that affect people's emotional and physical health; employment, unemployment, housing, homelessness, and racial harassment and violence.

Employment

Employment crucially affects people's income and living standards. In the UK, the 1976 Race Relations Act was expected to reduce the incidence of racial discrimination and create greater equality between black and white people in the labour market. In reality it has had little effect. Although there has been some improvement, research shows that skin colour is still a major determinant of employment opportunities.

Early immigrant workers were recruited to low-paying, low-status jobs in a small number of industries and public services. These employment patterns have changed very little. Ethnic minority workers, the majority of whom are now born in the UK, are still more likely to be working in low-paying manual occupations. (From Amin, 1992, by permission)

Even when they have the same experience and levels of qualification, there are considerable disparities in job levels, pay and working conditions between black and minority ethnic people and white people (Cheung-Judge, 1993). Within each occupational category they are likely to hold the lower-paid jobs (Employment Department, 1993). They are more likely to work shifts, less likely to receive occupational benefits, more likely to work in poor physical conditions, and less likely to have access to training (Amin, 1992; Breugel, 1989). Regardless of their qualifications, black and minority ethnic people are also more likely than white people to be in manual occupations (Brown, 1984).

Racial discrimination is not confined to manual or semi-skilled occupations; its existence has also been confirmed in the professions, including medicine, nursing, accountancy, the law and journalism (see also next chapter) (Ahmad, 1992; Cheung-Judge, 1993). Black and minority ethnic graduates find it more difficult than white graduates to get jobs, and, when they do find work, are more likely to have job levels below their qualifications and to receive lower salaries

(Cheung-Judge, 1993; CRE, 1990). Although there have been few studies into the experience of black managers in Britain, research in the USA finds that black managers continue to experience racial discrimination, sidelining into so-called 'black' jobs, negative stereotyping, lack of co-operation from white managers and exclusion from informal networks, and increased pressure to perform well because they are seen as 'representing' black people (Cheung-Judge, 1993).

No objective reasons have been found for the gross differences in employment patterns between black and minority ethnic people and white people with the same levels of experience and qualifications (Cheung-Judge, 1993). It appears that again and again simple racial hostility, as well as stereotypes about what the kinds of jobs they can do, prevents black people getting the jobs they are able and qualified to do, particularly in the more popular areas of the labour market.

Unemployment

Unemployment is a major cause of poverty. In spring 1994, unemployment rates for black and minority ethnic people were almost **three times as high** as for white people (OPCS, 1995a). Even when black and minority ethnic people are better qualified than white people they are more likely to be unemployed (Amin, 1992). The relative disparity in unemployment between black people and white people **increases** in groups with higher qualifications (Cheung-Judge, 1993; Newnham, 1986). When unemployment rises it rises even faster among black and minority ethnic groups (Brown, 1992). Rates of long-term unemployment are higher in most black and minority ethnic groups (Smaje, 1995).

Although there has been some increase in the employment of black and minority ethnic people over the years, this has largely been in the service and retail sectors where jobs are often low-paid, part-time and involve shifts (Wrench, 1989). Jobs have also been created in the growing 'ethnic businesses' (Ahmad, 1992). In many cases, people who have experienced repeated discrimination have become self-employed and set up their own business.

Housing

Decent housing is fundamental to physical and emotional health and to stable family life. Patterns of housing tenure differ between different ethnic groups (see Table 4.1). However, housing tenure on its own is not necessarily a guide to housing conditions. Black and minority ethnic people in all housing sectors are particularly likely to experience poor-quality housing and overcrowding (Brown, 1984; Sarre *et al.*, 1989).

- Black and minority ethnic owner-occupiers are more likely than white owner-occupiers to be in houses built before 1939, often in the poorest areas. Many local authorities exclude all owner-occupiers from council house waiting lists, however bad their housing conditions, because they are assumed not to be in 'housing need' (Amin, 1992).
- Black and minority ethnic people who cannot afford to buy and are not eligible for council accommodation face severe racial discrimination in the private sector and often get the worst accommodation in the most run-down areas (Brown, 1984).

Table 4.1   Housing tenure by ethnic group of head of household

	Owner-occupier	Local authority rented	Privately rented
White	64%	25%	10%
Indian	84%	8%	9%
Pakistani/Bangladeshi	67%	17%	17%
African-Caribbean	47%	42%	11%
Other ethnic minority or mixed	49%	21%	11%
All	64%	25%	11%

Reproduced from *Poverty in Black and White: Deprivation and Ethnic Minorities*, by Kaushika Amin with Carey Oppenheim, 1992, Child Poverty Action Group, by permission.

- Black and minority ethnic council tenants are more likely than white tenants to be in flats. Forty-six per cent of Bangladeshi households, compared with 8 per cent of the total UK population live in flats (HEA, 1994). People living in flats have been shown to face a number of specific health problems (Heginbotham, 1985).
- Various studies have found that some local authority housing departments discriminate, directly or indirectly, against black and minority ethnic households.

An investigation into Hackney's housing policies (by the Commission for Racial Equality in 1984) found that black applicants were given lower quality housing than white applicants. Discrimination occurred against those on the waiting list: black applicants were three times less likely to be offered a house – as opposed to a maisonette or flat – than white families in similar circumstances. In addition, white families were over eight times more likely to be offered a new property than black families. The investigation concluded that discrimination must have been the result of allocation officers differentiating between the ethnic origins of the applicants even though no formal ethnic monitoring system had been instituted at the time. (From Amin, 1992, by permission)

In the Health Education Authority's Health and Lifestyles Survey, significant proportions of the black and minority ethnic communities felt that their health was negatively affected by their housing (compared with only 2 per cent of the total UK population). Quality of housing was top of the list of the concerns of the Bangladeshi community, a large proportion of whom live in local authority flats; in particular, people mentioned dampness, lack of space, lack of heating and general poor maintenance (HEA, 1994; Hyndman, 1990).

Homelessness

Although there has been a shortage of accommodation in Britain since the Industrial Revolution, homelessness has re-emerged as a major problem relatively recently. In 1985 there were 15 000 statutorily homeless households living in temporary accommodation in England. In the first nine months of 1994 this figure had risen to 95,390 (Shelter, personal communication). Only about half of those homeless households who apply to local authorities are accepted by them as 'statutorily homeless'. Over two-thirds of homeless households are in London, but numbers are rising throughout the UK. Few authorities monitor the ethnic group of homeless households. However, the National Association of Citizens Advice Bureaux has estimated that black and minority ethnic households are four times as likely as white households to become homeless (NACAB, 1991).

Homeless people are often blamed for their situation, especially if they are black. But the reason most people are homeless is the lack of affordable accommodation. About half the homeless families in the UK are homeless because the parents, relatives or friends they were living with are no longer able or willing to house them. Others are homeless because of the break-up, often involving violence, of a relationship; because they have been evicted from private rented accommodation or have lost their service tenancy; or because they were unable to keep up mortgage or rental payments (LRC, 1990).

Among the Bangladeshi community, an additional factor causing home-lessness is that wives and children have recently come to Britain to join men who have been living and working here for twenty years or more. Their income is too low to buy or rent private accommodation, but councils will not put them on their housing waiting lists until the families arrive in Britain, even though many have been waiting years for government permission to come (Schott and Henley, 1992). In some cases these families have been considered 'intentionally homeless' once they arrive and so denied council help. It appears that white Britons in similar situations have been allocated priority housing (CRE, 1988; MacEwen, 1990). Asylum seekers often face similar problems of homelessness on arrival.

Racial harassment and violence

> *'I came to Britain in the 1960s at the invitation of a London teaching hospital that was recruiting nurses. When I first came people would admire my long hair and my sari and ask how to put a sari on. Now there are many places I won't wear a sari because I get spat at and called a dirty Paki.'*   Tamil nurse

Racial hostility, ranging from unfriendliness to harassment and violence, is a constant source of stress and anxiety for many black and minority ethnic people, affecting their daily lives and opportunities as well their emotional well-being. Persistent experience of racism can also affect a person's self-image and generate a sense of inferiority. It is recognised as contributing to mental health problems in some cases (Majid, 1992; Rack, 1991).

A survey of police forces in England and Wales showed that reported incidents of racial violence rose up to twenty-fold in some regions between 1992 and 1993. In London, where 40 per cent of all such incidents are reported, there were 3550 reported incidents of racial violence. There was a rise of nearly 300 per cent in the Isle of Dogs following the election of a British National Party candidate. Also in 1993 the Home Office Minister, Peter Lloyd, said that there could be as many as 140 000 racial incidents in Britain every year. Many people regard this as an underestimate (*Independent*, 18.3.94).

> A black cleaner was stabbed in the chest at a bus stop in Tottenham, north London, in what police believe was a racially motivated attack. The man, who had to be put into intensive care in North Middlesex Hospital, was in his 40s. He was abused by two white men and then stabbed. (*Guardian*, 15.11.93)

Local studies have confirmed that many black and minority ethnic people live in a climate of fear in which racial abuse and hostility are daily experiences. A study in Leeds in 1987 found that half the black and minority ethnic people interviewed had been forced to change their lives in some way because of racial attacks. Some said they lived like prisoners in their own homes because they were too afraid to go out (Gordon, 1990). A survey in Glasgow found that up to 90 per cent of South Asians and 16 per cent of Chinese residents had experienced racial abuse. Almost half the South Asian respondents had also been physically assaulted. The survey found that women bore the brunt of the harassment. Many South Asian women said they stayed at home most of the time, only went out with husbands and friends, and avoided certain streets and times of day (Gordon, 1990). Children are often kept in, not allowed to walk home from school alone or play in the park for fear of abuse or violence. Women keep the doors and windows locked when their husbands are at work (CRE, 1993).

'It's the children I'm frightened for. I don't want to teach them to be afraid all the time or to stay away from white people. But every time they go out of this house I'm frightened they won't come back. They're not even safe at school. And I don't like them to go out in the evenings. What kind of life is this for them? And what are they learning?' African mother

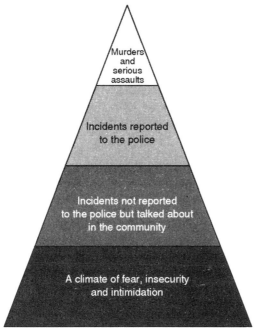

Figure 4.1 The racial violence pyramid. (Reproduced from *Multi-ethnic Britain: Facts and Trends*, 1994. Runnymede Trust by permission)

Racial violence and harassment can be pictured as a pyramid (see Figure 4.1):

- At the peak, there are incidents of murder and very serious violence. It is estimated that between 1970 and 1989 at least 84 black and minority ethnic people died as a result of racially motivated attacks (Gordon, 1990). Petrol bomb and arson attacks on black and minority ethnic people's homes and workplaces as well as other serious crimes of violence are increasing in number. Such incidents are usually reported in the mainstream media, though in much less detail and depth than in the minority ethnic press.

- The next level contains incidents which are reported to the police but not usually covered in the mainstream press and so are unknown to most white people. They include physical violence and assault, verbal abuse and criminal damage. They are widely discussed within the black and minority ethnic communities.
- The next level contains incidents which are not reported to the police but are intensely distressing and affect the behaviour and consciousness of the victims, their families and friends.
- At the base of the pyramid there is a climate of fear, insecurity and intimidation which cramps the lives of almost all black and minority ethnic people in our society. (After Runnymede Trust, 1994, by permission)

The whole pyramid exists in a society in which most black and minority ethnic people also see themselves as disadvantaged by exclusion and discrimination in most key areas including government and party politics and the criminal justice system.

5 Racial discrimination: health and health care

HEALTH SERVICE EMPLOYMENT

The National Health Service is the biggest employer in Europe and the largest employer of black and minority ethnic people in Britain (Ward, 1993). The establishment and growth of the NHS would not have been possible without the active recruitment of professionals and other staff from overseas, especially from the Caribbean and the Indian subcontinent. However, black and minority ethnic professionals have always been, and still are, regardless of their qualifications and experience, concentrated in the lower grades, the least popular specialties and hospitals, and on night shifts (Anwar and Ali, 1987; CRE, 1983; Smith, 1980; Ward, 1993). In some cases, the discriminatory processes that prevent black and minority ethnic people's access to jobs and training have even been formalised:

> An investigation into the computer program that helped pick candidates for selection interviews at St George's Medical School found that the program had been set up to weight the scores of female candidates and those with a 'foreign' name. (Ethnic group was not marked on the application forms.) The program increased the scores of these candidates and so reduced their chances of being selected for interview. (Candidates with the lowest scores were more likely to be called for interview.)
>
> It was found that the person who had programmed the computer had been instructed to develop a program that would mimic as closely as possible the judgements of the human selectors. He observed their judgements over a number of years, created the program and then fine-tuned it. He found that, in order to reproduce the selectors' judgements as closely as possible, he had to give a negative weighting to members of black and ethnic minority groups and to women.
>
> St George's Medical school immediately discontinued the programme and reviewed its selection and recruitment procedures. (CRE, 1987)

Although there is little current information available on the numbers of British-born numbers of black and minority ethnic employees nationally or locally within the NHS, nor on their distribution by occupation and grade, it appears that little has changed and that black health professionals continue to be undervalued and marginalised (Baxter, 1988; Ward, 1993). Evidence of racial discrimination has been found recently in, for example, the employment and promotion of nurses and doctors (see the formal and annual reports of the Commission for Racial Equality).

Apart from the personal injustice experienced by black and minority ethnic professionals who are denied the opportunity to use their skills and qualifications to the full, racial discrimination in employment is a major factor in preventing health services becoming more flexible and responsive to the needs of minority group clients. Senior professionals, managers, planners and trainers are still predominantly white, even in those places with a large minority ethnic population and/or a high proportion of minority ethnic staff in junior positions.

DISADVANTAGE AND THE OUTCOMES OF PREGNANCY

People's health is fundamentally affected by the socio-economic and environmental context in which they live. 'One would thus expect many Black Britons to suffer the health disadvantages of the working class. They endure working class health inequality and then some more' (Grimsley and Bhat, 1988).

Perinatal and infant mortality*

Statistical information on the outcome of pregnancy for black and minority ethnic women is limited. Up to the time of going to press only the country of birth of the parents was recorded on birth registration forms, not their ethnic group. This meant that no separate figures were available from birth registration forms for British-born black and minority ethnic women and their babies, and almost all published data were based on the parents' country of birth. This situation should change when ethnic monitoring becomes established.

In 1992, the lowest **stillbirth** rates occurred among babies whose mothers were born in the UK, the rest of Europe (including the Mediterranean), and the 'Old Commonwealth' (Australia, Canada and New Zealand). (Note that the legal definition of stillbirth in 1992 was still a fetal death after 28 weeks' of gestation.) Babies whose mothers were born in the Irish Republic had higher stillbirth rates, while rates for babies whose mothers were born in the 'New Commonwealth' (which includes India, Pakistan, Bangladesh, the African Commonwealth countries and the Caribbean Commonwealth countries) were even higher (see Table 5.1). The highest stillbirth rate was for babies whose mothers were born in Pakistan; this was more than twice the rate for babies whose mothers were born in the UK. Lethal congenital malformations are a major factor in the high perinatal and infant mortality rates among babies of Pakistani-born women (Parsons et al., 1993).

The lowest **neonatal death** rates occurred among babies whose mothers were born in the UK, the Irish Republic and the Old Commonwealth. Babies of mothers born in the New Commonwealth all had higher neonatal death rates. Neonatal death rates for babies of mothers born in Pakistan, Africa (excluding East Africa, from which most immigrants are of South Asian origin), the Caribbean and the remainder of the New Commonwealth were nearly twice the rate for the babies of UK-born mothers.

* Much of this section has been adapted and updated from Parsons, Macfarlane and Golding, 1993, by kind permission of the authors and HMSO.

Table 5.1 Stillbirth and infant mortality rates by mother's country of birth, England and Wales, 1992

Mother's country of birth	Stillbirths No.	Rate[a]	Neonatal deaths No.	Rate[b]	Postneonatal deaths No.	Rate[b]
All	2944	4.3	2911	4.2	1524	2.2
United Kingdom[c]	2469	4.0	2470	4.1	1317	2.2
Irish Republic	28	4.9	21	3.7	12	2.1
Australia, Canada and New Zealand	10	3.3	11	3.6	6	*2.0*
New Commonwealth	321	6.5	304	6.2	143	2.9
Bangladesh	41	7.4	29	5.2	12	2.2
India	43	5.6	41	5.3	15	*1.9*
Pakistan	111	8.6	102	8.0	56	4.4
East Africa	41	6.5	31	5.0	15	2.4
Rest of Africa	29	5.1	45	8.0	18	3.2
Caribbean	22	6.5	25	7.4	11	3.3
Mediterranean[d]	9	4.3	9	4.4	4	*1.9*
Rest of New Commonwealth	25	4.6	22	4.0	12	2.2
Rest of Europe	46	4.4	50	4.9	26	2.5
Other	64	4.5	55	4.0	20	1.4

[a] Per 1000 total births.
[b] Per 1000 live births.
[c] Includes the Isle of Man and Channel Islands.
[d] Cyprus, Gibraltar and Malta.
Rates in italics are based on very small numbers.

Definitions
Stillbirths: fetal deaths after 28 weeks of gestation. (Data collected before the legal definition was changed to 24 weeks of gestation.)
Neonatal deaths: deaths before the 28th day after live birth.
Post-neonatal deaths: deaths after the 28th day, but under one year after live birth.

Source: Mortality Statistics: Perinatal and Infant, 1992. OPCS, (HMSO, 1995). Crown Copyright, by permission.

Post-neonatal mortality rates showed a slightly different pattern but were again high for babies of mothers born in Pakistan, Commonwealth Africa (excluding East Africa) and the Caribbean.

The factors which lie behind the differences in mortality are multiple and often interlinked. They include socio-economic factors, differences in the provision and uptake of maternity care, mother's health, and patterns of marriage and childbirth. They may also include differences in immunity to teratogenic viruses, genetic make-up and differences in the uptake of screening and other services (Balarajan and Soni Raleigh, 1991).

Socio-economic factors

Within the total population of England and Wales, babies whose fathers are unskilled manual workers (OPCS Social Class V) have much higher rates of stillbirth, neonatal and infant death than those whose fathers are in professional occupations (Social Class I). The proportion of babies with very low birthweight born to fathers who are unskilled manual workers (Social Class V) is also far higher than that for babies whose fathers are in a professional occupation (OPCS, 1990). Although stillbirth and infant mortality rates have fallen over time, the ratios between the stillbirth and mortality rates for different social classes have changed little (Macfarlane and Mugford, 1984; Townsend et al., 1988).

Because the numbers of deaths are small, mortality rates are not usually tabulated by both ethnic group and social class. Recent research, however, shows that within overall higher rates of infant mortality among babies born to New Commonwealth-born mothers, rates also differ to some extent according to social class (Balarajan and Soni Raleigh, 1991; Parsons et al., 1993).

Births outside marriage

In the population as a whole, mortality rates are higher for births outside marriage. The infant mortality rate for babies whose mothers are unmarried and who register the birth of their baby alone is higher than that for babies of unmarried mothers jointly registered by both parents, which, in turn, is higher than that for babies born within marriage. These differences are more marked in the poorer social classes. Some of the difference in the rates between the different groups of mothers may however be partly explained by the fact that the mothers of babies born outside marriage are younger, on average, and therefore more at risk (OPCS, 1990).

Under the rules of the registration system, if a baby is born outside marriage, the father must attend the registration if the parents want his name on the birth certificate. About 70 per cent of fathers whose names appear on birth certificates also live at the same address as the baby's mother (OPCS, 1991). Single mothers who register the birth of their baby alone are more likely to be unsupported by the baby's father.

Although stillbirths and infant deaths inside and outside marriage are tabulated by mother's country of birth, differences between ethnic groups are difficult to interpret as the numbers of perinatal and infant deaths are relatively small.

Local differences

Mortality rates among babies of overseas-born women differ a good deal between different health districts within the UK. For example, in Sheffield the perinatal mortality rate among overseas-born mothers is more than double that among British-born mothers. In contrast, in Central Birmingham Health District, rates for the two groups are similar. The reasons for these differences are not clear but one factor appears to be differences in the way care is provided (see below) (Balarajan and Soni Raleigh, 1991).

Low birthweight

In general, there is a statistical association between low birthweight and stillbirth and infant mortality rates as well as the health of babies. The available data show that babies whose mothers were born in the New Commonwealth have higher rates of low birthweight than babies born to UK-born mothers. Mothers born in the Caribbean and in Africa (excluding East Africa) have a particularly high rate of low birthweight babies.

However, low birthweight is not associated to the same extent in all ethnic groups with perinatal mortality and morbidity. One study found that South Asian babies within each birthweight category required less intensive care, such as assisted ventilation, than 'non-South Asian' babies in the same birthweight category (Jivani, 1986). Stillbirth rates among babies under 1500 grams with mothers born in the Caribbean and Commonwealth Africa (excluding East Africa) are significantly lower than those among babies of UK-born mothers in the same weight group. But stillbirth rates among babies over 2500 grams with mothers born in the Caribbean and Commonwealth Africa (excluding East Africa) are much higher than those among babies in the same weight group with UK-born mothers (Parsons et al., 1993).

Birthweight distributions vary among different ethnic groups. The mean birthweights of babies of women born in Bangladesh, India and East Africa (mainly of South Asian origin) appear to be about 300 grams lower than those of babies born to UK-born women. Babies of women born in the Caribbean and Pakistan are on average 100 grams lighter (Parsons et al., 1993; Wilcox et al., 1993). Research also indicates that gestational age at spontaneous delivery may normally vary between ethnic groups. Women born in Pakistan and India, for example, appear to go into spontaneous labour on average five days earlier than women born in the UK and Ireland (Parsons et al., 1993). All this has implications for clinical practice and decision-making.

Maternal health

There are very few studies on the health status of mothers of different ethnic groups. One study found that black women who internalise rather than verbalise their responses to unfair treatment and gender discrimination are more likely to be hypertensive than those who express their views. In white respondents no link between gender discrimination and hypertension was demonstrated (Krieger, 1990). It has also been found that psychological distress in late pregnancy is associated with an increased risk of pre-term delivery (Hedegaard et al., 1993).

Because maternal deaths have become so rare, the possibility that women may die in childbirth tends to be forgotten. Maternal mortality rates are, however, higher for women born in the New Commonwealth. Reports on confidential enquiries into maternal deaths in the late 1970s and early 1980s drew attention to the risks associated with anaesthesia in women with dark skins among whom complications are said to be more easily missed (Parsons *et al.*, 1993). More recent reports have not discussed this topic explicitly.

Intervention rates

There are few data on maternity interventions related to ethnic group. However, from the data that are available it appears that induction rates at 42 weeks' or more gestation vary a good deal, ranging from 10 per cent for women born in Bangladesh to 18 per cent for women born in the UK and Ireland. The reasons for these differences are not clear (Parsons *et al.*, 1993).

Caesarean section rates also appear to vary according to ethnic group. Between 1982 and 1985 in the UK, women born in Africa (excluding East Africa) had caesarean rates of 16.2 per cent, and women born in Bangladesh caesarean rates of 13.2 per cent. In England in the same period the general caesarean rate was 10.1. Among women having their first child, Bangladeshi-born women had a caesarean rate of 20.9 per cent, compared with 11.1 per cent for UK-born women. Among women with four or more previous births, the caesarean rate for Bangladeshi-born women was 15 per cent, compared with 8.5 per cent for UK-born women. That for women born in Africa (excluding East Africa) was 23.6 per cent. Again, the reasons for these differences are not clear but the very high rates among certain groups are a cause for concern and further investigation (see also Chapters 18 and 19).

> While biological factors such as cephalo-pelvic disproportion could contribute to these differences, the high caesarean rates in primiparous women from Bangladesh, a group that contains a high proportion of non-English speaking women, suggests that communication problems may also play a part by hindering them from discussing decisions with staff. (From Parsons *et al.*, 1993)

HEALTH RESEARCH AND RACE

Most of the current research on the health of black and minority ethnic communities focuses on ethnicity or 'racial group' as the main variable. However, the categories of racial or ethnic group used are rarely clearly defined; they are used inconsistently and often overlap; and the way people are assigned to them is frequently arbitrary and confused. This makes useful comparisons and conclusions almost impossible (McKenzie and Crowcroft, 1994). The value of many such comparisons is anyway dubious, since they often assume a non-existent direct link between 'race', biology, genetic factors and culture (see Chapter 4). In much UK research, country of birth is also used as a proxy for ethnic group which means that British-born black and minority ethnic people are excluded or hidden (Amin, 1992).

In addition, much research on health outcomes in black and minority ethnic groups assumes that their culture and biology, as well as, in some cases, language barriers, are the main causes of any negative differences found. It largely ignores the importance of socio-economic factors, including racism (Ahmad *et al.*, 1989). Since culture, language and biology are in some ways the 'responsibility' of the client, or at least can be located in the client, society and the health service may be let off the hook.

> Thus, for example, at the turn of the century, high mortality rates in Glasgow were attributed to the racial stock of the Irish immigrants even though mortality rates in Ireland were a lot lower. The excess was the result of the poor social conditions in which migrant labour was placed. (From Sheldon and Parker, 1992, by permission)

Some researchers argue, therefore, that health research needs to incorporate racial discrimination as a key risk factor. They also argue that categories such as racial or ethnic group should only be used as variables when looking at the impact of racism, or at the impact of disadvantage due to cultural differences in the use and provision of health care (McKenzie and Crowcroft, 1994; Sheldon and Parker, 1991).

> My point is not that culture and genetics . . . are of no significance in health; it is simply that these are among a host of possible determinants and explanations. Through racialisation problems become redefined and a different range of explanations are applied to black than to white people. For black people this focus is almost exclusively on cultures and ethnicities, genetics and metabolisms, being different and therefore inferior. (From Ahmad, 1993, p.22, by permission)

It is clearly important for people wishing to inform their practice and the services they provide, to be aware of the pitfalls surrounding research in this area and to be very clear about what any research does or does not show.

INSTITUTIONAL RACISM AND HEALTH SERVICES

Health services and the people who work in them inevitably reflect the attitudes and practices of wider society. There is a growing body of evidence that black and minority ethnic people in Britain receive worse health care (Ahmad, 1993; McNaught 1985; Mohammed, 1991). The tangled combination of factors that cause such discrimination are often referred to as institutional racism. Institutional racism has three main planks:

- personal discrimination
- the culture of the organisation
- established organisational processes (Open College, 1992).

These form a powerful and poisonous combination, creating and maintaining inequalities in access to health care.

Personal discrimination

Racism is often described as prejudice plus power. Wherever people have the power to make a decision affecting other people, they also have the power to discriminate, whether consciously or unconsciously. In relation to clients and their families seeking maternity care, health professionals have enormous power. If professionals have prejudices about people of a different ethnic group, feel that the needs and preferences of black and minority ethnic clients are not as legitimate as those of white clients, or are hostile and resentful towards certain groups, these feelings must affect the many day-to-day decisions they make and the care they give.

Personal racism is often remarkably explicit. It includes racist comments and remarks, asides about clients to colleagues, sighs and gestures, off-hand treatment, ignoring clients' requests, even shouting and swearing (Currer, 1986).

'I think when you are young and go to hospital to have a baby, they should be more helpful, more concerned. This sister said to me 'You black people have too many babies'. As far as I was concerned I wasn't 'You black people', I was me. You don't forget something like that . . . She was supposed to be caring for me.' (From Larbie, 1985, by permission)

'I was very lonely in hospital. Even though my English isn't very good they could have tried to talk to me and also respected my culture and religion. They shouldn't have shown their dislike and they shouldn't have laughed at me.' Bengali woman

'In our antenatal clinic the clerk calls out people's names. The Asian names are sometimes wrong or she pronounces them wrongly so the women often don't realise they are being called. She usually calls a name twice and then puts it to the bottom of the pile. By the end of the clinic only the Asian women are still waiting, some of them have been there for hours. She said to me the other day that 'they' don't even know their own names!' Student midwife

Personal racism also leads to more subtle differences in behaviour, for example, health professionals may offer less explanation to black and minority ethnic clients or may take their symptoms and worries less seriously.

'I was with a Greek Cypriot woman who'd just had a baby. She was in obvious pain and I asked a midwife if she could do anything to help. The midwife replied that the woman was making a fuss about nothing. Then she said, "They're all like that, moaning and wingeing. You just have to learn to ignore it".' Interpreter

Some health professionals treat clients whose needs and lifestyles are different or unfamiliar as a nuisance or a problem, or consider them responsible for their own health problems, or for the failure of services to meet their needs (McNaught, 1985).

The view of many health professionals is that nothing is wrong with the services provided. It is 'those people', with 'special diets', 'strange religious practices', or 'funny maternity habits', who have the problem. (From Parsons *et al.*, 1993, by permission)

Colour and culture-blind approaches Some professionals feel that it is wrong to take account of 'race' or culture, and may adopt a 'colour-blind' approach which they see as neutral. In reality, however, the effects of such a 'colour-blind' approach are discriminatory. They maintain the status quo – provision based on the preferences and needs of the white majority population – and neglect or marginalise the needs of black and minority ethnic communities (Mohammed, 1991). In refusing to recognise the significance of culture and racism to many of their clients they are also failing to address clients' needs fully.

The culture of the organisation: 'the way things are done around here'

The culture of an organisation includes the values shared by the majority of its staff, its informal arrangements and the unstated beliefs that influence people's behaviour (Cheung-Judge and Henley, 1994). Part of health service culture includes ideas about the kind of client the organisation really exists to serve. Where clients do not fit these ideas, or have needs and wishes that may be different, they are often resented or simply not given the care they need.

> The judgmental attitude of some hospital and community staff towards young, black, unmarried women with unplanned pregnancies caused much concern for these particular women. It demanded particular courage to attend clinics, the punitive response from staff often acting as a deterrent. (Larbie, 1985, by permission)

If managers and professionals are unaware of their own culture and the culture of their organisation, and of how these affect their assumptions and practice, they are unlikely to see the need for change and greater flexibility.

> *'We must not view people of different cultures and ethnic groups as a problem. We are the problem if we do not adapt care to meet their needs. We are contracted to provide a service. The service exists for the community, not for us health professionals. If we are not providing it then we are the problem.'*   Director of midwifery education

Established organisational processes

Much of the discrimination that occurs within organisations is due to established organisational policies, practices and procedures. Many of these appear to work well and to be non-discriminatory. But often, apparently neutral policies shut out black and minority ethnic clients.

> If the service does not reflect the local population, and if it projects an image of mainly white staff, its black clients will surely find it hard to relate to it. Moreover, midwives' services are often based on what would be acceptable to their own community. Women from other ethnic groups may interpret this as racial prejudice and become reluctant to avail themselves of this care, no matter how good the midwives' intentions. (From Kroll, 1990, by permission)

Most of us automatically plan and provide services largely on the basis of our own experience and understanding of what is needed. It takes careful consultation and listening to do anything else. There is also a tendency in all organisations to meet the needs of the organisation and those who work for it, rather than the needs of the people it exists to serve.

Take a few minutes to imagine how different an antenatal clinic in your hospital might be if it was planned and managed by non-English speaking women.

- How might it look different?
- What practical things might be organised differently?
- How might you feel if you went there for an antenatal appointment? What would you be worried about?
- What could the people running the clinic do to make you feel welcome?

Organisational inertia is also a factor. It is easier and less risky to go on running things the way they have always been run than to try to change them. The status quo often has a spurious authority. Asking people to adapt services or make them more flexible so that they meet the real needs of the current population may be resented. It may be seen as 'special provision' or 'bending over backwards' rather than as part of the normal process of ensuring that services evolve to meet changing needs and circumstances.

> *'Health authorities are not being asked to do something extra or special. They are simply being asked to make up for existing deficiencies in their service.'*   Health education officer

Change in a complex and hierarchical institution is always slow and difficult, especially when the people in whose interests the change is required have little power and may be resented.

HOW DOES INSTITUTIONAL RACISM AFFECT HEALTH CARE?*

Examples of discriminatory services include:

- Services that are **unattractive or off-putting** to members of black and minority ethnic groups. For example, if a clinic appears, through its posters and notices, to be aimed only at white or English-speaking people, or if certain staff are known to be hostile to black and minority ethnic clients or to clients who do not speak English well.
- Services that are **unacceptable** to certain members of black and minority ethnic groups. For example, no female doctors available for those women who cannot, for religious or cultural reasons, be examined by male doctors; hospital food or washing facilities that are unsuitable for religious or cultural reasons.
- Services that are **useless** to certain members of minority ethnic groups. For example, if the only language spoken in a clinic is English, or if important leaflets are only available in English, failing to provide trained interpreters in an area where many women speak little or no English.
- Services that are **inflexible** and culturally unacceptable to members of certain black and minority ethnic groups. For example, rules that only a husband or male partner can accompany a woman in labour, or that only two visitors are allowed at a time.
- Services that may be particularly required by members of certain black and minority ethnic groups **not made available**. For example, screening and counselling for sickle cell disorder, thalassaemia or Tay–Sachs disease.
- **Care based on stereotypes** about the characteristics or needs of certain groups. For example, assuming that women of African descent are more likely to be HIV positive and taking special precautions with them rather than applying universal infection control precautions; offering limited contraceptive, antenatal or other choices to minority ethnic women because of prejudices or stereotypes about their preferences or what is 'best' for them.
- Lack of training for professionals in the **skills** they need to provide care to all clients and families whatever their ethnic origin, culture and personal

---

* Much of this section is adapted from Henley, 1991, by permission of the National Extension College.

preferences. They may know little about possible cultural variations, for example, around the time of birth or death and may fail or ask the right questions or offer appropriate care.

- **Lack of training** for professionals about particular aspects of **practical care** in a multiracial population. For example, how to recognise jaundice and cyanosis in dark skins, how to deal with different naming systems and how to address and file people's names correctly, how to give dietary advice that is useful in terms of people's own dietary preferences and habits.
- **Lack of training** for staff about the reality and the effects of **racism** in society, or how it operates within the health service. Professionals may be uncertain how to recognise racism and how to react to it.

Take some time to think about the attitudes and practices in your workplace.

- Is there an equal access to services policy? If yes, how is it implemented?
- Is there an equal opportunities in employment policy? If yes, how does it work in practice?
- How aware are you and your colleagues of the possible needs of different minority groups?
- How effectively do you and your colleagues identify and meet varying needs?
- How easily can the service be adapted to meet the differing needs of clients and their families?
- What training and education have you received on:
    The law in relation to racial discrimination?
    Equal access to health services?
    Potential cultural and religious variations in relation to health care needs?
    Health issues which specifically affect minority groups?

In the next chapter we look at ways of challenging institutional racism and ensuring equality of access to services for all communities.

6 Challenging inequalities

Equal access

Equal access means ensuring that everyone, whatever their 'race', colour, creed, national origin, gender, marital status, class, disability or sexuality has equal and full access to the health care that is available, and that no one receives less favourable treatment on these grounds.

> *'Nobody should get worse care or be cut off from care because of their colour or culture or because they do not speak English. Each individual should get the best we can give them.'* Director of midwifery services

Equal access does not mean **offering** the same service to everyone and assuming that each person will therefore **receive** the same service. It means providing flexible responsive services in which differing needs are identified and accommodated so that each person **benefits** equally.

Flexible services

> The needs of black and minority ethnic women are not dramatically different from those of other consumers. It must be recognised, however, that if their needs are to be adequately and sensitively met in the ethnically and culturally diverse Britain of today, the services themselves cannot be uniformly and narrowly defined. The NHS has to improve its services and increase flexibility to make services more sensitive to the needs of those women to whom the predominantly eurocentric models do not apply. (From NAHAT, 1990, with permission)

Minority communities and their 'cultures' are often blamed for the lack of uptake of services, when the real reasons may be, for example, inflexible services, lack of information about services, poor communication, and lack of respect for individuals' needs and wishes. These are things to which everybody has a right. Where they are not available some people may not use the services. But this is not because of their culture, it is because the services are inappropriate (BHAN, 1991).

> A study comparing Bangladeshi and English women's experiences of maternity care in Tower Hamlets found that the two groups had much the same wishes and complaints. Both groups wanted more privacy and more explanations during antenatal check-ups, shorter waiting times and a crèche in the antenatal clinic, better preparation for labour and childbirth, more help with looking after the baby, more home visits by community midwives and health visitors, and to be re-housed. In addition, the Bangladeshi women

wanted an interpreter, women doctors, and staff who spoke Bengali. They also wanted to be able to eat with their fingers and to wear saris in hospital, and to observe their religious and cultural requirements, such as saying prayers and resting after the birth, without being ridiculed. (Grant, 1987)

In general, it is not different services, but more flexible and responsive services that are needed to ensure equal access. Providing different services to different communities on the basis of narrow definitions of their cultures, customs and traditions, can simply result in the creation of new stereotypes and is not usually necessary.

Equal access to services cannot be achieved by ad hoc measures or by individuals working alone. It must be a fundamental policy of the organisation, understood and implemented by everyone responsible for managing and providing care, and backed up by training and practical support. Combating institutional racism is an essential part of achieving equal access to services.

COMBATING INSTITUTIONAL RACISM

Combating institutional racism (see Chapter 5) is a key part of ensuring genuinely equal access to services for all clients and their families. But it can be hard and take a long time because:

- It can be difficult to see precisely how the discrimination is occurring, even when the effects are visible.
- Many of the processes involved are well established and appear neutral.
- The negative emotions aroused by discussion of racism can stop people listening properly and thinking clearly.
- People are often reluctant to see that their own actions, even though unconsciously, may be contributing to discrimination.
- Many people dislike change, especially if they are afraid that it will disadvantage them or make them more vulnerable (Open College, 1992).

If the culture of the organisation does not encourage flexibility, or is professional-centred rather than client-centred, it can also be hard for individual staff to achieve changes that will meet clients' needs.

Dismantling discriminatory practices and providing a service that genuinely meets the needs of all ethnic groups requires careful thought and planning. Good communication is essential; everyone involved in delivering the service must understand the legal, moral and service basis for change and know what they are trying to achieve. They need safe opportunities to talk through their fears and doubts about change and what it will mean for them. They also need information, training and practical and emotional support, their successes acknowledged and celebrated, and their mistakes and failures accepted and seen as part of the learning process (Cheung-Judge and Henley, 1994).

Why are people racially prejudiced?

Discriminatory attitudes and beliefs are a mixture of misinformation and lack of information. Nobody is born with racist attitudes and beliefs. No child acquires racist or other misinformation by his or her own free choice. Prejudices and racist myths and attitudes are passed down the generations and handed on to children by the people they most love and trust. Once prejudices are formed, people go on to interpret what they see and hear in the light of those prejudices and so reinforce them. Prejudices and racist beliefs damage white people as well as black, dividing and isolating people from each other on the basis of false information, distorting their understanding of reality and creating fear, resentment, guilt and hatred.

The situation is not hopeless. People can learn and change, even though the process of learning and changing is often painful. People will usually change their minds about deeply held convictions if:

- **they are not being blamed for having been misinformed**
- the new idea is presented in a way that makes sense to them
- they trust the person giving it.

Take some time to think about the following. You may find it helpful to jot down your thoughts and feelings as they surface.

> Think back to your childhood:
>
> ■ What is your earliest memory of hearing about people whose skin colour was different from your own?
> ■ What is your earliest memory of seeing a person with a skin colour different from your own?
> ■ What do you remember about the responses of the people around you?

How would you like it to have been different? Tackling racism and racial inequality is difficult and stressful. Many people feel uncertain where to begin. The rest of this chapter contains some guidelines. Think through the implications of each for your practice. You may like to discuss them with your colleagues.

Challenge racist remarks and behaviour

Many racist remarks and incidents of racist behaviour are inadvertent or unconscious. Others are conscious and intentional. Either way they cause offence and can be extremely damaging. To assess whether something is offensive ask yourself whether you would make the same remark, ask an equivalent question, or behave in the same way towards a person whom you consider to be the same as yourself. If the answer is no, the remark, question or action is likely to be racist.

Challenging prejudice and discrimination is not easy. Many of us have painful memories of times when we have failed to act in the face of racism, or when we have not achieved as much as we wanted. It is important to think about why challenging racism can be difficult, and how to do it more effectively, without blaming ourselves or becoming discouraged. It takes time to develop approaches that work, but any action we take, however small, to counteract discrimination is important and positive.

- Begin by noticing how and when you and other people generalise, make assumptions or act differently towards people because of the group they 'belong' to.

- Then decide to stop and not to collude with other people when they do these things.
- Finally, challenge people firmly and politely when they make assumptions or generalisations or discriminate against clients or colleagues.

Racial discrimination and abuse are unprofessional and unacceptable in the health service. Health professionals have a right to their own attitudes but they do not have a right to behave unacceptably or to express their prejudices when they are at work. They have a responsibility to be equally welcoming and responsive to everyone, whatever their colour or ethnic group. If black and minority ethnic women and their families are alienated or insulted by the treatment they receive, they are less likely to make use of services when they need them. The health of people who are already disadvantaged will be compromised still further. If necessary, or if the behaviour continues, you may wish to complain to your own manager or to the personnel department. Your employer's equal opportunities policy should support you.

Find out about racism

If you are white, you may need to find out more about the reality of racism. Discuss racism with black and white colleagues and clients. An open and sensitive discussion that accepts the reality of racism can break down barriers and reduce tension. Most black people have experienced the denial or trivialisation of racism from white people. Make it clear to black and minority ethnic clients and colleagues that you respect and would like to hear their experience and views. White and black people usually live in very different worlds. Try to find out more about the experience of black and minority ethnic people in society. One way to start is by reading black and minority ethnic newspapers.

Support black and minority ethnic colleagues

Recognise the special contribution that black and minority ethnic colleagues can make in helping to plan and provide care for clients whose culture or religion they share, and in helping all staff better understand the possible needs of such clients. At the same time, it is important not to push black and minority ethnic staff into caring always or only for clients whose backgrounds they share, and, if there is a language barrier, not to use them routinely as interpreters rather than as professionals in their own right. Both these are exploitative, undervalue the contribution of black and minority ethnic professionals, and may damage their career progress by limiting the breadth of their experience. It is also important not to assume that all black and minority ethnic clients are experts in this field simply because of their membership of a minority group (Tilki *et al.*, 1994).

Black and minority ethnic health professionals can also be the targets of racism from clients.

A senior midwife who was born in the West Indies described how clients had rubbed her skin 'to see if the black comes off'. Other clients asked her such things as 'Why didn't you stay in your own country?', 'Do you have to send food parcels home?' and 'How big are the trees you live in?'

It is important to have a clear policy for dealing with racism directed by clients against health professionals as well as against other clients. This must include making it clear that such remarks or behaviour are unacceptable, and open and strong support for the person at whom the racism was directed.

Become an effective agent of change

Think carefully about how best to achieve lasting change in the area of equal access to services and what skills and information you need. Good communication skills and a clear understanding of the issues are essential if you are to persuade people to rethink their attitudes and practices in this difficult area. It is also important to listen to people with respect and to be prepared to argue rationally for change. Although aggressive campaigning is effective in politics it can be counterproductive within an organisation (Cheung-Judge and Henley, 1994).

Recognise the positive influence you can have as a role model for junior and other staff in challenging discrimination and providing care that meets the needs of all clients.

Organise strong support for yourself both at and outside work. Ensure that you have somewhere to go to let off steam. Be reasonable about what you can achieve in the short-term. Celebrate your successes.

Develop a vision of what genuinely equal access services would be like

Develop, with your colleagues, a vision of what care would be like if it was more flexible and equally accessible and effective for clients of all ethnic groups. Incorporate equal access into the standards you set for your own practice, your ward, department clinic, unit or team. Make sure you and your colleagues have the information, training and support you need to deliver such a service.

Push for equal access and equal opportunities policies throughout your organisation to cover service provision and employment, and for action to implement them. Although individuals can make a difference, it should be everybody's business to work towards equality and the changes should be led and supported by senior management. A strong equal access policy can also give you some of the support and legitimacy you need to demand change successfully.

References, further reading and useful addresses

CULTURE: CHAPTERS 1–3

Ballard, C. (1979) Conflict, continuity and change: second generation South Asians. In *Minority Families in Britain: Support and Stress* (ed. V. S. Khan), Macmillan, London

Bloomsbury Health Authority (1984) *The Health Care Needs of Chinese People in Bloomsbury Health District: the Report of a Survey* Bloomsbury Health Authority, London

Bowler, I. (1993) Stereotypes of women of Asian descent in midwifery: some evidence. *Midwifery*, **9**, 7–16

Coombe, V. and Little, A. (eds) (1986) *Race and Social Work: a Guide to Training*, Tavistock, London

Currer, C. (1986) *Health Concepts and Illness Behaviour: the Care of Pathan Mothers in Bradford.* Unpublished PhD thesis, Department of Sociology, University of Warwick

Enkin, M., Keirse, M. J. N. C. and Chalmers, I. (1989) *A Guide to Effective Care in Pregnancy and Childbirth*, Oxford University Press, Oxford

Furnham, A. and Bochner, S. (1986) *Culture Shock: Psychological Reactions to Unfamiliar Environments*, Routledge, London

Green, J., Kitzinger, J. V. and Coupland, V. A. (1990) Stereotypes of childbearing women: a look at some evidence. *Midwifery*, **6**, 125–32

HEA (1994) *Health and Lifestyles: Black and Minority Ethnic Groups in England*, Health Education Authority, London

Helman, C. (1986) *Culture, Health and Illness*, Wright, Bristol

Hoecklin, L. A. (1993) *Managing Cultural Differences for Competitive Advantage*, The Economist Intelligence Unit, London

Hofstede, G. (1991) *Cultures and Organisations – Software of the Mind*, McGraw-Hill Book Company, London

Keesing, R. M. (1981) *Cultural Anthropology: a Contemporary Perspective*, Holt Rinehart and Winston, New York

Littlewood, R. and Lipsedge, M. (1989) *Aliens and Alienists: Ethnic Minorities and Psychiatry* Unwin Hyman, London

Lupton, D. (1994) *Medicine as Culture: Illness, Disease and the Body in Western Societies*, Sage, London

Mares, P., Henley, A. and Baxter, C. (1985) *Health Care in Multiracial Britain*, National Extension College, Cambridge

Milner, D. (1975) *Children and Race*, Penguin, Harmondsworth

Modood, T. (1990) Colour, class and culture: the three Cs of race. *Equal Opportunities Review*, **30**, 31–33

NAHAT (1988) *Action not Words: a Strategy to Improve Health Services for Black and Ethnic Minority Groups*, National Association of Health Authorities and Trusts, Birmingham

OPCS (1993) *1991 Census: Ethnic Group and Country of Birth – Great Britain (CEN 91 TM EGCB)*, Office of Population Censuses and Surveys, London

Payer, L (1989) *Medicine and Culture: Varieties of Treatment in the United States, England, West Germany and France*, Victor Gollancz, London

Phoenix, A. (1990) Black women and the maternity services. In *The Politics of Maternity Care: Services for Childbearing Women in Twentieth-century Britain* (eds J. Garcia, R. Kilpatrick and M. Richards), Clarendon Press, Oxford

Rack, P. (1991) *Race, Culture and Mental Disorder*, Routledge, London

Reber, A. (1985) *Dictionary of Psychology*, Penguin, London

Roberts, C. (1977) *Asians in Kenya and Tanzania with Reference to Immigration to Britain*, National Centre for Industrial Language Training, Southall, Middlesex, (out of print)

Roberts, C. (1985) *The Interview Game and How It's Played*, BBC Publications, London

Scambler, G. (1991) *Sociology as Applied to Medicine*, Baillière Tindall, London

Seelye, H. N. (1993) *Teaching Culture: Strategies for Intercultural Communication*, National Textbook Company, Lincolnwood, Ill.

Smaje, C. (1995) *Health, 'Race' and Ethnicity: Making Sense of the Evidence*, King's Fund Institute, London

Trompenaars, F. (1993) *Riding the Waves of Culture – Understanding Cultural Diversity in Business*, Nicholas Brealey Publishing, London

Walmsley, J. (1986) *Brit-think, Ameri-think: A Transatlantic Survival Guide*, Harrap, Edinburgh

RACIAL DISCRIMINATION AND EQUAL ACCESS: CHAPTERS 4 TO 6

Ahmad, W. I. U. (1992) 'Race', disadvantage and discourse: contextualising black people's ill health. In *The Politics of 'Race' and Health* (ed. W. I. U. Ahmad), Race Relations Research Unit, University of Bradford

Ahmad, W. I. U. (1993) Making black people sick: 'race' ideology and health research. In *'Race' and Health in Contemporary Britain* (ed. W. I. U. Ahmad), Open University Press, Buckingham

Ahmad, W. I. U., Kernohan, E. E. M. and Baker, M. R. (1989) Influence of ethnicity and unemployment on the perceived health of a sample of general practice attenders. *Community Medicine*, **11**, 148–56

Amin, K., with Oppenheim, C. (1992) *Poverty in Black and White: Deprivation and Ethnic Minorities*, Child Poverty Action Group, London

Anwar, M. and Ali, A. (1987) *Overseas Doctors: Experiences and Expectations*, Commission for Racial Equality, London

Balarajan, R. and Soni Raleigh, V. (1991) *Perinatal Health and Ethnic Minorities*, Institute of Public Health, University of Surrey

Baxter, C. (1988) *The Black Nurse: an Endangered Species*, National Extension College, Cambridge

BHAN (1991) *AIDS and the Black Communities*, Black HIV and AIDS Network, London WC1N 3XX

Breugel, I. (1989) Sex and race in the labour market. *Feminist Review 32*, Summer, 49–68

Brown, C. (1984) *Black and White in Britain*, Heinemann, London

Brown, C. (1985) *Racial Discrimination: 17 Years after the Act* Policy Studies Institute, London

Brown, C. (1992) 'Same difference': the persistence of racial disadvantage in the British employment market. In *Racism and Anti-Racism: Inequalities, Opportunities and Policies* (eds P. Braham, A. Rattansi and R. Skellington), Sage, London

Cheung-Judge, L. M. (1993) *Equal Opportunities in Management Education and Development*, Q & E Consultancy Services, 18–24 Middle Way, Oxford

Cheung-Judge, M. Y. and Henley, A. (1994) *Equality in Action: Introducing Equal Opportunities in Voluntary Organisations*, NCVO Publications, London

CRE (1983) *Ethnic Minority Hospital Staff*, Commission for Racial Equality, London

CRE (1987) *Report of a Formal Investigation into St George's Hospital Medical School*, Commission for Racial Equality, London

CRE (1988) *Homelessness and Discrimination: Report of a Formal Investigation into the London Borough of Tower Hamlets*, Commission for Racial Equality, London

CRE (1989) *Indirect Discrimination in Employment: a Practical Guide*, Commission for Racial Equality, London

CRE (1990) *Ethnic Minorities and the Graduate Labour Market*, Commission for Racial Equality, London

CRE (1990) *Ethnic Minorities and the Graduate Labour Market*, Commission for Racial Equality, London

CRE (1991) *Race Relations Code of Practice in Employment*, Commission for Racial Equality, London

CRE (1992) *Race Relations Code Of Practice in Primary Health Care*, Commission for Racial Equality, London

CRE (1993) *The Sorrow in My Heart: Sixteen Asian Women Speak About Depression*, Commission for Racial Equality, London

CRE (1994) *Race Relations Code of Practice in Maternity Services*, Commission for Racial Equality, London

Currer, C. (1986) *Health Concepts and Illness Behaviour: the Care of Pathan Mothers in Bradford*. Unpublished PhD thesis, Department of Sociology, University of Warwick

Employment Department (1993) Analysis of Labour Force Survey Data 1988–1991, *Employment Gazette*, February, HMSO, London

Friedman, D. and Pawson, H. (1989) *One in Every Hundred: a Study of Households Accepted as Homeless in London*, London Housing Unit/London Research Centre

Godrej, D. (1994) Race: unlocking prejudice. *New Internationalist*, October, 4–7, (New Internationalist Trust, Oxford)

Gordon, P. (1990) *Racial Violence and Harassment*, (rev. edn.,) Runnymede Trust, London

Government Statistical Service (1992) *Social Trends, 1992*, HMSO, London

Grant, J. (1987) Getting it right. *Medicine and Society*, 13(2), 21–5

Grimsley, M. and Bhat, A. (1988) Health. In *Britain's Black Population: a New Perspective* (ed. A. Bhat *et al.*), Gower, London

HEA (1994) *Health and Lifestyles: Black and Minority Ethnic Groups in England*, Health Education Authority, London

Hedegaard, M., Henriksen, T. B., Sabroe, S. *et al.* (1993) Psychological stress in pregnancy and preterm delivery. *British Medical Journal*, **307**, 234–8

Heginbotham, C. (1985) Health and housing. *Hospital and Health Services Review*, September, 218–20

Henley, A. (1991) *Caring for Everyone: Ensuring Standards of Care for Black and Ethnic Minority Patients*, National Extension College, Cambridge

Hyndman, S. J. (1990) Housing, dampness and health among British Bengalis in East London. *Social Science and Medicine*, **30**(1) 131–41

Jivani, S. (1986) Asian neonatal mortality in Blackburn. *Archives of Disease in Childhood*, **61**, 510–12

Joseph Rowntree Foundation (1995) *Income and Wealth*, Joseph Rowntree Foundation, York

Kierse, M. J. N. (1994) Maternal mortality: stalemate or stagnant? *British Medical Journal*, **308**, 354–5

Klug, F. and Gordon, P. (1983) *Different Worlds: Racism and Discrimination in Britain*, Runnymede Trust, London

Krieger, N. (1990) Racial and gender discrimination: Risk factors for high blood pressure? *Social Science Medicine*, **30**(12), 1273–81

Kroll, D. (1990) Equal access to care? *Nursing Times*, **86**(23), 72–3

Larbie, J. (1985) *Black Women and the Maternity Services*, National Extension College, Cambridge (out of print)

Lee-Cunin, M. (1989) *Daughters of Seacole*, West Yorkshire Low Pay Unit, Batley, West Yorkshire

LRC (1990) *Housing Need and the Supply of Rented Housing in London*, London Research Centre

MacEwen, M. (1990) Homelessness, race and the law, *New Community*, **16**(4), July

Macfarlane, A. and Mugford, M. (1984) *Birth Counts: Statistics of Pregnancy and Childbirth*, HMSO, London

McKenzie, K. J. and Crowcroft, N. S. (1994) Race, ethnicity, culture and science *British Medical Journal*, **309**, 286

McNaught, A. (1985) *Race and Health Care in the United Kingdom*, Health Education Council, London

Majid, A. (1992) The mental dilemma of innocents abroad. *Hospital Doctor*, 12 November, p. 46

Mares, P., Henley, A. and Baxter, C. (1985) *Health care in Multiracial Britain*, National Extension College, Cambridge

Mohammed, S. (1991) Improving health services for black populations. *SHARE Newsletter*, Issue 1, (King's Fund, London)

NACAB (1991) *Barriers to Benefit: Black Claimants and Social Security*, National Association of Citizens Advice Bureaux, London

NAHAT (1988) *Action Not Words – a Strategy to Improve Health Services for Black and Ethnic Minority Groups*, National Association of Health Authorities and Trusts, Birmingham

NAHAT (1990) *Words About Action: Bulletin No. 2: Maternity Services*, June 1990, National Association of Health Authorities and Trusts, Birmingham

Newnham, A. (1986) *Employment, Unemployment and Black People* Runnymede Trust, London

OPCS (1990) *1987 Mortality Statistics, Perinatal and Infant: Social and Biological Factors*, Series DH3, No. 21, HMSO, London

OPCS (1991) *1988 Mortality Statistics, Perinatal and Infant: Social and Biological Factors*, Series DH3, No. 22, HMSO, London

OPCS (1995a) *Social Trends, 1994*, HMSO, London

OPCS (1995b) *Mortality Statistics, Perinatal and Infant, 1992*, HMSO, London

Open College (1992) *Managing in Diversity: Understanding Discrimination*, Open College, Manchester

Parsons, L., Macfarlane, A. and Golding, J. (1993) Pregnancy, birth and maternity care. In *'Race' and health in contemporary Britain* (ed. W. I. U. Ahmad), Open University Press, Buckingham

Rack, P. (1991) *Race, Culture and Mental Disorder*, Routledge, London

Runnymede Trust (1994) *Multi-Ethnic Britain: Facts and Trends*, Runnymede Trust, London

Sarre, P., Philips, D. and Skellington, R. (1989) *Ethnic Minority Housing: Explanations and Policy*, Avebury

Schott, J. and Henley, A. (1992) *Breaking the Barriers: a Training Package on Equal Access to Maternity Services*, Obstetric Hospital, University College London Hospitals NHS Trust, London

Senior, P. A. and Bhopal, R. (1994) Ethnicity as a variable in epidemiological Research. *British Medical Journal*, **309**, 327–30

Sheldon, T. and Parker, H. (1991) Ethnicity and race – a cautionary note. *SHARE Newsletter*, Issue 1, pp. 3–4 (King's Fund, London)

Sheldon, T. and Parker, H. (1992) The use of 'ethnicity' and 'race' in health research: a cautionary note. In *The Politics of 'Race' and Health* (ed. W. I. U. Ahmad), Race Relations Research Unit, University of Bradford

Sheldon, T. and Parker, H. (1993) Race and ethnicity in health research. *Journal of Public Health Medicine*, **14**(2), 104–10

Shelter (1991) *Building for the Future*, Shelter, London

Smaje, C. (1995) *Health, 'Race' and Ethnicity: Making Sense of the Evidence*, King's Fund, London

Smith, D. J. (1980) *Overseas Doctors in the National Health Service* Policy Studies Institute, London

Tilki, M., Papadopoulos, I. and Alleyne, J. (1994) Learning from colleagues of different cultures. *British Journal of Nursing*, **3**(21), 1118–24

Townsend, P., Davidson, N. and Whitehead, M. (eds) (1988) *Inequalities in Health*, Penguin, Harmondsworth

Ward, L. (1993) Race equality and employment in the National Health Service. In *'Race' and Health in Contemporary Britain* (ed. W. I. U. Ahmad), Open University Press, Buckingham

Wilcox, M., Gardosi, J., Mongelli, M. *et al.* (1993) Birth weight from pregnancies dated by ultrasonography in a multicultural British population. *British Medical Journal,* **307**, 588–91

Wrench, J. (1989) Unemployment and the labour market. *New Community,* **15**(2), 261–8

USEFUL ADDRESSES

Commission for Racial Equality
Elliot House
10–12 Allington Street
London SW1E 5EH

Maternity Alliance
15 Britannia Street
London WC1X 9JP

National Perinatal Epidemiology Unit
Radcliffe Infirmary
Woodstock Road
Oxford OX2 6HE

NHS Ethnic Health Unit
7 Belmont Grove
Leeds LS2 9NP

Office of Population Censuses and Surveys
St Catherine's House
10 Kingsway
London WC2B 6JP

SHARE – Sharing black and ethnic minority health information
The King's Fund Centre
11–13 Cavendish Square
London W1M 0AN

Part Two **Communication**

Communication in a multiracial society

Communication lies at the heart of health care delivery. To be effective it must be a two way process; the service must give patients the information they want and need and it must listen and respond to them. And it must do this, as far as possible, in a way that is tailored to the individual's . . . unique blend of beliefs, understanding, expectations and ability to communicate.

Audit Commission, 1993 (Crown copyright)

THE IMPORTANCE OF COMMUNICATION

Communication is probably the single most important component of effective maternity care. It underpins everything else. Good communication enables clients to understand and participate fully and confidently in their own care. It enables professionals to offer information, intervention and support at the right time and in the way that is most acceptable and useful to the client. It maximises the effective use of resources and minimises wasted time and energy.

Every expectant and new parent faces a host of new experiences and decisions as they take on what is probably the greatest responsibility of their lives. They are uniquely sensitive and vulnerable at this time. Every interaction that a health professional has with parents is therefore also a chance either to enhance or to undermine their confidence and self-esteem. Insensitive communication alienates parents, increases stress and can have adverse physical as well as emotional effects. Research shows that giving people information about their treatment and care positively affects their physical well-being and reactions. A study of patients undergoing surgery showed that understanding what was happening to them reduced their stress, improved their tolerance of pain, helped healing and lowered postoperative infection rates (Hayward, 1975).

From the clients' point of view, excellent physical care can often be completely negated by poor communication. Poor communication is the commonest cause of dissatisfaction with health services, and can lead to inappropriate treatment, to clients rejecting beneficial advice, and to complaints and litigation (Audit Commission, 1993; Heavey, 1988).

Communication in maternity care

Communication in maternity care has often fallen short of women's needs and expectations. It has frequently been a one-way process in which health professionals have set the agenda, women have been treated like children and expected to obey, and so-called reassurance has taken the place of meaningful discussion. Much of the language used has been over-technical, or euphemistic and patronising (Kirkham, 1988; Leap, 1992; Magill-Cuerdon, 1992). Women have generally been expected to be satisfied with the advice and information selected for them and to supply the information required of them.

Growing pressure from consumers and the publication of, for example, the Winterton Report (House of Commons, 1992) and Changing Childbirth (Department of Health, 1993) have resulted in moves to put women back at the centre of their own care. These have highlighted the need to re-think communication with women and families during pregnancy, birth and the early days of parenthood. Informed choice and participation in one's own care require good two-way communication.

But how much still needs to change? Women who understand the system of health care and who know something about the issues are more likely to get the information they require and to be able to exercise their right to informed choice, but this is not true for everyone. Women who are unfamiliar with the issues, who are reticent about speaking out or asking questions, or who do not speak fluent English are less likely to be given the information and support they need to make their own choices. Racism also plays a part. Women from minority groups who ask questions or say what they want often find that they are not treated with respect or taken seriously. They may also find that their motives are misinterpreted (Alibhai, 1988).

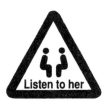

THE BASIC PRINCIPLES OF GOOD COMMUNICATION

The principles outlined here apply to **all** encounters with **all** clients and their families, irrespective of their culture, religion or lifestyle. If a woman has a different family heritage from your own, speaks English as her second language, or speaks very little English, there may also be other factors to consider. We say more about these in the rest of this section.

Good manners

Fundamental to good communication are good manners, behaving towards people with courtesy and respect. Good manners reduce clients' feelings of vulnerability and uncertainty in an unfamiliar environment, and enable them to manage the experience better. It is easy to forget good manners in busy hospitals and clinics where large numbers of women and their families attend for the same routines over and over again. It is also easy to abandon them if they are not modelled by those in authority.

Good manners include:

- Introducing yourself clearly and being ready to explain what you do.
- Finding out how women and their partners would like to be addressed and then remembering (this requires special attention with people who have different naming systems, see also Chapter 14).
- Explaining things that are commonplace and everyday to you, but may be strange and unfamiliar to them.
- Making sure that people know what to expect and where to go.
- Using everyday language that people can understand and identify with. This includes signposting.

'I was told to go for a blood test. I couldn't find the right department and wandered about feeling rather a fool. Eventually someone told me to go through a door labelled Phlebotomy. They might as well have put up a sign to Timbuctoo for all the sense that made to me.' First-time mother

Bad manners destroy the mutual respect, trust and exchange of information that are essential to good maternity care.

'I lay there on the couch almost naked while three doctors discussed across my stomach whether my baby was too small, too large, or just right for its dates. I felt like a discarded bin liner. I was so angry and humiliated I couldn't ask any of the questions I had come with. When I got up I couldn't speak.' Mother of two

Communicating to meet clients' needs

If women and families are really to be partners in their own care, health professionals need to establish genuine and open two-way communication and to respond appropriately to each person in terms of their own circumstances and needs.

This means:

- Creating an environment in which clients feel able to talk about what really matters to them, showing complete and respectful attention to the client, both verbally and non-verbally, and maintaining privacy and confidentiality.
- Listening attentively.
- Finding out and building on what clients already know.
- Giving balanced, objective information at an appropriate pace and level.
- Using language that enhances clients' autonomy and self-esteem.
- Picking up clients' verbal and non-verbal cues and, as appropriate, helping them explore their thoughts and discover what they really need to talk about.
- Asking questions sensitively and being ready to explain the reasons for asking. For example, a question about family origins may be asked in order to assess potential genetic risks, but may be perceived as racist or as querying the person's immigration status.
- Acknowledging and dealing calmly with strong feelings.
- Enabling people to make choices, recognising that they may then need additional support since increased choice often increases dilemmas.

- Breaking bad news sensitively and supporting people through the painful aftermath.
- Supporting people when things do not go as they had planned and hoped for.
- Understanding the particular needs and perspectives of fathers and other close family members in order to communicate effectively with them.

Communicating with fathers

In most cases, the father of a new baby is deeply involved in and affected by his partner's pregnancy and the birth. Although health professionals may have little contact with him during the pregnancy, he is experiencing the changes in his partner at home, has hopes and fears about what is happening and about the new baby, and is taking on, at whatever level, new emotional, practical and financial responsibilities. His responses to these changes, and how he shows them, will vary from culture to culture and from individual to individual, but he is a crucial part of the equation, and the support and acknowledgement he gets may affect both the support he is able to give the mother, and his future involvement with the baby. Nowadays, he is also expected to be present at the birth, and is likely to need preparation, support and understanding in his own right during what can be a difficult as well as a positive experience.

The practical involvement of fathers in the medical processes of care during pregnancy and childbirth in Western Europe is relatively recent. It has meant that professionals in the maternity services, who have traditionally related almost exclusively to women, have had to adapt to include fathers in antenatal classes, in clinics and on labour wards.

In order to communicate effectively with fathers, health professionals need to develop an understanding of and empathy with men's particular perspectives, needs and feelings. This can be particularly difficult for female health professionals who may have few opportunities to learn about what men really need and feel, and may be reticent about asking. Assumptions are often made about the father's role in maternity care and men's real needs and feelings are frequently ignored. The ways in which men are culturally conditioned can also make it hard for some fathers to express feelings and anxieties, particularly in situations where they feel they must protect and support their partners. When a man does not exhibit emotion it does not mean that he is not feeling anything nor that he does not care.

It is important to bear the following issues in mind when communicating with fathers in a multiracial, multicultural society:

- The involvement of men in pregnancy and childbirth is mainly a Western idea. In many cultures such matters are exclusively the concern of women. Some men brought up within such a tradition may find the idea of any involvement unnatural and unacceptable. Others, depending on their experience, may wish to be more involved. For every man, whatever his background, the degree of involvement should be a matter of individual choice. It is important to find out what each father and couple want and not to make assumptions.

- Most men rely on their partners to explain and guide them through antenatal clinics and hospitals. Where both are unfamiliar with the system they are likely to need extra explanation and guidance.
- Men in some cultures are unused to relating to women in professional or authority roles. They expect to discuss important issues with other men. The idea of a midwife as a trained professional in her own right in charge of the management of pregnancy and childbirth may also be unfamiliar. In some cases, female health professionals may need to explain their status, role and responsibilities. Some men may find it difficult to accept the status and authority of female professionals.
- In some cultures eye contact between men and women is seen as flirtatious or threatening. Men who do not make eye contact with women when being introduced or during interviews are not usually being rude or evasive, but respectful.
- In some cultures it is unacceptable to discuss intimate matters with a member of the opposite sex. Female staff may need to be sensitive about what they say to fathers and how they say it. If necessary a male member of staff should be available to speak to the father.

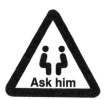

Training in communication skills

Although some people seem to be more skilled at communicating than others, the ability to communicate effectively is rarely innate. Since health professionals are generally regarded as authority figures they rarely get feedback from clients on the way they communicate or on their behaviour or effectiveness. All health professionals need opportunities for sensitive experiential training away from the workplace to enable them to develop the wide range of communication skills they require, especially in a multiracial, multicultural society. They also need safe opportunities to understand their own style of communication, to be able to adapt it to suit different people and different situations, and to discover how the way they communicate is perceived by others.

COMMUNICATION IN A MULTIRACIAL SOCIETY

Expectations and attitudes

In general, the more similar people are in terms of background, culture, experience and outlook the easier it is for them to communicate. They are likely to bring similar expectations, knowledge, assumptions and ways of communicating to the conversation. They are also likely to feel more positive about each other and to assume basic goodwill, overlooking things that could be irritating (Tannen, 1992).

However, where there are differences in background and experience, it is often more difficult for communication to flow smoothly and automatically, **even when both parties speak English as their first language**. Differences in class, 'race', gender, age, occupation and family heritage may all influence the values, assumptions and ways of communicating that each person brings to the encounter. One or both people may also have negative expectations of the other which affect the way they interpret any difficulties in communication. For example, past experience of being patronised or ignored by professionals, or of rudeness and racism from people in authority, may make some clients anxious, suspicious or hostile. Stereotypes and uncertainty about, for example, young black people's attitudes to white people may make white health professionals nervous and particularly sensitive to anything that seems like hostility. In such situations, health professionals need to take conscious steps to overcome barriers and to recreate mutual confidence.

Communicating across cultural barriers

Communicating across cultural barriers is often very rewarding. Finding the underlying similarities between your own culture and values and someone else's, and achieving genuine rapport is exhilarating. The sensitivity and openness required to understand someone of another culture can create special bonds.

However, cross-cultural communication can also be frustrating and difficult. It requires a positive will and effort to understand and a clear suspension of ethnocentric judgements. It is tiring to **really** listen and to keep listening, without resorting to shortcuts and snap judgements. Questions that you think are important may draw only a vague and unsatisfying response from the client. In the field of maternity care where so much is extremely sensitive and personal, clients may find your detailed questions intrusive and impertinent. It may be difficult to find out exactly what a client needs without seeming prurient or inquisitive. It may also be difficult to hide your response to those things that from your cultural perspective are upsetting, unacceptable or simply odd (see also Chapter 15).

Difficult interviews

Sometimes clients who have been on the receiving end of stereotyping and prejudice do not wish to expose themselves to yet more judgement, particularly from someone whom they see as having power and authority. Some may not be particularly interested in helping you understand them. In such a situation it is easy to feel uncomfortable, vulnerable and frustrated, and to turn these negative feelings against the client or the community they 'represent'.

Here is an account by a health professional of her feelings during a difficult interview with three members of a minority ethnic group. Everyone spoke English as their first language.

'I felt that we were not really making contact, but I did not understand why. So I kept quiet in order not to lose face or look a fool. I just felt I had to plough on and hope for the best, keeping at bay my feelings of discomfort, frustration and being out of my depth.

'When I asked what seemed to me a straightforward question, the reply was often vague and off the point. I am used to getting fairly direct answers to direct questions but with them I didn't. They seemed puzzled by my interest in certain things. In retrospect perhaps I should have found out what they felt about what I was asking, but I didn't.

'Looking back, they were quite different from my stereotype of how they would be. Also their agenda was totally different from mine though I could not see this at the time. My questions and concerns were a mystery to them. Their ideas about what is important are entirely different. I still don't really know what they were thinking, but I know there are fundamental differences. We were on different planets. The experience was hard because I'm supposed to understand people's needs and wants. It's part of my job and one of the skills I most value.

'Also, they did not seem at all concerned whether I understood or not, they were certainly not falling over themselves to be helpful or to please. I was dismayed to be confronted with my unconscious expectations about how people will respond to me. I had to accept that they were not particularly keen to communicate with me and were certainly not grateful for my efforts.

'It was a challenging, unsettling and exhausting experience. It has taken me two weeks to digest it to a point where I can begin to understand it. I can see why I felt tempted to deal with my discomfort by being brisk and backing off. It would have been easier to dismiss them as unimportant, to think, if they don't want to be clear with me, why should I bother to be clear with them? It would have been easier to give up and to label them as a problem, difficult, uncommunicative, unco-operative, aggressive, all potential steps towards a psychiatric label and excuses for my not listening or persevering.

'In psycho-analytical terms I suppose what tends to happen when cross-cultural encounters between health professionals and clients go badly is that the professionals feel confronted, aggressive or inadequate but cannot tolerate these feelings because 'nice' health professionals shouldn't feel them. So because the health professionals have the power, they project the confrontation and aggression onto the client. Of course, in reality the client is not the problem, the communication gap and our inability to bridge it are the problems.'

Managing cross-cultural communication well

Successful communication across cultural barriers can take time, especially while you are building up a relationship, sorting out basic facts, and establishing ways of discussing cultural issues together. Here are some suggestions.

- Do what you can to put the client at ease. Try to create an atmosphere of emotional warmth.
- Show your genuine concern and interest. Listen with wide open ears and a wide open mind to everything. Be aware of your assumptions and stereotypes and try to suspend them. Check if necessary that you have really understood.
- Make it clear verbally and non-verbally that you respect and trust the client and that it is your job to understand her needs and meet them as far as possible.
- Spell out your assumptions or those of the organisation where necessary. Explain who you are and what you do. Explain the purpose and structure of the interview.

- When you are asking questions about what people would like, make sure they have enough information to make a properly informed decision. Ask specific questions, for example, 'Would you feel comfortable wearing this gown (show it) in the delivery room?', rather than, 'What are your views about modesty?'.
- The current Western European cultural assumption is that a woman has a right to be in sole, overall charge of her pregnancy and birth and that she is the only person you need to talk to. But in some cultures maternity care and the choices involved are concern of all the adult women in the family. Some women may wish to have other, possibly older, female relatives present at the interview, or may want to get their advice and permission before agreeing to certain procedures. For some women it may be important for their husband or, where he is not available, another close male relative to agree and give permission. It is necessary to take each mother's needs and expectations into account in managing the interview.
- Try to meet your client more than half way. Notice what you have in common as well as what is different. Look at things from her point of view and listen to her priorities, anxieties and responsibilities.
- Do not give the impression that you think the way you do things or the way things are done here is necessarily better.

'We had a group of musicians to stay from Rumania. We felt like bountiful hosts and assumed that they would be impressed and grateful. We even felt a little embarrassed about our standard of living in comparison to theirs. One musician watched me washing up and said, 'We don't have taps like that'. I assumed he had no running water and felt sorry and perhaps a little superior. I asked what he did have and he said, 'Mixer taps'!' English woman

- Bear in mind that most people are not used to discussing culture or to seeing their own behaviour and preferences within a cultural framework any more than you are. You may need to work on this together.
- Allow more time. You are likely to get responses you didn't expect expressed in unfamiliar ways. It may take longer to get to know the other person.

When things go wrong

If there are difficulties, make it clear that you are not blaming the client, and see if, between you, you can try to sort it out. Resist the temptation to back off. Acknowledge that the situation is difficult, frustrating and tiring for both of you. Explain why you are asking certain questions. Offer the client a gentle invitation to say what she is thinking and feeling. Find ways to build bridges.

Try to avoid blaming or labelling the client. She is not the problem. She is also having a hard time and is probably doing the best she can. She is in a far more vulnerable position than you are and it is in her interests not to antagonise you. Try to set your own feelings aside for the moment.

Try also to avoid blaming yourself. Afterwards, find someone who will respect your confidentiality and with whom you can let off steam (see also Chapter 15). Once you have unloaded your frustration, anger and so on, reflect on what you did well and on what you would like to do differently next time.

8 Language and culture

'I was simple enough to think that the British people were all the same, all speaking the same sort of language, the language which I learnt at English school in India. I was surprised I couldn't understand the English nurse and was even more surprised because she did not understand English – my English!'   Indian husband (from Ahmed and Watt, 1986, by permission)

Every language is part of a culture and has its own cultural features. It is often assumed that it is easy to communicate with clients whose first language is not English but who speak English well. In fact, people who retain features of their mother tongue that clash with those of English often unintentionally cause offence or give the wrong impression. Such misunderstandings can be difficult to overcome because they are often subtle and unrecognised.

Similar problems sometimes occur when people speak another variety of English as their first language (or one of their first languages), for example, Indian English, Caribbean English or West African English. Each of these forms of English has been influenced by other languages and has developed aspects of its own grammar, intonation, rhythm, accent and vocabulary. Sometimes these clash with the conventions of British English and give rise to misunderstandings. Some people in the UK also assume that these different forms of English are in some way inferior and limited and that those who speak them are intellectually slow or under-educated. They do not realise that each is a complete and fully developed language in its own right (d'Ardenne and Mahtani, 1989).

LANGUAGE IS MORE THAN JUST WORDS

Paralinguistic features

On the surface language consists simply of words, linked by certain grammatical rules to convey meaning. In fact, there are many devices which help indicate meaning, including intonation, emphasis, pauses, volume, rhythm and pace. These 'paralinguistic features' are generally used unconsciously but are a crucial part of the way we indicate, for example, our attitude to what we are saying and to the person we are speaking to (Mares *et al.*, 1985).

> To see how paralinguistic features work, try saying this sentence, 'She says she's been in agony for three hours', in the following four different ways:
>
> 1 As a straight statement.
> 2 As a question.
> 3 Indicating that you don't believe her.
> 4 Indicating that you are shocked that this has been allowed to happen.

Notice how your intonation, emphasis, timing and pace differed in each sentence, so that although you used exactly the same words and grammar, you conveyed very different meanings. In British English, though not in all languages, paralinguistic features are an important way of indicating politeness, anger, resentment, uncertainty, interest or lack of it, apology, excitement, disagreement and so on.

Emphasis and pace   British English uses emphasis to signal important or new information, for example, 'I told her to take it **three** times a day', 'Mrs Smith **is** coming on Monday'. Speakers of other languages or of other forms of English may not realise that a specific meaning is being indicated, or may themselves use emphasis differently to indicate something which British English speakers fail to grasp. In British English emphasis is also used to indicate emotions such as anger or excitement. In other languages it may simply indicate that what is being said is very important. Alternatively, in some languages people show that something important is being said by speaking faster; in other languages they slow down and lower their voices (Mares *et al.*, 1985).

Linguistic tunes   Each language has its own intonation or tune. In tonal languages such as Chinese and Thai, the tune or tone is part of each word. Changing the tone to high, low, falling or rising actually changes the word. So, for example, the sound 'ma' in Mandarin Chinese means 'old woman', 'horse', 'hemp', or 'to scold', depending on the tone used. People have to get the tone absolutely right in order to be understood.

In British English, tone does not change the meaning of individual words but is often used to modify the meaning of a phrase or sentence. For example, a raised tone at the end of a statement can turn it into a question; 'You've done your urine sample?'. But raising the tone of the **whole** sentence is often associated with intense emotion such as anger, shock or excitement; 'You've won the Nobel prize!', 'You've flooded the whole ground floor!'. In other languages a raised tone over the whole sentence may instead indicate its importance, or the friendly intentions of the speaker.

British English and other northern European languages use a relatively limited range of tones in normal speech: some other languages and some other forms of English use a far greater range. To British English speakers, speakers of these languages often sound excitable and excessively emotional. To them, British English speakers sound flat, bored or depressed. It is easy for neutral linguistic features to be misconstrued as indicating something about the personality or intentions of the person concerned.

Volume   Acceptable volume for normal conversation differs; British English speakers tend to speak relatively quietly and may feel disconcerted or threatened by someone in whose culture it is normal to speak more loudly. People who speak 'too loudly' may be incorrectly perceived as angry, excitable, over-emotional or dangerous.

Structuring conversation   In most European languages it is common to state the main point in an argument first, and then to illustrate or expand upon it. In many other languages it is common to set out the preliminary arguments and illustrations first, working up to the main point as a conclusion. British English speakers, who are used to hearing the main point early on, may become bored and impatient when listening to a client or colleague who uses the other system. They may conclude that he or she has nothing important to say and switch off before the main point is reached (Roberts, 1985).

Conversation generally requires people to take turns. But different languages use different conventions to indicate when one person has finished and another can begin. For example, the first speaker may lower her voice and slow down; she may indicate the next person's turn by beginning to repeat herself; she may pause and leave a space for the second person to begin. The length of this pause varies; for example, people from Latin America generally take and expect very short pauses; English speakers from North America take slightly longer pauses; British English speakers take still longer pauses (Tannen, 1992).

In British English, though not in all languages, it is considered normal and polite for only one person to speak at a time and for people to pause to allow each other to speak. It is also important to indicate that you are listening by nodding, making eye contact and encouraging noises. In some languages it is not necessary to do anything at all to show that you are listening.

In some cultures talking at the same time as another person and talking over them ('high-involvement style') is regarded as friendly and polite, and proof that you are really listening; in northern Europe it is generally regarded as aggressive and pushy (Tannen, 1991).

Misunderstandings and blame

The key point about paralinguistic features is that most of us assume that they are universal and that they tell us something reliable about a person's behaviour, intentions or personality. If a client raises her voice and talks faster, for example, we may conclude that she is angry. If her voice goes up and down a lot we may conclude that she is excited or indignant, or we may simply be puzzled. Problems also arise when people use different turn-taking signals. Person A may never get a chance to talk and feel cut out; Person B may wonder why Person A isn't saying anything. They may then label each other pushy, shy, or unfriendly. But since paralinguistic features and the way they are used differ in different languages and different forms of English, such conclusions are often unreliable (Tannen, 1992).

The paralinguistic features of a different language or a different form of one's own language are the most difficult thing to learn. Native speakers of the language are generally unaware of them and rarely explain them. People speaking a second language almost always carry over some of the paralinguistic features of their mother tongue, even if they speak the new language fluently. Few second-language speakers therefore have the same control over the way they are perceived.

NON-VERBAL SIGNALS

Non-verbal signals are another important part of the way we communicate. Professionals and clients may misinterpret each other's intentions if the non-verbal signals they use are based on different conventions. For example, there may be differences in the meaning people of different cultures attach to:

- eye contact
- facial expressions
- head and body movements and posture
- gestures
- touch
- physical distance from the other speaker.

Some cultures use a lot of physical gestures and movements when talking; others do not. The significance of different gestures varies. In some cultures, for example, 'yes' is indicated by moving the head up and down, in others by moving it from side to side, in others by dipping it sharply downwards (Collett, 1993). Movements and gestures such as shrugging the shoulders, making a fist or clicking the tongue may be perfectly acceptable in some cultures and very offensive in others.

Physical distance   Physical distance between speakers varies in different cultures and situations. In English culture, partners, and parents and children are generally comfortable at much closer distances than friends. Acquaintances usually stand even further apart. People from Northern Europe tend to stand further apart than people from the Middle East, Greece or Turkey (Morain, 1986). When conversing, most people try to maintain the distance they find comfortable; if their cultural conventions differ this may mean that one speaker constantly moves backwards to try to gain space, while the other 'pursues' him or her to get closer.

Eye contact   The degree of acceptable eye contact also differs. In most cultures there are different rules for eye contact between members of the same sex and between members of the opposite sex. In some cultures, looking people in the eye is taken to indicate honesty and straightforwardness; in many others it is seen as challenging and rude. Most people in Arab cultures, for example, share a great deal of eye contact and may regard too little as disrespectful (Argyle, 1975). In English culture, a certain amount of eye contact is required, but too much makes many people uncomfortable. Most English people make eye contact at the beginning and then look away periodically to avoid 'staring the other person out'.

In South Asian culture direct eye contact is generally regarded as aggressive and disrespectful. This can cause problems, for example, for some overseas-trained South Asian doctors taking oral examinations in Britain. Lowering their eyes as a sign of respect may be wrongly interpreted as a sign of not knowing the answer. They may also have to overcome other cultural prohibitions such as calling older people by their first name and holding the hand of a patient of the opposite sex to express sympathy and concern (Sami, 1989).

> 'I trained in Switzerland and I was astonished when a Swiss doctor told me that I would be considered to be telling a lie if I did not look straight into a person's eyes.'
> Pakistani doctor

Physical posture and touch   All cultures also have clear conventions about certain aspects of physical posture.

> In Thai culture it is deeply offensive to point the soles of one's feet at people, for example when sitting. People of lower status should also try to keep their heads below those of people of higher status, if necessary by bending the knees. It is extremely rude to pass between two adults who are talking without bending down so that one's head is below theirs. In British culture none of this is an issue and most British people in Thailand give terrible offence without ever intending to or realising it.

Cultural rules about posture often differ between men and women. It may be completely acceptable, for example, for men to sit with their legs apart but not for women. Different cultures also decree which parts of the body should be covered. In some cultures the legs and upper arms must always be covered; in others almost everything can be exposed. In some cultures men must cover their heads; in others, women. Rules of acceptable touch are also gender- and situation-based. In some cultures it is unacceptable for members of the same sex to touch each other in public; in others it is unacceptable for members of the opposite sex. The amount of touch expected also varies. In a study of the number of times heterosexual couples touched each other in cafes, it was found that in Puerto Rico they touched 180 times per hour, in Paris 110 times, and in London, about 200 miles away, not at all (Argyle, 1975). In some cultures certain kinds of touch are acceptable, for example in a medical situation, which would not normally be acceptable except in the closest relationships.

Misunderstandings and blame

All these non-verbal conventions are culture-based, acquired in childhood and then used unconsciously. As with paralinguistic features, we usually only notice non-verbal behaviour when it feels wrong or makes us uncomfortable. We often then judge the person who makes us feel this way and dislike them. However, it is very difficult to master the non-verbal conventions of a new culture. Non-verbal conventions are absolutely ingrained in each of us and hard to change, they are rarely made explicit or taught, and inappropriate non-verbal behaviour is generally regarded as intentional and therefore not pointed out.

CULTURAL CONVENTIONS ABOUT POLITENESS

Each culture has rules of polite behaviour which enable people to get on together. The importance of formal politeness varies; some cultures value it more highly than others. Once again, failure to follow the local rules of polite behaviour is usually construed as intentional bad manners.

Please and thank you   In British English the words 'please' and 'thank you' are extremely important. Although the amount they are used differs to some extent between men and women and in different situations, people who do not say 'please' and 'thank you' are regarded as arrogant and intentionally rude. 'Please' and 'thank you' are particularly important between people of different status and in formal situations.

In other cultures, politeness may be managed differently. For example, instead of the formulaic 'please' and 'thank you' it may be indicated by a different choice of verb form or pronoun (like *tu* or *vous* in French), or by a different tone of voice. In some cultures, 'please' and 'thank you' are not used when people are simply doing their job; omitting them is not regarded by either side as at all impolite (Bowler, 1993). Here again, people who are used to one particular convention often feel offended or angry when faced by a different one.

'In trying to speak English, the women frequently offended the midwives. Their main complaint was that the women did not say "please" or "thank you" and that they "gave orders". Although Urdu has words equivalent to "please" and "thank you" these are rarely used. Instead there is a polite form of the imperative with the "please" built into the verb. The use of the imperative (fetch my bottle, bring my breakfast) without 'please' is indeed very rude in English, but was not intended as such by the women.'   Hospital midwife (from Bowler, 1993, by permission)

While working in a foreign country an Englishman noted that the words 'please' and 'thank you' were seldom used to accompany requests or instructions. Curious about this and not believing that the whole country was rude, he asked someone of the host culture about this.

'The trouble is, Colin,' he was told, 'you use please and thank you far too often. How can people believe that you are sincere when you use the words so often that they lose their meaning? If a person of my country says thank you, they really mean it.'

'So do I,' protested the Englishman.

'Then use them less,' said the other man.

Saying no   Conventions of politeness also clash over the word 'no'. In some cultures saying no directly, particularly to a person of higher status, is offensive and unpleasant. There are other indirect but polite ways which are understood by both sides and which a person can use to refuse a request or answer a question negatively. Unfortunately it can be difficult to translate these into English and when people try they are often misunderstood.

It is particularly impolite to answer 'no' to someone older or of higher status than oneself. In the Vietnamese language there is an expression which avoids this – *da khong* (South), or *thua khong* (North). It translates literally as 'yes, no' but it is used in the sense of 'I'm afraid not' or 'I'm sorry to say no'. (From Mares, 1982, by permission)

In other cultures, people who avoid saying no directly are regarded as hypocritical or devious. Directness is valued and is thought to indicate honesty and straightforwardness.

English culture lies somewhere in the middle, and, like all cultures, contains variations on the basis of class and gender. In general, however, English culture is relatively indirect, expecting people to understand unstated messages, especially when there is any awkwardness. People tend to avoid conflict and often try to defuse situations by avoiding or changing a difficult subject, giving a non-committal reply or making a joke. This can seem deceitful and confusing to people of other cultures.

Anger   Many English people also tend to avoid anger; overt anger is usually reserved for very serious or intolerable situations, often as a last resort. It often leaves deep scars. In other cultures anger may be more lightly expressed, received and forgotten. Argument and confrontation may be seen as a positive sign of friendliness and engagement. Here again there is a good deal of opportunity for misunderstanding and mutual resentment.

> *'I find the English deceitful. If you say that you are angry about something they all agree, but when you want to go and confront the person responsible they melt away.'* .Belgian woman

Greetings   Different societies have different norms about how people should behave when they meet, and how they say hello and goodbye. People who do not behave as expected are often perceived as intentionally bad mannered.

> *'We have some Californian neighbours and the children come round to our house a lot. They never greet me when they walk in. They simply say 'Where are the cookies?'. I see red immediately and feel like throwing them out. And if I give them a biscuit they never say thank you. When I discussed it with their mother she said their behaviour was perfectly polite and in fact I should be pleased because it indicates how at home they feel with me!'* English mother

It is important not to assume that people intend to cause offence or are in some way deficient if they do not conform to your own expectations of polite behaviour.

Take a moment to think about your own behaviour. If you found yourself living in a culture where your normal behaviour was unacceptable:

- What sort of reactions would you get from others?
- How would you feel?
- How would you react?

- Would you be willing to change your behaviour to fit in?
- For how long?
- How much would you be willing to change?
- What would be the long-term effect on you?

Embarrassing words

Every language has a range of polite and impolite words for most different bodily functions and parts of the body. In British English, words of Latin origin are generally more acceptable in polite conversation than words of Anglo-Saxon origin. There are also a large number of euphemisms and words regarded as bad or derogatory which may vary in different parts of the country. Certain words, such as stool and urine, are usually only used in a medical context. For people whose first language is not English all this can pose major problems. It can be embarrassing and difficult to find out the acceptable words for these things (see also Chapter 11).

SUSPENDING AUTOMATIC RESPONSES

Our reactions to the way people speak and behave are largely automatic and often difficult to control. Misunderstandings about other people's personality or intentions are inevitable when we have different linguistic and cultural conventions. There are no easy solutions. It is, however, always important:

- to be aware of the reasons why things may go wrong;
- to monitor and try to suspend your automatic responses; and
- to assume, at least until other clear evidence emerges, that the person does not wish to irritate or offend you. **Try to remember that they may not mean what you heard them say** (Tannen, 1991).

If you can, check out any judgements tactfully with the person concerned or with other people from their community. Where you have developed a relationship of mutual trust, it may also be possible to discuss your reactions with the client, find out whether they realise how they appear, and respectfully suggest modifications in their approach. This may be helpful to them in the long term. Try to find out also whether there are things that you automatically do that cause offence to some of your clients and how you can adapt.

9

The language barrier

CLIENTS AND THE LANGUAGE BARRIER

The NHS Patient's Charter on Maternity Services stresses women's right to information from professionals about local maternity services, the different types of care they can choose, the tests available during pregnancy, possible treatments and their benefits and risks, pain relief during labour, infant feeding and more (Department of Health, 1994). But where client and professional cannot ask questions, understand replies, outline choices, or discuss problems and anxieties, maternity care is often reduced to the most basic physical minimum. This is a transcript of a real antenatal interview between a midwife and a Bangladeshi woman who does not speak or understand any English.

Midwife: *Baby moving? Baby kicking?* (Woman doesn't understand)

Midwife: *Date of last period?* (Woman doesn't understand)

Midwife: *Are you well? All right?* (Woman nods)

Midwife: *Have you got one of these?* (Shows hospital card) (Woman offers envelope with forms, etc.)

Midwife: *I'll give you one. This card you take to hospital with you.* (Gestures) *You bring here.* (Gestures)

Midwife: *OK? Your husband OK?* (Woman nods)

Midwife: *Baby kick?* (Woman doesn't understand) *Take your coat off.* (Woman doesn't understand) *Take your coat off.* (Woman doesn't understand) (Midwife gestures, woman takes coat off) *Sit down.* (Woman sits down. Midwife takes blood pressure)

Midwife: *Pop up on the scale.* (Gestures. Woman gets onto scales)

Midwife: (Gestures to bed: *OK.* (Woman lies on bed)

Midwife: (Palpates woman's stomach) *It's growing.* (Woman winces) *Does it hurt?* (Woman doesn't understand) *Pain?* (Woman doesn't understand. Midwife makes noise of someone in pain by breathing in sharply. Woman interprets this as an instruction and starts saying '*schoo, schoo*'...)

Woman: *Very pain here.*

Midwife: *You see doctor. You go tonight. Go see Dr W.* (Midwife repeats this twice but woman doesn't seem to understand)

Woman: *Finish?*

Midwife: (Nods) *Sit down.* (Woman gets off bed. Sits down)

(From Shackman, 1984, by permission)

Reduced information and choices

Research confirms that women who speak little or no English are generally given less information and offered fewer choices (Bowler, 1993; Currer, 1986; Homans and Satow, 1982). The care they receive is less flexible and often paternalistic, not attuned to their emotional and medical needs. They are often unable to understand what is done to them and why. They cannot ask questions, voice worries or ask for what they want. They cannot give genuinely informed consent (Windsor-Richards and Gillies, 1988).

One survey (see Tables 9.1 and 9.2) found that South Asian women received a good deal less information about where they could have their baby and were less likely to have discussed important issues with health professionals beforehand. At least part of the reason for this is likely to be that a number of women of childbearing age in these communities speak little or no English.

The medical treatment given to women who speak little or no English may also be limited by the lack of communication. Watson (1986), for example, quotes a doctor who said she had prescribed a contraceptive method to a non-English speaking woman, 'not because she judged it to be the most efficacious or the most suitable medication for the patient, but because the others were too complex to describe'.

Table 9.1   Percentage of women who were aware of birth options

	All women (%)	*Indian women (%)*	*Pakistani women (%)*	*Bangladeshi women (%)*
Domino scheme	33	3	6	3
GP unit	22	1	7	4
Home birth	47	14	13	3

Source: MORI/Department of Health, *Changing Childbirth: a Survey of Women's Experiences of Childbirth* (unpublished), conducted for the Expert Maternity Group, 1993, Department of Health, by permission.

Table 9.2   Percentage of women who had discussed issues with health professionals

	All women (%)	*Indian women (%)*	*Pakistani women (%)*	*Bangladeshi women (%)*
Events during labour and birth	33	3	6	3
Who would be present at the birth	22	1	7	4
Pain relief	47	14	13	3

Source: MORI/Department of Health, *Changing Childbirth: a Survey of Women's Experiences of Childbirth* (unpublished), conducted for the Expert Maternity Group, 1993, Department of Health, by permission.

In some cases non-English speaking clients may become the targets of anger and resentment from professional staff.

They think you are a burden because you don't speak English, or simply because you are different.'   Hindu mother (Alibhai, 1988)

'Please understand us better and don't shout at us so much. Some staff are really rude to us.'   Somali woman

Bowler (1993), in her study of the delivery of maternity care to a number of South Asian women, found that communication difficulties were common. Women who spoke little or no English found it difficult to develop personal relationships with midwives and vice versa. Midwives tended to perceive the women as unresponsive, rude and unintelligent, and to rely on stereotypes in place of communication to decide what they needed. The South Asian women in the survey were unlikely to know about the choices available, such as the option of a female supporter in labour rather than their husband, or the kinds of pain control they could have. In several cases women were assumed to speak no English simply because they were Asian. In fact many spoke a little English and understood more but were shy.

Currer (1986) found that none of the Pathan women she interviewed, all of whom had had at least one baby in the UK, were sure whether they could ask for analgesia if they wanted it during labour. Most of the women had not liked to ask or had been unable to. One woman had said no to everything she did not understand including the offer of analgesia. Women who did not speak good English but who tried to ask questions about procedures or their baby's condition had often been ignored or rebuffed.

Clinical dangers

Health professionals base their decisions about care and treatment on the woman's medical and obstetric history as well as on the presenting symptoms and signs. If she speaks little or no English the required information may be either unavailable or inaccurate. This is bound to affect clinical care (Parsons and Day, 1992). It must also mean that professionals sometimes fail to identify problems during the pregnancy or birth and that the necessary action is not taken or is taken too late. Higher rates of perinatal mortality and morbidity within some communities may therefore be due in part to the language barrier.

In a letter to the *Lancet* in 1988 six bilingual obstetricians and gynaecologists stated that they knew of several cases where well-developed fetuses had died unnecessarily during the intrapartum period because of failures of communication with mothers who spoke little English (Samra *et al.*, 1988).

The language barrier also affects the overall quality of planning and provision for particular minority groups, and reinforces their marginalisation. General attempts to improve communication between professionals and clients, such as client-held notes, become meaningless.

Patients who do not speak English find it hard to talk to professional staff and managers about their experience of a hospital, or to make suggestions or to voice complaints. Very few hospitals advertise complaints procedures in anything other than English, and most obtain feedback in ways that only accommodate people who can read English. (Audit Commission, 1993, Crown copyright)

HEALTH PROFESSIONALS AND THE LANGUAGE BARRIER

Health professionals are clearly not in the same dependent and vulnerable situation as clients. Nevertheless, language barriers are often extremely frustrating and difficult. Many professionals feel that they cannot use their skills to the full and that their jobs in consequence are far less satisfying. Many miss the rewards of a good relationship with their clients and feel that they are unable to give the same level of care, support and comfort. Many feel guilty, furious, ineffective and stressed (Bowler, 1993; Murphy and Macleod-Clark, 1993).

Working across a language barrier also takes a good deal more time. When people are already very hard-pressed this may feel like the last straw. Some professionals turn their frustration against their clients. In some cases anger, frustration and pressure can lead to panic and extraordinary and unprofessional behaviour.

'If women can't speak English they cannot communicate their fear and must be left with some degree of emotional trauma. I've seen doctors and midwives being rough and brutal and shouting at women who are terrified of being examined, often because they don't understand what is going on.'   Community midwife

Take a moment to ask yourself the following question:

- When a woman who does not speak much English arrives at an antenatal clinic, how do you feel?
- How do you react?

Most professionals feel dismayed, irritated, angry or inadequate, or all of these. They know that to do this client justice they will have to give her more time, and time is always short. Some feel angry because the woman has not learnt English. If there are no interpreters available, useful discussion will be almost impossible. One midwife said, 'I just grit my teeth and get on with what has to be done and get it over as quickly as possible.' In the absence of communication it may be easier for professionals to accept widely held myths that allow them a way out such as 'Asian women make a fuss about nothing' (Alibhai, 1988) because they *cannot* find out what is wrong.

However much we try to hide our supposedly internal reactions, they always influence how we approach and care for clients. Non-verbal signals are hard to conceal and people who do not understand what is being said are often particularly sensitive to them. Clients easily sense discomfort or hostility on the part of professionals. These add to their own feelings of inadequacy, vulnerability and frustration. A woman in such a situation may assume that you do not like her or that something is wrong with her pregnancy. She may simply decide that you are racist.

In some circumstances she may also decide not to accept any advice or treatment or not to come back to the clinic. The risk of undetected problems and complications is increased.

WHY DO SOME PEOPLE NOT LEARN ENGLISH?

Many health professionals, especially those who are themselves multilingual, understand the problems facing adult immigrants who speak little or no English. However, some see learning English as a simple moral issue, and regard a client's failure to do so as evidence of idleness and stupidity. They may see the provision of interpreters as an unfair and unnecessary cost. Some professionals vent their frustration on non-English speaking clients and tell interpreters to tell them to learn English. A few cases have been reported of professionals refusing to treat clients until they learn English, or not to have another baby until their English is better (Watson, 1986).

> 'You know, in this country if you don't know English they make you feel you are nothing and that attitude makes you feel small and insignificant. No matter how much you know in your home and with your family, outside you are zero – you are utterly insignificant.'   Sikh woman (from Ahmed and Watt, 1986, by permission)

There is no doubt that caring for people across a language barrier is frustrating, difficult and time-consuming. It is also clear that non-English speaking clients would usually get better care if they spoke English and so it is in their own interests to learn the English they need for encounters with the Health Service. However, most clients are only too aware of this. They understand very well the problems caused by their lack of English. They would speak it if they could. Adding to the pressure they already feel in this situation only makes matters worse.

Learning a language as an adult

Many adult immigrants who speak little or no English find it very difficult to learn more. Many are trapped in a kind of vicious circle in which the less English they speak the fewer opportunities they have to meet English people and learn the language. Most people's domestic and work responsibilities leave them little or no time. Women with small children and a home to look after, for example, are very unlikely to have any chance to learn English informally, to practise it or to get out to English classes. In any case, they may see learning English as selfish and not as a priority in terms of their duties: the day-to-day needs of their family and their home come first. People in paid employment tend to get jobs that require little English and may have no opportunity to learn more. They often work unsocial hours and shifts. Precisely because people's English is poor, they are also unlikely to develop the kinds of relationships with English speakers that will enable them to learn more (Currer, 1986; Li, 1992).

> In fact, most women did express a desire to learn English and most saw that it would be an advantage to them. Their husbands were even more keen that they should do so, as they bore many of the burdens of their wives' lack of ability to communicate when necessary. But the incentives were not sufficient to overcome the difficulties of an overbusy daily routine of housework and childcare. (From Currer, 1986, by permission)

Language is a tool. Research into adult learning shows that most adults learn only what they need urgently to fulfil their short-term responsibilities (Rogers, 1989). Even for people with a high level of academic achievement and confidence, simply living in a country where a different language is spoken does not mean that one learns the language. The key issue is whether one needs to use the language frequently.

In the day-to-day lives of many non-English speakers there is little real need for English. Most have also developed strategies for managing without. If they live in an area with other members of their own community they can generally get help when necessary from people who speak English better than they do. They can shop in supermarkets where English is hardly needed, or in shops run by people who speak their language.

> *'My husband goes out to work so he speaks English much better than me. I speak very little English and I am very shy about it. So when I have to go anywhere I always try to take him with me and he can do all the talking. I would feel a fool speaking my bad English when he can say all the things much more clearly for me. Especially when it's really important and the people are so busy and in such a hurry always.'*   Punjabi woman (from Mares *et al.*, 1985, by permission)

A survey in 1993 looked at the level of English among South Asian women in the UK aged 16–35. Respondents assessed their own levels of English.

Table 9.3   Percentages of South Asian women in the UK aged 16–35 who do not speak English

Women	Non-English speakers (%)
Indian	13
Pakistani	29
Bangladeshi	42

Source: MORI/Department of Health, *Changing Childbirth: a Survey of Women's Experiences of Childbirth* (unpublished), conducted for the Expert Maternity Group, 1993, Department of Health, by permission.

Motivation and confidence

A major factor in learning is motivation, in this case the wish to learn the language in order to speak it to people. The experience of hostility or impatience from English speakers can destroy people's wish to communicate as well as their confidence in their ability to do so. People with little formal education may also lack the confidence to attend language classes and may find it difficult to learn in an academic environment (Mares *et al.*, 1985).

Paradoxically, the longer that people have been used to operating and fulfilling their daily responsibilities without English, the more going to classes can seem irrelevant and even pointless. People may then only really need English in exceptional and particularly difficult circumstances for which it is unlikely that any classes can equip them. It is in these highly stressful situations that health professionals often encounter them. In such situations both professionals and clients should have access to trained interpreters who can help them overcome the language barrier. (For more about working with professional interpreters, see Chapter 11.)

Table 9.4 Factors that help or hinder people from learning English

Factors that help people learn English	*Factors that prevent people learning English*
Completed secondary or higher education	Little formal education
Relatively new in the country	In the country for several years
Younger	Older
Responsibilities that require contact with outsiders	Heavy domestic or work responsibilities
Self-confidence	Low self-confidence and shyness
Accessible, suitable classes	Inaccessible classes, unsuitable approach, irrelevant vocabulary
Urgent, immediate and frequent need for English	English rarely needed except in occasional, stressful situations
Lots of opportunities for practice	Few opportunities for practice
Nobody available to interpret	Family member who speaks better English
Frequent, positive, regular contact with English speakers	Little contact with English speakers, fear of hostility and racism

10

Communicating across a language barrier*

STRESS AND LANGUAGE

Trying to communicate across a language barrier, especially with people in authority or in frightening situations, dramatically affects the way many people behave. It is important to bear this in mind when working with clients who speak little English, or whose English is adversely affected by stress or illness. Beware of making judgements from the other side of the language barrier.

Think back to a time when you were having difficulty understanding and being understood by someone in authority, possibly in a language you did not speak well.

- How did you feel? Physically? Emotionally?
- How did you cope?
- How did you react to that person at the time? If you met them again later?

In situations like this people commonly find that they:

- Feel nervous and less able to think clearly, get upset easily.
- Become very sensitive to people's non-verbal signals; body language, tone of voice, gestures.
- Smile a lot and try to show that although they cannot communicate they want to be helpful.
- Become quickly exhausted and understand less and less.
- Remain passive and silent, avoid eye contact and avoid initiating or prolonging conversations.
- Give simple, though inaccurate, answers or explanations because they cannot explain things as they want to.
- Give the impression of understanding more than they do to avoid irritating the other person and making the situation more difficult.

---

* Much of this chapter is adapted from Henley (1987) by permission of Bloomsbury Health Authority and Henley (1991) by permission of the National Extension College.

- Avoid situations and discussions they feel they cannot cope with. With health professionals they may, for example, describe specific physical symptoms rather than attempting to explain intangible chronic complaints or complex emotional problems.

Conversations across a language barrier are also wearing for health professionals. You may have noticed how hard you have to concentrate to try to understand someone whose English is not very good, how tiring it is, and how tempting to give up. You may also have noticed that you cut down the amount you try to communicate and settle for the bare minimum.

Reducing unnecessary stress

Emotional and physical stress and anxiety can seriously affect people's confidence and language ability even in their mother tongue. If you can cut down on the stress she is experiencing, a client's language ability may dramatically improve. **The more you can create a respectful, non-judgemental partnership in which both of you openly acknowledge the difficulties of the situation and encourage each other, the more successful the conversation is likely to be.** However, even with these techniques, communication with many clients will remain inadequate. You will need a professional interpreter for all important conversations (see Chapter 11).

To reduce stress:

- Make sure you have got the client's name right and are using and pronouncing it correctly (see also Chapter 14).
- Allow more time. If time is short, try not to show it. Signs of pressure or impatience increase the stress on the client and may reduce even further the amount you can achieve. If you have not got much time now, try to arrange another appointment.
- Try to convey sympathy and positive regard rather than irritation. If necessary, take time to let off steam in private later. Most non-English-speaking clients are only too aware that many professionals are irritated and frustrated by them.

  Women did not even look for success in communication. They did, however, notice whether or not people tried and whether or not they seemed to care. (From Currer, 1986, by permission)

- If the client does not understand verbal reassurance, concentrate on non-verbal signals such as smiles, eye contact, touch (if appropriate) and a sympathetic calm manner. A reassuring tone of voice can help even if people do not understand the words.

  'A Bangladeshi women came and asked specially for me to look after her, because I had looked after her sister when she was in labour. Her sister spoke no English so I couldn't communicate with her at all. All I had been able to do was stay with her throughout her labour and to hold her hand all the time. I had no idea that such a little thing had been so important and helpful to her.' Community midwife

- Watch for signs of weariness in your client and do not carry on too long. You too may become tired and less able to communicate clearly.

- In carrying out any procedure always say what you are doing or going to do next. Never maintain total silence or give the impression that you are ignoring the client. A reassuring tone of voice is much better than silence.
- Try to ensure continuity of care. The difficulties of establishing good relationships are even greater across a language barrier. For clients, getting to know individual health professionals helps reduce stress and makes communication easier. Keep good notes so that different professionals do not have to keep asking the same questions.
- Try to learn a few words of the client's language. 'Good morning', 'goodbye', 'yes', 'no', and a few other helpful words can make a great difference to your relationship with the client. Trying to speak her language also puts you on the same footing and enables you to understand some of her feelings of embarrassment and the difficulty of remembering even simple words in a foreign language.
- Non-English speaking clients often find that health professionals spend less time with them because they cannot communicate easily with them. Although this may be understandable it is also hurtful. On the ward, make a point of stopping to speak to non-English speaking clients as often as to English-speaking clients. If there are two women who speak the same language ask whether they would like to be in neighbouring beds. Loneliness is often a major problem.

SIMPLIFYING YOUR LANGUAGE

You may also be able to modify your language to make it easier for the client to understand. Listen to yourself, or get a colleague to listen and give you feedback. Become aware of areas that need more work. The guidelines below offer some ideas.

All the suggestions below must be used sensitively and judiciously. Never assume that a client does not speak English on the basis of their name or appearance. If there is a language barrier, listen and watch carefully to gauge how far you need to modify your normal way of speaking.

- Listen to and watch the client and assess her ability in English.
- Listen for the words she uses and try to use them too.

Are you speaking plain English?

- Speak slowly if necessary and try not to get louder.
- Do not use 'pidgin' English; it is not easier to understand and sounds patronising and insulting.
- Avoid hospital and clinical jargon and euphemisms. Use plain, everyday words as far as possible.

  Terms such as 'waterworks', 'down there', 'the other end', 'tummy' and 'dizzy' are difficult even for those Asian women who are competent in English. (Bowler, 1993)

- Try to be succinct and clear but do not condense what you want to say. This simply makes it more difficult to understand.
- Wherever possible, demonstrate things or point them out on a picture rather than simply relying on the spoken word.

Are you saying things in the right order?

If you have a complicated matter to explain, stop and think first:

- Plan what you are going to say and in what order.
- Stick to one subject at a time.
- If you need to give instructions, give them in the order in which they need to be done. For example, 'First I'll take your blood pressure and weigh you, then you need to do a urine sample, then the doctor will see you', is a lot easier to follow than 'Just hop on the couch so that the doctor can see you, but first I need a urine sample, oh, and I'll do your blood pressure and let's weigh you.'
- When you have dealt with the subject, pause and check that the client has understood. Then introduce a new subject as necessary.

Are you observing your client's reactions carefully?

It is sometimes possible to tell from their non-verbal signals when people do not understand or are so tired that they have simply switched off. If this happens try to reduce the pressure a little. Move on to another subject that you know the client can cope with. Or stop and go back a bit, trying to choose simpler words. If the client has completely run out of energy, it may be helpful to end the interview politely and in a friendly manner, and to fix another time. Alternatively, suggest taking a break and resuming later. The client may feel better once she has had a snack and a rest.

Do you always check that the client understands?

Encourage the client to stop you if she does not understand what you are saying. Make it clear that you want to know and that you will not become impatient.

If it is important to know whether the client has understood, try to avoid questions that can be answered with 'yes'. 'Yes' is probably the first word that anyone learns in a new language, but it does not necessarily mean they have understood or that they agree. It is more likely to mean something like:

- 'Yes, I'm listening and I'm trying to understand.'
- 'Yes, I want to be helpful even though I don't understand.'
- 'Yes, I'm listening but I'm too tired and confused to take in what you are saying even though I know you mean well.'
- 'Yes, I'm listening, I don't understand you but I don't think I ever will and if I say yes we might be able to end this conversation.'

It can be humiliating and upsetting not to understand what is said and difficult to deal with the consequences of admitting we have not understood. Most people when they are trying to communicate in a language they do not speak well, use 'yes' a lot to show that they are really trying to understand. It can be dangerous to assume that 'yes' means they have actually understood and agreed.

Try to ask questions that actually check out a client's understanding. For example, ask her to show you or to tell you what she will do.

Do you avoid overestimating the amount a client understands?

Many people who have learnt English informally through hearing it spoken are very good at social conversation and at topics they use a lot. They may seem fluent in English, but may get completely stuck when trying to discuss unfamiliar topics with special vocabulary such as screening, pregnancy, or contraception. Bear in mind that the concentration required to try to understand another language can seriously affect a client's ability to remember what was said.

Write down important points about treatment, drugs and so on in simple English for the client to take away. Even if she cannot read it herself she will have a relative or friend who can.

11 Working with professional interpreters

No agency can provide an effective service to people with whom it cannot communicate.

Shackman, 1984

'Proficiency in English should not be a requirement for access to maternity care.' Hospital midwife

Where health professionals and clients do not share a common language, someone is needed to interpret. In order to ensure good two-way communication and clear mutual understanding this person must:

- be trained and experienced;
- be fluent in both English and the client's mother tongue;
- understand medical and midwifery terminology; and
- be someone whom both the health professional and the client can trust (Henley, 1991).

The current situation is that in many places there is still no formal interpreting provision. Where provision exists it is often inadequate in terms of numbers of people employed, the training, management and support they receive, and the range of languages covered. It is very rare for interpreters to be provided out of hours when many labours and births as well as other cases of urgent need occur. Smaller linguistic communities or those which are geographically scattered are rarely provided for (Audit Commission 1993; Warrier, 1995).

The benefits of trained, professional interpreters

Most interpreter provision is not evaluated and it can be difficult to separate the effects of interpreter services from other influences on maternity outcomes. Nevertheless, the results of those evaluations that have been carried out show that the provision of trained, professional health interpreters has major benefits for clients, professionals and for the service. These include:

- Greater continuity of care and emotional support for clients.
- Better-informed clients.
- Reduced stress for both clients and professionals.
- Greater job satisfaction for professionals (Warrier, 1995).

- Improved practical provision in terms of clients' cultural needs and preferences, for example, longer dressing gowns in antenatal clinics, facilities for private prayers, more appropriate hospital food, improved information about procedures, health education leaflets in appropriate languages, and women-only antenatal classes for South Asian women in more suitable community settings (Rocheron and Dickinson, 1990).
- Shorter antenatal stays.
- Reduced rates of induction and caesarean section (Parsons and Day, 1992).
- Happier pregnancies.
- Greater health awareness among clients.
- Reduced use of analgesia during labour.
- Reduced maternal morbidity (Warrier, 1995).

In a control study of linkworkers in East Birmingham, the group of women who had access to linkworkers had babies with a mean birthweight of 226.12 grams heavier than women in the control group (Warrier, 1995).

> If a health advocacy scheme can reduce interventions while increasing patient satisfaction it is a 'good buy' for health authorities and a good investment for maternity units. (From Parsons and Day, 1992, by permission)

Interpreters and the law

Under the Race Relations Act 1976 it is illegal for anyone involved in providing a service to discriminate against a person on racial grounds by refusing, or deliberately failing, to provide them with services, by providing them with poorer services, or by treating them less favourably (see also Chapter 4).

It is illegal, therefore, knowingly to provide an inferior quality of care to a particular racial minority group. An example of this is the failure to provide maternity interpreters for a minority group, many of whose female members are known to speak little English. Although no hospital, health authority or trust has yet been challenged on this aspect of discrimination, such a challenge is always possible.

The need for more black and ethnic minority health professionals

Communication through an interpreter, however good, is never likely to be as effective as direct communication between a health professional and a client who share the same language and cultural background. It is important, therefore, that authorities serving a multilingual population also employ black and ethnic minority health professionals at all levels and in all fields. The recruitment and use of interpreters must go hand in hand with a properly implemented equal opportunities policy on employment (Shackman, 1984).

Terminology

Many titles are used to describe people who provide language support for non-English-speaking clients. These include interpreter, health aide, maternity aide, linkworker, language aide, patient adviser and health advocate. The variety of terms reflects the current lack of clarity about the responsibilities of the job and its generally low status in the hierarchy. In this book we use the term interpreter, while being fully aware of the breadth and complexity of the role of a health interpreter, the responsibilities she carries, her importance in ensuring that clients get the care they need, and the status she should be accorded.

We have referred to the interpreter throughout as she. In some cases it may also be necessary to provide a male interpreter to discuss personal issues with a husband or male partner.

WORKING WELL WITH A PROFESSIONAL INTERPRETER*

For health professionals, working well with an interpreter involves a difficult balance between:

- retaining overall responsibility for the discussion and for the care the client receives;
- ensuring that the client gets the care she needs and wants; and
- helping the interpreter to work effectively using her skills to the full.

This requires conscious and careful management. Below are some suggestions.

Beforehand

If this is the first time you and the interpreter have worked together, discuss how to handle the conversation. Make it clear to the interpreter that you value her as an interpreter and a colleague. Ask her to alert you to any cultural issues that arise, and to stop you if she or the client have difficulties. Encourage her to tell you if you talk too fast or do not pause often enough. Check that she understands the importance of keeping both you and the client fully informed of what is going on. For example, if she needs to have a longer conversation with one of you, she should always tell the other person briefly what she is doing.

Make sure that you are both clear about the purpose of the session and discuss any particular concerns. If there are likely to be difficulties, it is useful to consider in advance how the interpreter should respond. Discuss what she might do, for example, if the client becomes upset or does not want to be interrupted. It is very difficult for an interpreter to ignore a client's distress and simply to continue translating. It may be better for her to concentrate on listening and on supporting the client, and to summarise what has been said to you both at the end.

Ask her how to pronounce and use the client's name correctly.

At the beginning

Check, if necessary, that the interpreter really speaks the client's language and (if appropriate) dialect. Not all the South Asian languages spoken in Britain are mutually comprehensible (see Table 34.1). People who speak one Chinese dialect do not necessarily speak another.

* Much of the following is adapted from Henley, 1991, by permission of the National Extension College.

Try to check that your client feels able to talk openly through the interpreter. Is there any reason why she might not trust or feel comfortable with the interpreter? Check with the interpreter whether she knows of any reason why the client may feel awkward or worried about talking to her. It is important that you can honestly assure the client that everything she says will be treated in total confidence (see also Chapter 12). There may be particular issues of security if the client is a refugee from government oppression in her own country.

Allow more time. You probably need at least twice as long as usual because everything has to go through the interpreter in both directions. If the subject is complicated or new the interpreter may have to do a lot of explaining. Unexpected issues and queries may also need to be discussed.

The interpreter and the client may also need time to get to know each other if they have not met before. People in many cultures find it discourteous to go straight into an interview, even a medical one. Your client may need to know a bit about the interpreter and what kind of person she is before she reveals intimate personal and medical details. If you can, introduce them and leave them alone for a few minutes.

During the conversation

You are still responsible for the care and well-being of the client. Do all the things you normally do. Greet the client. Sit facing her, and speak directly to her using normal gestures and expressions. Look at her most of the time. Try not to draw back physically or emotionally from her because you are working with an interpreter.

Use all your normal communications skills, listening, observing, responding, explaining and checking. Try to keep your English simple and jargon-free so that it is as easy as possible for the interpreter to translate it correctly and clearly.

Everyone always understands more of a foreign language than they speak. The more simply and clearly you speak, the more likely the client is to understand some of what you say or at least to follow the direction of the conversation. It also makes the interpreter's task easier. If the client's English is fairly good, you could agree to converse in English and ask the interpreter to listen for and help with any misunderstandings.

Break up what you say into manageable chunks for the interpreter to translate. Ask her to stop you if there is anything she does not understand.

Beware of putting a clinical burden on the interpreter. Except in very exceptional circumstances and with a clear protocol, never leave an interpreter alone to give clinical advice. Although many interpreters are excellent and experienced, they are not normally qualified midwives or doctors and are not responsible for the care of the client. It is your responsibility, for example, to check that the client understands, that she is not left with any unanswered questions, and that she knows what will happen next.

Although most of your attention should be on the client, remember the interpreter's need for acknowledgement and support. Show that you respect her expertise and judgement. Give her the time she needs. Try not to look impatient while she and the client are talking together.

Afterwards

Encourage the interpreter to talk generally to the client to find out if she has any other worries or problems.

Talk to the interpreter about how the session went. Ask for any insights or information the interpreter was unable to give you at the time. Ask her if there is anything you can do to make her job easier next time. Be prepared to spend time with her if she has had to give bad news or to deal with a difficult situation. She always bears the brunt of the client's emotions.

Every so often, after working with an interpreter, take time to note down for yourself what was hard and what you did well, and then celebrate your successes.

If a client holds her own notes the interpreter may need to translate them for her. Try to ensure in hospital that an interpreter visits each non-English-speaking client on the wards at least once a day. She can use this time to find out if the client has any unanswered needs or worries. Make sure that the interpreter knows where to refer anything that needs action and that her importance as the client's advocate and supporter is recognised by all staff.

If you are not satisfied with the interpreter provision you have, discuss this with the person in charge and ask for improvements. You should have access to a competent, trained, professional interpreter whenever you need one.

WHAT AN INTERPRETER DOES

Imagine that you are an interpreter working in a busy antenatal clinic in north-eastern China where there are a large number of English women who do not speak the local language. The doctor is a middle-aged Chinese man. You have to interpret in the following situations in one morning. What would you do in each situation?

Mrs Brown is four months pregnant and very tense. This is her fourth pregnancy. Her first two ended in miscarriages at 12 weeks. Her third ended in a stillbirth at term. After he has examined her internally the doctor says 'Can you ask Mrs Brown to come for a scan. I think there's something wrong.'

■ How do you feel? What do you say to Mrs. Brown? What are your responsibilities in such a situation? What will your responsibilities be during and after the scan? How will you manage?

Mrs Jackson comes to the antenatal clinic pregnant with her fifth child. Her fourth is only six months old. The doctor is annoyed because she had serious complications with her last pregnancy, and he spent a long time with her after the birth discussing what she should do and finally persuaded her to go on the pill. He cannot understand why she is pregnant again. She tells you she didn't take the pill but insists that you do not tell the doctor.

■ How do you feel? What are your responsibilities in such a situation? What do you do?

Mrs Hayes has two small children and is pregnant again. She is overweight and says she is frightened of putting on too much weight in this pregnancy. The doctor advises her to cut down on fried noodles and eat more steamed vegetables and durian. She says yes but you think she probably eats an English diet and that this advice is irrelevant to her.

■ What do you do? What are your responsibilities in such a situation?

Mrs Buonomo is pregnant with her first child. She is Italian and speaks no English. She is also very nervous and has been having some vaginal bleeding. You do not speak Italian. There is no Italian interpreter. When you tell the doctor you cannot translate for Mrs Buonomo he says, 'Come on, it's important. I know you Europeans all understand each others' languages. Please have a go.' Mrs Buonomo is obviously very upset and pours out her worries to you in Italian. You don't understand what she is saying but you can't stop her.

■ How do you feel? What do you say? What are your responsibilities in such a situation?

Interpreting in the field of health care is never straightforward. In none of the situations above will your client get good care if you simply translate words from one language to another, even where that is possible. Often the interpreter is the only person who has the complete picture of what is going on and the only one who can communicate with and help both sides. She understands more about the maternity care system, how it works, and what kind of care it should provide than the client. She understands more about the client's fears, personality, situation, needs, culture and likely expectations than the health professional. She has responsibilities to both parties and she alone is in a position to assess how things are going. Her task is therefore extremely complicated. It includes:

● Translating as accurately as possible everything that health professional and client say.
● Helping the professional make an accurate assessment of the full situation.
● Encouraging the client to ask questions where she does not understand or needs more information.
● Providing emotional support and encouragement for the client.
● Ensuring that both parties have the information they need to make informed decisions, and that both feel fully involved.
● Explaining treatments, tests and other aspects of maternity care that the client is not familiar with.
● Explaining cultural factors that may be important for both sides to understand.
● Acting as a supporter for the client, helping to ensure that she gets the treatment and care she has a right to.
● Challenging negative stereotypes, racism and discriminatory practices.

At the same time, the interpreter must keep pushing the responsibility and the control of the discussion back to the health professional and to the client. Part of the interpreter's role is to limit the client's dependence on her by providing her with information, language and self-advocacy skills so that eventually, in theory at least, she can manage the discussion on her own (Baylav, 1994).

The task of translation

Given the list of responsibilities above, the actual translation of words from one language to another could be seen as the easiest part of a health interpreter's job. In fact it is never straightforward. No two languages use exactly the same grammatical structures, or express things in exactly the same way. Even if two words appear to be the same, there may be a subtle difference in meaning. Word order and the order in which ideas are sequenced differ. Sometimes an interpreter needs several sentences to translate a single word; sometimes a single word will convey several sentences. The more different the roots and structures of the two languages, for example, Bengali and English, the more difficult the interpreter's job (Schott and Henley, 1992).

The vocabulary and concepts in each language reflect the culture and key concerns of the people who speak it. Western medical and health care terminology can cause particular difficulties for interpreters since there may be no equivalent in the client's language. The Health and Lifestyles Survey (HEA, 1994) found that a wide range of English health-related terms had no equivalent in some South Asian languages, and were not generally understood in some communities. These included 'stress', 'personal space' and 'healthy foods' as well as many medical terms. Often the concepts were untranslatable. People who were familiar with the concepts tended to use the English word for them.

Even if a word exists in the client's language, she may not be familiar with it. Words such as amniocentesis, show, virus, antenatal classes, consultant, discharge, genetic, and labour ward may all need explanations, often lengthy. An interpreter may have to choose between simply translating the word, knowing that it makes no sense to the client, or taking the time to give a detailed explanation, checking also that the client has understood, and answering her questions.

In many languages there are no socially acceptable words for the female or male private parts or for sexual activities. These words have only developed even in Western Europe since the nineteenth century, with the medicalisation of sexuality and of sexual behaviour (Khan, 1994) (see also Chapter 26). Interpreters may have to develop and explain their own translations for such words to clients. They may have to find other acceptable ways of explaining what they mean. They may also have to deal with their own and the client's embarrassment and reticence.

Problems over the lack of equivalent words also work in the other direction: English and most other European languages, for example, have very few words to describe anything but the closest family relationships. More distant relationships are simply not important in most European cultures. In Hebrew, South Asian and many other Eastern languages there are precise one-word terms for, for example, 'my child's spouse's mother', 'my child's spouse's father, and 'my child's spouse's parents'.

An interpreter also has to make continual on-the-spot decisions about, for example, each speaker's intentions and the implications behind questions or answers, and to convey these as best she can. The more complex the ideas, and the more difficult or upsetting the issues being discussed, the harder the task is for the interpreter and the more time she needs.

THE ROLE AND STATUS OF INTERPRETERS

'It's very pressurised. The midwife wants me to translate everything as fast as I can, to make the interview go well and to make the client comply. The client wants to make sure I understand her situation, explain it fully to the midwife, and get her the care she needs. Both of them want me to solve their problems, and if things go wrong I'm often the one who gets the blame.'   Maternity interpreter

For professionals

Many health professionals who work with interpreters understand and value the contribution they make and the responsibilities they carry, involving them completely in the care of the client (Warrier, 1995). However, others feel strongly that interpreters should act only as word-for-word translators. They may feel threatened if the interpreter acts as an advocate or supporter for the client. The evaluation of the Asian Mother and Baby Campaign confirmed that many health professionals used linkworkers, who were intended to have a much wider role, simply as interpreters. 'In practice the role of the linkworker was defined first by the health professional to whom she was accountable, and second by her client' (Rocheron and Dickinson, 1990).

Many health professionals also find it frustrating and difficult to work with an interpreter, however skilful she is. They may feel de-skilled, out of control, inadequate and embarrassed. They may not know how to handle the session or may feel redundant. They may be unsure whether what they want to say is really getting through. It is helpful for professionals to take time to think through the pressures on each person in the interpreting triangle, to understand the full extent of the interpreter's task, and to think about how best to manage the interaction and to support both the interpreter and the client.

For clients

From the client's point of view, the interpreter's advocacy and help are often crucial. The interpreter can encourage her to ask questions, or can ask them on her behalf. She also has the experience to know how the consultation should go and to help steer it so that the client gets the care she needs.

Obstetrician to expectant mother: *'I think we will have to induce the labour.'*
Linkworker to mother (in mother's language): *'He wants to induce labour. Ask him why.'* (Ahmad, 1989)

The interpreter also acts as a supporter and a companion at a time when many women are anxious and vulnerable.

Doctors, nurses and midwives were generally perceived as being 'too busy'. Linkworkers and advocates, on the other hand, generally had enough time to communicate with the women in their own language, to listen to their views and feed them back to professional care providers and to seek answers for their anxieties.

More importantly, it wasn't what linkworkers did but **how** they did it, which appeared to matter to their clients. The emotional reassurance provided by their linkworker/advocate was valued as much, if not more, than the information or health education and advice they gave. (From Warrier, 1995, by permission)

If the interpreter's role is restricted merely to that of a literal translator of words and meanings, the client will not get the care she needs. To ensure a fully satisfactory consultation, and to compensate not only for the client's lack of English but also for her lack of knowledge and for her dependence in the medical situation, interpreters must help ensure the greatest possible participation of the client in her own care, and the best possible care.

It is particularly important for managers and colleagues to be clear about and support the advocacy role of the interpreter. This role sometimes causes resentment and conflict, particularly where interpreters challenge the behaviour of health professionals or practices which, whether intentionally or not, are discriminatory.

Feeding comments and criticisms back to the service

Interpreters have a unique understanding of the care that non-English-speaking women are receiving and the problems they face. This understanding should be fed back to service providers so that provision can be improved. Unless there is a formal route for such feedback, interpreters inevitably absorb and, in effect, silence the legitimate demands and complaints of non-English speakers about the service they receive. If managers and policy-makers never hear the views of non-English-speaking clients, they cannot respond to them (Shackman, 1984).

The interpreters should also be able to help individual women and families complain about poor service. Where clients themselves are reluctant to complain, the interpreters need ways of feeding back gross cases of poor service in confidence to managers. They require strong support from managers in such situations.

Support for interpreters

Most health interpreters have little status, recognition or support. This makes it difficult for them to take a stand, where necessary, to ensure that clients get the care they need and have a right to. Interpreters face high levels of need and high expectations from their clients and their community. They often also experience or witness impatience and racism from professionals.

> Linkworkers frequently heard comments made by staff which revealed a remarkable degree of insensitivity and intolerance towards linkworkers and their clients. Racist stereotyping was not infrequent. (Rocheron and Dickinson, 1990)

To be effective, interpreters need the support of their health professional colleagues, especially those in senior positions. They must be recognised as professionals and as partners in providing care and improving services for non-English-speaking women. Their training, management, pay, conditions and so on should reflect and support their professional status. All staff should understand the interpreters' role, the pressures they face and the responsibilities they carry.

> Often when a new group of junior doctors arrive, they object to a lay black women telling them that their behaviour is not acceptable. Senior staff must explain and

support, and, if the doctor's or nurse's behaviour was not acceptable, make that clear to the professional without delay . . . Equally important is the support of staff who work alongside the health workers – midwives and ward sisters. In some instances staff have supported the workers in complaining about behaviour and have spoken to their colleagues on the workers' behalf. More often it has been covert support, telling them they are right, suggesting that something is wrong and they ought to ask questions, alerting them to problems. (From City and Hackney CHC, 1988, by permission)

Despite the importance of the interpreter's role, the power structure and culture of the health service, and the low status that clients are accorded by some professionals, especially if they are black and speak no English, can easily lead to interpreters being marginalised and misused. Some, especially if they are not well supported, may respond by distancing themselves from their clients. They may come to identify with the higher-status health professionals and not carry out that part of their role that relates to the support and empowering of clients, thus adding to the problems they are meant to solve.

'We have an interpreter. But I am never quite sure that she tells the women everything I say. She seems to make a lot of decisions for them. She wears a white coat and feels, I think, very much one of us. Her husband is a teacher and sometimes I feel she looks down on the women as uneducated and stupid and feels she knows better than they do.' Community midwife

Training for interpreters

The work of a health interpreter is demanding. Considerable linguistic skills and knowledge are required. Interpreters are expected to convey clinical information, a task that even doctors and midwives often find difficult. Without specific training they inevitably piece together their own understanding of medical procedures and vocabulary, and pass this understanding on to clients (Audit Commission, 1993). They must also make difficult decisions all the time about what and whether to explain, whether and how to intervene, and how to help both sides manage the consultation as well as possible, particularly under time pressure.

Interpreters also have to provide emotional support to clients who are often anxious, confused and distressed. Their success depends to some extent on the relationship they develop with the women; this too can be emotionally draining. Supporting women in labour requires understanding, strength, judgement and empathy. When bad news has to be broken it is usually the interpreter, rather than the professional, who has to prepare the woman to receive it, to translate it, and to be on hand to support her and her family. Where there is rudeness or racism, the interpreter bears the brunt of it, and also has to decide how and whether to handle it, and whether and how to take it further. Simply knowing how to speak two languages is therefore not enough. Interpreters need regular training and opportunities to discuss difficult issues away from the workplace.

Initial training should cover, for example, the main physiological processes involved in pregnancy, birth and postnatally, and the key terms used; the aims and processes of maternity care, including tests and treatments, and the key terms used; detailed discussion of the role and responsibilities of an interpreter, practice in the linguistic and other skills needed to interpret accurately; training in dealing with difficult interpreting situations, including, for example, breaking bad news, interpreting where there is conflict, and handling racism assertively.

Interpreters, like other health professionals, also need time to examine their own attitudes and feelings in order to be able to provide more effective support. They may need experiential training on, for example, dealing with loss and grief, counselling skills, working with clients who are HIV positive or have AIDS, working with homeless people and so on. In such situations interpreters face exactly the same difficulties as health professionals and must have similar training (BHAN, 1991).

Training for professionals

Training is also required for all professionals who work with interpreters. This should include an understanding of what is involved in health interpreting, including linguistic and other issues; an understanding of the pressures and difficulties affecting each party in the interpreting triangle and how to help manage the conversation as well as possible; how to deal with difficulties and conflicts; how to maintain as good a relationship as possible with clients when an interpreter is present, and how to support the interpreter. Training should also include discussion of cultural issues and how to work across cultural barriers, and of racism, how it works, and how to challenge it.

Other management issues

Interpreters must be strongly managed, preferably by someone who is not part of the midwifery or medical hierarchy, or who is outside the organisation altogether, and who has status and power. Conflicts can then be openly discussed and resolved in the interests of clients and the community (Warrier, 1995). In City and Hackney Health Authority, for example, the health advocates are funded by the health authority but managed by the Community Health Council (City and Hackney CHC, 1988).

Health interpreting requires special personal qualities and experience as well as linguistic and other skills. It is very important therefore to select people who share as many characteristics as possible with the people for whom they work, taking into account factors such as age, life experience, standing within the community and personal attitudes (City and Hackney CHC, 1988). A clear job description is essential. Lack of clarity about the interpreter's role and responsibilities, combined with the conflicts and pressures inherent in the job, can lead to difficulties for interpreters, for the service and, ultimately, for clients.

12 Informal interpreters: a short-term measure

USING FRIENDS AND RELATIVES TO INTERPRET

'Wherever I went my husband was with me. When he couldn't accompany me a lady member of the family used to go with me to explain things to me. But it was not always possible for them to accompany me, so I had to skip two appointments. I was scared to go on my own because of the language.'   Bengali woman

In most situations where there is a clear need for a trained interpreter none is provided. Health professionals and clients have to struggle through, with stress and frustration on both sides, and achieving very little. In many places clients are asked or expected to bring someone to interpret for them. But a relative or friend is unlikely to be familiar with antenatal and other procedures or to understand the terms used. The translation is likely to be inaccurate and unreliable.

A study in Leicester of four medical interviews with Gujarati-speaking patients using family members who were thought to be fluent in both languages to interpret, found an alarmingly high proportion of mistranslations, misunderstandings and words that were not translated at all. In each interview the English-speaking doctor thought it had gone reasonably normally.

The study found that simple questions were translated best, though still with mistakes. Complex questions proved more difficult, and serial questions the most difficult of all. In one interview over half the serial questions were mistranslated or not translated. Many terms were also mistranslated.

In the 143 questions and answers, there were more than 80 words or phrases which were mistranslated, misunderstood or not translated by at least one interpreter. These included anatomical terms – for example, leg used for ankle; back teeth for jaw; neck for tonsil; and chest for ribs. Symptoms caused more difficulties – such as laxative used for diarrhoea; watery faeces for passing water; and getting fat for swelling. Technical terms were often mistranslated, with breathlessness used for asthma and being mad for epileptic fit. Words such as gynaecological, waterworks and gallstones were not translated at all ... .Children found it embarrassing to translate questions about menstruation or bowel movements to their parents, and there was a general tendency for questions about bodily functions to be ignored. (From Ebden *et al.*, 1988, p.347, by permission)

Depending on the relationship between client and 'interpreter' there may also be bias and distortion in the interpreting. The 'interpreter' may not feel happy translating some of what is said; the client may not feel able to answer questions honestly or voice any worries. Both may be very embarrassed by certain questions or procedures. One study found that over a third of patients who used informal interpreters reported difficulties, including inhibitions about discussing women's health issues via their husband, son or daughter, as well as problems with inaccurate interpretation (HEA, 1994).

The 'interpreter' is also unlikely to be able to explain important cultural issues in either direction, or to give the client any information she needs about maternity services and how to get what she needs. In addition, if family members or friends need to take time off work to accompany women to clinics, their own jobs and the family's income may be put at risk (Shackman, 1984). Where non-family interpreters are used, confidentiality may be a problem, especially in a tightly knit community.

> Some people used as interpreters do not understand exactly what you want them to do, or that they are supposed to translate everything that is said in both directions. They may just have a conversation with the client and relay what seems useful. They may answer a lot of your questions themselves. This often happens with family members since they usually know many of the answers to your questions without having to ask your client. They may see no point in asking when they already know the answer perfectly well. (From Shackman, 1984, by permission)

Using a relative or friend or even possibly an acquaintance to interpret is clearly unsatisfactory and poses major problems both for the client and for the health professional. Both sides need and deserve the level of proper communication that can usually only be achieved through a trained interpreter. However, in some situations it is impossible to avoid using a relative or friend as a short-term emergency measure. We say more about ways of managing this as well as possible below.

CHILDREN

In some cases children are used as interpreters. This is always completely unacceptable.

> Under no circumstances should children be asked to interpret medical details for their parents. It appears to us to be unethical, unprofessional, uncivilised and totally unacceptable. (Rack, 1991)

All the problems outlined above apply in the case of children, but are likely to be even more acute. There are aspects of maternity care, contraception and so on that many women do not want their children to learn about until they are older. Using children to translate matters that are distressing or highly personal can cause serious long-term damage both to the children and to family relationships. Parents are placed in a dependent role and children given power, responsibility and knowledge that they should not have. Most parents also try to shield their children as far as they can from distressing or sensitive information and so are unlikely to answer difficult or sensitive questions honestly or to tell you everything you need to know. Most children anyway do not speak both languages equally well and are unlikely to be able to translate important medical terms accurately or reliably. In addition, using children to interpret usually means keeping them away from school.

> Many English-speaking professionals believe that ethnic-minority parents do not mind using their children to interpret in such cases. Our experience indicates that they generally mind intensely but do not know what else to do. (Shackman, 1984)

STAFF LISTS

Some hospitals use lists of staff who speak one or more other languages to interpret, sometimes paying them a small fee. While this may be useful in emergencies and in other exceptional situations, it is inadequate and undesirable as part of a general communications policy. In the case of non-professional staff, such as cooks and cleaners, many of the same issues arise as with relatives and friends, with additional major problems of suitability, confidentiality and trust.

> *'They wouldn't be happy to give you an amateur doctor or nurse if you were ill. So why an amateur interpreter? It's just the same.'*   Community worker (from Shackman, 1984)

When minority ethnic health professionals are used as interpreters, issues such as confidentiality, professional standards and the ability to understand and translate medical terminology are not a problem but other factors need to be considered. Taking health professionals away from their normal work on a regular basis may adversely affect them and their work and put them under serious pressure. It also wastes and ignores their professional skills, places them in a subordinate position to their colleagues, and may affect their career development and prospects (Shackman, 1984). Where it is policy to use health professionals to interpret on a regular basis, it is important to discuss the implications for everyone concerned and to make sure that the professionals concerned are happy with the situation.

WORKING WITH INFORMAL INTERPRETERS: MINIMISING THE PROBLEMS*

There are inevitably occasions when it is impossible to get a trained interpreter immediately and health professionals have to work with a client's relative or friend to translate. This can be difficult for everyone but there are ways to minimise problems and distress and some very important things to bear in mind.

How much can you expect the person to translate?

Many people with patchy English end up having to interpret for friends and relatives because there is no one else. Listen carefully to the person's command of English and decide how much you can expect him or her to translate. You may

---

* Adapted from Henley, 1991, by permission of the National Extension College.

decide to communicate only the essential details for now and to leave the important issues until you can get a trained interpreter. You may even decide that you can communicate better directly with the client than through the interpreter you have available.

What is the interpreter's relationship to the client?

It is often very difficult for clients to find sympathetic people who speak good English, whom they feel comfortable using as interpreters, and who are able to accompany them to clinics or spend time with them in hospital. The person the client brings to translate for her may be a husband, partner, child, close relative, distant relative, friend, acquaintance, community worker, or someone who charges a fee for interpreting. Find out what the interpreter's relationship is with the client as this will affect what you can ask them to translate.

> 'There are no interpreters at this hospital and patients who don't speak English have to resort to desperate measures to get treatment and to communicate with professionals. In the Oncology Department a woman brought her six-year-old daughter to translate for her. The girl had to tell her mother that she had to have both breasts removed. A Portuguese couple brought a man to help them discuss what kind of breast prosthesis the wife might have after her operation. It later emerged that he just worked in the local electrical shop. They didn't know him at all well but he had kindly agreed to come along and help them because they were desperate.'   Researcher

Confidentiality

Confidentiality is vital in all health interpreting. Be aware that your client may not want the interpreter to know everything about her. Clients need to be absolutely sure that everything they say will be kept totally confidential and that nothing will be repeated to anyone outside. This may be particularly important in a small community where most people know each other and news travels fast. Where there is a social stigma attached to, for example, a pregnancy outside marriage, miscarriage or fetal abnormality, confidentiality may be even more important. Failures of confidentiality can have serious consequences not only for the client herself but, in some cases, for her whole family. If a client does not feel comfortable or safe with the person acting as an interpreter, she may not wish to answer all questions fully or truthfully. You must therefore be able to assure the client in good faith and with complete confidence that the person who is interpreting will not mention the interview to anyone, will not say anything to anyone about what has been said or has happened during the interview, and will not discuss the interview or anything said in it with the client at any later date unless she herself wishes to discuss it.

It is almost impossible to respect clients' confidentiality when you are using a non-professional interpreter. Even with a husband or partner, there may be things that the woman does not want to tell anyone but a health professional. In cultures where topics such as menstruation, pregnancy and childbirth are largely women's matters, wives and husbands may not feel able to discuss these issues together. In some cases men may know very little about such matters and may not know the relevant words either in English or in their first language. Where a couple wish to be seen together, it is important not to assume that the man wishes or is able to act as interpreter for the woman.

Take a minute to think about how you would feel if you had to talk to a doctor through an interpreter about your symptoms. Suppose you had haemorrhoids or a vaginal discharge.

■ Who would you prefer to translate for you:
  Your husband/wife/partner?
  Your son or daughter?
  A friend?
  A hospital cleaner?
  A man or woman waiting in the surgery?
  A neighbour?
  A trained interpreter?

Help the interpreter to do as good a job as possible

Find out whether the interpreter feels able to interpret everything you need. A relative or friend may be too embarrassed to discuss some things with the client, may disagree strongly with some of what you want translated, or may find the information so distressing that they cannot bear to tell it to the client.

Try to assess whether the interpreter is worried about translating in this situation. Spend time explaining what you want and finding out if there are problems. Try to give the interpreter the confidence to tell you if there are things they do not understand or are not sure how to translate. Make it clear that you are grateful for their help and realise that the situation is not ideal. Do not blame them for having come along to translate nor resent the fact that they cannot do it better. Be aware that a non-professional interpreter may become upset when seeing or discussing medical procedures and may themselves need support.

Unless you are completely happy with your interpreter's fluency, suitability and reliability, **you need to find a professional interpreter as soon a possible to check out what has been said**. Mistranslations can have serious or even fatal consequences and can cause great distress to clients and their families.

Any written material is only effective if:

- It takes into account the values, assumptions, knowledge, lifestyles and preferences of its target audience, and also reflects the possible diversity of expectations and attitudes.
- The information it contains is useful, relevant and applicable.
- It is in simple, straightforward language and contains a clear message.
- It is respectful and non-patronising.

In a multiracial and multicultural community all these criteria remain important, but it is essential to consider their implications in relation to the particular group or groups for whom material is intended. In addition all material must be non-racist and must not imply, for example, that English ways are 'better'.

Where local communities have very different traditions and expectations, it may be more useful to produce separate leaflets. For example, information on healthy eating during pregnancy must be relevant to the people for whom it is intended. Advice to people eating a traditional African-Caribbean or Somali diet may need to be different from that given to people eating a traditional English diet. People living in bed and breakfast hostels are likely to need information and advice that takes their very restricted options into account.

Consultation with professionals working in the community, with community workers and representatives, and with consumers of services is always essential. It is important that scarce resources are not wasted on producing materials that are irrelevant, misdirected, unclear or offensive.

MATERIALS IN OTHER LANGUAGES

In many areas information and health education materials are needed in languages other than English. Producing really good material in other languages can be time-consuming and expensive so it is important to think through the process carefully before you begin and to be well-informed both about the languages read by local people, and about their particular concerns in relation to the subject matter.

What languages do people read?

Different communities have different levels of literacy in English and in their first language. Levels of literacy also vary according to age. In some communities, the older people are, the less likely they are to read either their own first language or English. In communities where women traditionally have had little access to formal education, women may be less likely to be literate than men. Nevertheless, in all communities, most people read their first language and everybody has access to someone who can read if they themselves cannot.

In some cases bilingual materials, in English and the community language, are most useful. People can then read whichever language they find easiest. English-speaking professionals also know exactly what is in any material that they hand out.

In choosing the languages and scripts in which material should be produced, it is important to understand what people in the target group actually read. For example:

- Younger people in almost all communities are more likely to have been educated in Britain and to have English as their main language of reading and writing. Nevertheless, there are women of childbearing age in many communities who read their own language but not English.
- Among the Vietnamese community in Britain, most people of ethnic Vietnamese origin read Vietnamese. Many people of ethnic Chinese origin read both Vietnamese and Chinese. Chinese is written in ideographs. Vietnamese is written in the Vietnamese script (Mares, 1982). It is important to find out whether both are needed in your area.
- The mother tongue of most Pakistani immigrants in Britain is Punjabi. But the language of education in Pakistan is Urdu, written in the Arabic script. Although Punjabi can be written in the Arabic script, it very rarely is. The most useful language for material intended for the Pakistani community is therefore Urdu (HEA, 1994).
- The mother tongues of most people from India (and of Indian origin from East Africa) are Punjabi and Gujarati.

  - Many Punjabis of Indian origin in Britain read and write Punjabi, usually in the Gurmukhi script.
  - People from Gujarat, or of Gujarati origin from East Africa, are most likely to read Gujarati written in the Devnagri script.

- Most Bangladeshis in Britain speak Sylheti, a dialect of Bengali. Sylheti has no written form; the language of education in Bangladesh is Bengali written in the Devnagri script. The Health Education Authority 'Health and Lifestyles' survey used Bengali to communicate in writing with Bangladeshi respondents but was careful to use 'the terms closest to those which would be used by Sylheti-speakers wherever possible' (HEA, 1994).

The HEA survey, published in 1994, asked people of South Asian origin what language they preferred to read. The resulted are presented in Table 13.1.

It is also necessary to carry out local research before making final decisions on language and content. As with the majority population, minority communities in different parts of the country may have different concerns or needs for

Table 13.1   Preferred reading languages of South Asian women

Ethnic group	Language	Age 16–29 (%)	Age 30–49(%)
Indian	English	75	36
	Gujarati	18	35
	Punjabi (G)	6	16
	Hindi	0	2
	illiterate	0	4
Pakistani	English	63	7
	Urdu	21	46
	Punjabi (U)	2	10
	illiterate	11	31
Bangladeshi	Bengali	57	73
	English	42	1
	illiterate	0	24

Punjabi (G) = Punjabi written in the Gurmukhi script; Punjabi (U) = Punjabi written in the Urdu or Arabic script.

Source: Adapted from *Health and Lifestyles: Black and Minority Ethnic Groups in England*, 1994, Health Education Authority, by permission.

information on particular topics. Levels of English and literacy in their first language may also differ, depending on the age of the community and other factors.

PRODUCING MATERIALS IN OTHER LANGUAGES

Producing material which is culturally relevant to the target group will not come naturally to someone who does not share that culture. (Lovell, 1990)

Good written material is based on the real interests, priorities, knowledge and attitudes of the people for whom it is intended. Information about maternity services, for example, should take into account what readers are already likely to know, what they need or want to know more about, which terms they are familiar with and which need explaining, what their main worries are likely to be, and so on. When material is intended for members of a particular community, it is necessary to take their likely interests, priorities, knowledge and attitudes into account. It is essential always to work closely with members of the group or community for whom the material is intended.

Translating existing materials

In some cases it may be possible to begin with an existing English version and get it translated, discussing carefully any cultural and other adjustments that are needed.

● The meaning of the English original must be absolutely clear and the language as straightforward and simple as possible. A complicated, unclear or badly worded English text will usually be made worse by translation.
● The message must be clearly defined and must be understood by everyone involved in the translation and discussion. An unclear message can easily be

obscured or lost altogether in the complex process of drafting, consulting and checking across cultural and language barriers (Lovell, 1990).

- It is also very important to choose people who write both well and colloquially in the target language; being able to speak a language does not necessarily mean that one writes it well. In some languages it is customary to use a very formal written style; in health-related materials for a wide readership an accessible, colloquial style is clearly more appropriate (Mares, 1982).
- Translation is a difficult skill. It is important to find experienced translators, if possible with a portfolio of past work which can be assessed, and to be prepared to pay them a professional fee for their services.

The language and subject of the leaflet should always be clearly marked in English. If the material is not bilingual it must at least state somewhere, in English, the title and language.

Producing materials from scratch

Producing good written material about highly sensitive issues with major social and cultural implications, such as antenatal screening or HIV and AIDS, requires careful thought and skill in any language. Producing such material across language and cultural barriers is even harder.

It is important to find and work closely with community members and/or translators who understand the needs, expectations and concerns of the people for whom the material is intended. Often the best solution is to ask them to draft the material from scratch in their own language after extensive discussion. In some subject areas suitable terms either do not exist, or the terms that do exist are offensive or unacceptable to many people. Detailed explanations or new forms of words may be needed (see also Chapter 11).

Where possible, people who were not involved in producing the material should be asked to comment on clarity and style and to check if these and the content are appropriate for the community. The material must also be carefully re-checked at every stage of production. Faulty or inappropriate translation can make the material useless. BHAN (1991), for example, cites an example of an HIV/AIDS leaflet in which the phrase 'oral sex' in the English original was translated into 'verbal sex' in the Hindi leaflet. Beware if the typesetter does not understand what he or she is setting. Labels under illustrations in Urdu materials, for example, have sometimes been transposed because the Arabic script runs from right to left.

Illustrations and pictorial conventions

Any illustrations must be carefully considered and the views of users sought before a final decision is reached. Cartoons can easily offend, even if unintentionally. Drawings of people of different communities can also cause offence. Pictorial conventions and symbols such as ticks, crosses, arrows, things crossed out, speech bubbles, thought bubbles, cartoons, outline maps and so on, are often assumed to be a way of communicating on paper with people who cannot read. In fact they are usually linked to literacy; people who cannot read may not understand them (Mares et al., 1985).

The importance of names

Recording people's names correctly, so that files can be retrieved easily and accurately, and so that test results, treatments and medication can all be linked to the right person, is absolutely vital to the smooth and safe delivery of clinical care. Lost, confused or duplicated records always cause delays and frustration and waste money. In some cases they can also be very dangerous: The results of vital tests or screening may become attached to the wrong set of notes, the wrong woman may be treated or not treated for a serious illness. In some cases confusion over notes may lead to litigation.

Addressing people correctly and in such a way that they recognise their own name is also a fundamental part of good health care. Names matter. Wilful or careless misuse of names is alienating and insulting and is unlikely to enable the development of good caring relationships.

> *'It upsets me really – I can pronounce English names. Why is it so difficult to get a Vietnamese person's name right? What if I always called you by the wrong name. How would you feel?'* Vietnamese man (from Mares, 1982)

The British naming system

The British naming system is only one of many in the world, but it is the one that health professionals use automatically and the one on which records and retrieval systems are based. Records rely on the following assumptions.

- Everyone has a personal name and a surname.
- The order of the names indicates their usage: the personal name always comes first and the surname always comes last.
- Some people have a number of middle names.
- Most first names are recognisably either male or female.
- Surnames are not male or female; they are gender-neutral family names handed down through the generations.
- The formal form of address is title plus surname.
- The informal form of address is first name.
- There is a limited range of possible spellings for any name.

Also, to help link mothers and babies, and members of the same family:

● most women take their husband's surname when they marry;
● most children share their surname with one, if not both, of their parents; and
● in most families all the children share the same surname.

Health service record and filing systems automatically use the last name as the primary identifying point, then the first and the middle names, and the date of birth. With familiar names, health professionals and clerical staff can normally tell when something 'doesn't make sense' or looks wrong, and can usually sort it out with the client.

Other naming systems

None of the assumptions on which the British records system are based, however, is universal. Although everyone has a personal name, it does not always come first. Titles may come either before the name, as in the British system, or after it. Sometimes they are part of the name. Some people have a religious name which must never be used on its own. Not all systems have a family name. In some systems none of the family members shares a name. In some systems the family name comes first instead of last. For example:

● In the traditional **Chinese naming system** the family name comes first, followed by a two-part personal name always used together (or occasionally a single personal). In many families the first part of the personal name is shared by all the sons, and another by all the daughters. A woman does not change her name on marriage. She usually adds her husband's family name before her own (see Table 14.1). Chinese Christians may have a Christian personal name as well.

Table 14.1   Example of a Chinese family using the traditional naming system

Family member	Name
Husband	Cheung Koon-Sung
Wife	Cheung-Ng Wai-Yung
Sons	Cheung Chi-Wah
	Cheung Chi-Kong
Daughters	Cheung Mee-Ling
	Cheung Mee-Tuan

● The **Vietnamese naming system** is similar to the Chinese. There are about 25 common family names in Vietnam, shared by a large number of families.

● In the **South Asian Muslim naming system** (used in Pakistan, Bangladesh and India), there is no tradition of a family name shared between men and women (see Table 14.2); all names are either male or female.

    Most **South Asian Muslim women** traditionally have a personal name, usually followed by a title (for example, Bano, Bi, Bibi, Begum, Khanum,

Khatoon, Sultana). There are also a few common second personal names which may be used instead of a title, for example, Akhtar, Jan, Un-Nessa and Kausar. Women do not traditionally share a last name with their husbands, fathers or children. Baby girls are not usually given their title for some time, and initially have only one name.

Most **South Asian Muslim men** traditionally have a religious name (the most sacred are Mohammed, Allah and -Ullah). The religious name usually comes first (except -Ullah, the form of Allah which follows another name). The religious name is often regarded as the most important part of the name and should **never** be used alone. The religious name and the personal name are usually used together in formal situations; in some cases separating them makes nonsense of the name. Many men have only these two names. Some men have a two-part personal name instead of or as well as a religious name; again these parts should not be separated.

Some men have another name which comes last. This may be a male title (e.g. Miah), or a clan or village name (e.g. Chaudry, Khan, Ansari) or their fathers' first name. These names are sometimes shared with other male members of the family but this is a matter of family custom and personal choice. Since clan and village names are male names they are not normally used by women. In some cases male titles come first instead of last.

Table 14.2   Example of a Pakistani family using the traditional naming system

Family member	Name
Husband	Abdul Rahman
Wife	Fatma Jan
Sons	Mohammed Ra'uf
	Mohammed Riasa
	Mohammed Rashid
Daughters	Salamet Bibi
	Mehr-un-Nessa

- The **naming systems of Muslims in other parts of the world** vary. For example, in the Middle East it is perfectly acceptable to use Mohammed, alone or with another name, as the personal name of a Muslim man.

- In the traditional **Somali naming system** the personal name comes first, followed by either the family name or the grandfather's name. A woman does not take her husband's last name on marriage, but keeps her father's last name. Children are given their father's last name. Mother and children do not therefore usually share a last name. It is acceptable to use the title plus last name to address someone formally.

  Great offence may be caused if a baby is given the mother's family name. For example, the new baby of Mrs Amina Ali and Mr Ahmed Abdillahi should be called 'Baby Abdillahi', **not** 'Baby Ali'.

- The traditional **Sikh naming system** is based on a religious ruling which requires people not to use a family name and to use only a first name plus a male or female title. Women have a personal name followed by the title Kaur.

Table 14.3   Example of a Sikh family using the traditional naming system

Family member	Name
Husband	Kushwant Singh
Wife	Daljeet Kaur
Sons	Ranjeet Singh
	Jaswinder Singh
	Joginder Singh
Daughters	Dilvinder Kaur
	Davinder Kaur

Men have a personal name followed by the title Singh (see Table 14.3). Most Sikh first names can be used for men or women. Devout Sikhs may find it unacceptable to use a family name (see Chapter 41).

- In the traditional **Greek Cypriot naming system** some women use their husband's last name as a surname, and some use their husband's first name. But the male name is changed to the female form, for example, Marcos becomes Marcou, Andreas becomes Andreou.

- In the traditional **Turkish naming system** most people have two names. When a women marries she adopts her husband's first name as her last name. Children traditionally take their father's first name as their last name. The father does not, traditionally, share a last name with his wife or children.

- In the traditional **Hindu naming system** used in north-western India, most people have three names, a personal and a complementary name, often used together, followed by a family name. The most common female complementary names are Behn, Devi, Gowri, Kumari, Lakshmi and Rani. The most common male complementary names are Bhai, Chand, Das, Dev, Kant, Kumar, Lal, Nat and Pal. Occasionally people's complementary names are changed, for example, when they marry. Since most of the Hindu families in the UK originated in Gujarat, certain Gujarati family names, such as Patel, are very common.

    Most women traditionally take their husband's family name when they marry, and children have their father's family name. But the family name is not normally used when talking to people. Instead people use and give only their first name and their complementary name. This can cause problems if a complementary name is recorded as a surname.

Changing names and adopting family names

Many immigrants change their names or their children's names to try to fit in with the British system once they realise that it is different and that the differences are leading to confusion and difficulties. But for most of us our name is part of our identity. People are often very reluctant to change their names, especially if the new name sounds unnatural or ludicrous in terms of their own system.

Some women adopt, formally or informally, their husband's last name as a British-style surname. Occasionally they are assigned their husband's last name by a clerical officer or health professional. But in some naming systems there is no suitable 'surname' available. Simply adopting the husband's or father's last name may be unacceptable or pointless.

- If a Bangladeshi woman whose husband's last 'name' is the Bangladeshi male title, Miah, adopts this as a surname, she becomes Mrs Miah, equivalent to Mrs Mr. This is both ridiculous and not helpful for identification. Similarly, many Sikh women object to being called Mrs Singh.
- If Fatma Jan, in Table 14.2 above, adopts or is given her husband's last name, Rahman (in fact his personal name) she becomes Mrs Rahman under the British system. This is like calling the wife of Fred Brown, Mrs Fred. It may be unpleasant and unacceptable for many women, particularly in a community which is traditionally sexually segregated.

The decision to change one's name is often very difficult; many people feel quite unable to do so. Changing one's name can also sometimes cause major problems, particularly for people whose status in the UK is often questioned and who may be accused of being illegal immigrants if their documents contain different names.

In some families, some members have changed their names and adopted a British-style surname, others have not. For example, in some Sikh families some members have re-adopted the family surname. For other family members this may be out of the question on religious grounds. In South Asian Muslim families it may be more acceptable for the sons to take on their father's personal name as a surname than for the wife and daughters. In some families members born in the UK are registered under a family surname; overseas-born members are not.

Even where people want to change their names to fit in with the conventions of the British naming system it is not always easy. For example, Leung Kar-Po, who is Chinese, changed her name to Kar-Po Leung, so that her family name now comes last. But she was not able to explain what she was doing, and ended up with two unconnected sets of records. People who try to change their names also frequently meet with hostility and suspicion, especially if they are 'foreign' or speak little English.

Spelling

The spelling of some names in English varies a good deal, particularly where they are transliterated from another alphabet. A search in one set of hospital records, for example, found 15 ways of spelling the South Asian Muslim name that is pronounced K'reshi and is normally written in the Arabic script. These included Qureshi, Kuraishi, Kureshi, Qurayshi, Qrashi, Qureschi, Qurraishy and others; all attempts to write down the sound correctly, but all filed in different places. Since there is no 'correct' spelling, the same person may have the name spelled in several different ways on different documents. Asking for passports in an attempt to sort out the problem is more likely to damage the professional-client relationship than to provide a definitive spelling, since the passport reflects only one possible way of spelling the name, and may even have been spelled that way by the official who issued the passport rather than by the client.

The important thing is to try to make sure that each client's names are recorded and spelt the same way on all her records. Use the spelling the client gives you. If her name is spelt in different ways on different documents, find out which one she wishes to use and explain, if necessary, the importance of always giving the same spelling. If appropriate, give her a card with the chosen spelling for future use. Make sure that all her health records are amended to match.

Dates of birth

Dates of birth are often used as an additional means of identifying records, especially when people have common or unfamiliar names. Birthdays and their celebration are nowadays an extremely important part of Western culture, and a person's date of birth is an important part of their identity. But in many cultures birthdays are not traditionally celebrated. People may celebrate saints' days instead, or may not have any individual celebrations. In less bureaucratized countries, births and deaths are not always registered and there may be no reason to note or remember people's date of birth. People born in these countries may never have had their date of birth recorded. They may not know it, and **may not realise that it is a crucial part of their identity as far as health services are concerned and that they must give a consistent date of birth, however fictional, in all official situations**.

Many people who do not know their date of birth but realise its importance, choose, for ease of memory, the first of January of the year in which they were, or think they were, born. As a result, there may be a large number of women in some areas with their 'date of birth' as January 1st. Health professionals do not always understand the significance of this.

> One midwife, in all innocence, remarked how surprising it was that 'all these women' are born then. This reflects how incomprehensible it is to western people that someone should not know their birthday; it is more likely [to western people] that a high percentage of Asian women should be born on the same day. (From Bowler, 1993, by permission)

IDENTIFYING, RECORDING AND USING NAMES CORRECTLY

> '*When I go to the doctor and a name is called I watch to see if anyone else moves. If no one else gets up, then I go and ask if it's me they've called. Otherwise I could sit there all morning and never find out. People are always getting the wrong bit of your name, or pronouncing it so you can't recognise it.*'   Vietnamese patient (from Mares, 1982, by permission)

Differences in naming systems and in people's assumptions about how names work frequently cause major problems and frustrations for both clients and professionals. With so many variations in naming systems, health professionals cannot rely on everyone producing a first name, a surname and a date of birth.

Nor can they assume that people are happy to be called by their first name and can be filed under their last. For clients whose last name is a title, such as Kaur, Begum or Miah, the traditional British system of address, Mrs Kaur, Mrs Begum or Mr Miah, is meaningless. Even if a woman does not mind being called Mrs Kaur, her husband is certainly never Mr Kaur nor her new-born son Baby Kaur. Write on the baby's identity bracelet, for example, 'Son of Swinder Kaur' of Son of Swinder Kaur and Harpal Singh'.

None of us likes having our names constantly mispronounced or misused, let alone changed by other people. It is clearly necessary to take more care over identifying and recording people's names in order to avoid confusion, offence and possibly serious damage.

Recording the full name and how it should be used

For each client, ask:

- What is your name?
- What would you like us to call you?
- What is your husband's/partner's name?
- What would he like us to call him?
- What is your baby's name (if appropriate)?
- What would you like us to call him/her?

If the name is unfamiliar, indicate the personal name with a (p) and the family name, if there is one, with an (f). If the last name is very common or is a title and there are likely to be problems with the correct identification and retrieval of records, test results and so on, it is essential to get extra identifying information. It may be helpful to note the names of other family members, purely for records purposes:

Fatma Jan (wife of Abdul Rahman)
Mohammed Ra'uf (son of Abdul Rahman)
Salamet Bibi (daughter of Abdul Rahman)

Pronunciation and usage

If a name should be pronounced very differently from the way it is spelled, write down the correct pronunciation in brackets in the notes as indicated below. Underline the stressed syllables if necessary. Note how the name should be used if this is not clear. As a general rule it is safest and most helpful to clients to use their full name if you are not sure.

Jahanara Bibi (Jahanara Bibi – use full name)

Dilvinder Kaur (Dilvinder Kor – use full name)

Cheung-Ng Wai-Yung (Use Mrs Ng or full name)

Shahida Begum Ditta (Shaheeda Baygum Ditta – use full name or first two names, not Mrs Ditta)

Lew Sapieha (Leff Sapiayha – Mr Sapieha)

Mohammed Yunus Miah (Muhamad Yoonus Meeah – use full name, or first two names together)

Sometimes a client's name is obviously wrong in terms of her traditional naming system. Many people have come to terms with the adaptation or misuse of their name over the years and may be using this as their official name. In such a complicated situation it is important not to be too purist or, for example, to refuse to accept a name that appears to be the result of earlier misunderstandings or compromises. The important thing for records is consistency. Ask the client what name she wants to use, explain to her, if necessary, the importance of giving this name in all contacts with the health service, and check that this is the name in all her documentation.

FULL NAME	
Preferred form of address	
File under	
HUSBAND/PARTNER'S NAME	
Preferred form of address	
INFANT'S NAME	
Preferred form of address	
File under	

Figure 14.1 Sample form for recording clients' names correctly

Developing appropriate systems

Once a name has been recorded correctly, make sure that it is used on all records, notes and labels. It may be necessary to redesign forms to provide extra spaces and to alter computer programs to provide sufficient fields to help with the identification of individuals. For example, booking forms, notes and computer packages could be amended as shown in Figure 14.1.

References and further reading

Ahmad, W. I. U. (1989) Policies, pills and political will: a critique of policies to improve the health of ethnic minorities. *Lancet*, i, 148–50

Ahmed, G. and Watt, S. (1986) Understanding Asian women in pregnancy and confinement. *Midwives Chronicle and Nursing Notes*, **99**, May, 98–101

Alibhai, Y. (1988) Maternity care: Black women speak out. *New Society*, 1 April

Argyle, M. (1975) *Bodily Communication*, International Universities Press, New York

Audit Commission (1993) *What Seems to be the Matter: Communication between Hospitals and Patients. National Health Service Report No. 12*, HMSO, London

Baylav, A. (1994) Advocacy in primary health care. *SHARE Newsletter*, Issue 9, pp. 3–4, (King's Fund, London)

BHAN (1991) *AIDS and the Black Communities*, Black HIV anbd AIDS Network London WC1N–3XX

Bowler, I. (1993) Stereotypes of women of Asian descent in midwifery: some evidence. *Midwifery*, **9**, 7–16

City and Hackney CHC (1988) *Experiments in Health Advocacy*, City and Hackney Community Health Council

Collett, P. (1993) *Foreign Bodies: a Guide to European Mannerisms*, Simon & Schuster, London

CRE (1994) *Race Relations Code of Practice in Maternity Services*, Commission for Racial Equality, London

Currer, C. (1986) *Health Concepts and Illness Behaviour: the Care of Pathan Mothers in Bradford*. Unpublished PhD thesis, Department of Sociology, University of Warwick, UK

Dance, J. (1987) *A Social Intervention by Linkworkers to Pakistani Women and Pregnancy Outcome*. Unpublished paper, East Birmingham Health Authority

d'Ardenne, P. and Mahtani, A. (1989) *Transcultural Counselling In Action*, Sage, London

Department of Health (1993) *Changing Childbirth: Report of the Expert Maternity Group*, HMSO, London

Department of Health (1994) *NHS: The Patient's Charter: Maternity Services*, Department of Health, London

Ebden, P., Bhatt, A. Carey, O. J. and Harrison, B. (1988) The bilingual consultation. *Lancet*, i, 347

Hayward, J. (1975) *Information – a Prescription Against Pain*, Royal College of Nursing, London

HEA (1990) *Health Education For Ethnic Minorities*, Health Education Authority, London

HEA (1994) *Health and Lifestyles: Black and Minority Ethnic Groups in England*, Health Education Authority, London

Heavey, A. (1988) Learning to talk with patients. *British Journal of Hospital Medicine*, May, pp. 433–39

Henley, A. (1980) (out of print) *Asian Names and Records: a Training Pack*, National Extension College, Cambridge

Henley, A. (1987) *Caring in a Multiracial Society*, Bloomsbury Health Authority, London

Henley, A. (1991) *Caring for Everyone: Ensuring Standards of Care for Black and Ethnic Minority Patients*, National Extension College, Cambridge

Homans, H. and Satow, A. (1982) Can you hear me? Cultural variations in communication. *Journal of Community Nursing*, January, pp. 16–18

House of Commons (1992) *Health Committee Report on Maternity Services*, HMSO, London

Khan, S. (1994) *Contexts: Race, Culture and Sexuality*, The NAZ Project, Palingswick House, 241 King Street, London W6 9LP

Kirkham, M. (1988) Don't worry. *Nursing Times*, **84**, 15 June, 63–4

Kochman, T. (1981) *Black and White Styles in conflict*, University of Chicago Press, Ill.

Leap, N. (1992) The power of words. *Nursing Times*, **88**, 21 May, pp. 60–1

Li, P.-L. (1992) Health needs of the Chinese population. In *The Politics of 'Race' and Health* (ed. W. I. U. Ahmad), Race Relations Research Unit, University of Bradford

Lovell, S. (1990) *Health in Any Language*, North East Thames Regional Health Authority, London

Magill-Cuerdon, J. (1992) A question of communication. *Modern Midwife*, November/December, pp. 4–5

Mares, P. (1982) *The Vietnamese in Britain: a Handbook for Health Workers*, National Extension College, Cambridge

Mares, P., Henley, A. and Baxter, C. (1985) *Health Care In Multiracial Britain*, National Extension College, Cambridge

Morain, G. G. (1986) Kinesics and cross-cultural understanding. In *Culture Bound: Bridging the Cultural Gap in Language Teaching* (ed. J. M. Valdes), Cambridge University Press, Cambridge

Murphy, K. and Macleod-Clark, J. (1993) Nurses' experience of caring for ethnic minority clients. *Journal of Advanced Nursing*, B18, **3**, 442–50

Parsons, L. and Day, S. (1992) Improving obstetric outcomes in ethnic minorities: an evaluation of health advocacy. *Journal of Public Health Medicine*, **14**(2), 183–91

Rack, P. (1991) *Race, Culture and Mental Disorder*. Routledge, London

Roberts, C. (1985) *The Interview Game and How It's Played*, BBC Publications, London

Rocheron, Y. and Dickinson, R. (1990) The Asian Mother and Baby Campaign: a way forward in health promotion for Asian women? *Health Education Journal*, **49**(3), 128–33

Rogers, J. (1989) *Adults Learning*, Open University Press, Milton Keynes

Sami, A. R. (1989) Letter. *British Medical Journal*, **298**, 1523

Samra, J. S., Iqbal, P. K., Tang, L. C. H. *et al.* (1988) Letter: bilingual consultation. *Lancet*, **1**, 648

Schott, S. and Henley, A. (1992) *Breaking the Barriers: a Training Package on Equal Access To Maternity Services*, Obstetric Hospital, University College London Hospitals NHS Trust, London

Shackman, J. (1984) *The Right to be Understood: a Handbook on Working with, Employing and Training Community Interpreters*. Available from J. Shackman, c/o 96 Grafton Road, London, NW5 3EJ

Tannen, D. (1991) *You Just Don't Understand: Women and Men in Conversation*, Virago, London

Tannen, D. (1992) *That's Not What I Meant*, Virago, London

Training in Health and Race (1985) *Bilingual Fieldworkers: a Vietnamese Case Study*, National Extension College, Cambridge

Warrier, S. (1995) *Consumer Empowerment: an Evaluation of Linkworker and Advocacy Services for non-English Speaking Users of Maternity Services*, The Maternity Alliance, London

Watson, P. (1986) Towers of Babel, *Nursing Times*, 3 December, 1986, 40–1

Windsor-Richards, K. and Gillies, P. (1988) Racial grouping and women's experience of giving birth in hospital. *Midwifery*, **4**, 171–76

Part Three

Implications for Practice

INTRODUCTION

This section looks at the influence of culture and religion on daily life and on attitudes to childbearing and maternity care. It includes examples from a variety of religions and cultures, and examines some of their implications for maternity care.

Throughout this section there are opportunities for reflection. Our own attitudes colour our perceptions and can have a profound effect on the way we view others, and on our ability to listen and to respond with empathy and respect. It is important, therefore, to be aware of our own attitudes and values, and to reflect on how they may influence us in certain situations.

How to use this section

You can work through the reflections by yourself. It may, however, be more useful to work through them with a trusted friend or colleague, especially someone of a different background and culture from your own.

If you decide to work with someone else, you need time and privacy. Divide the time and take equal turns to listen to each other with complete attention and respect. Agree that everything you say will be in confidence. Without these conditions neither of you is likely to feel able to say what you really think and feel. Agree to listen without interrupting, and to discuss respectfully and without arguing. Listen to the **differences** between you as well as to the similarities. Although it is often much easier to listen to someone who shares our views and experiences, it is the differences between us that add richness and variety and from which we can learn the most.

15

Finding out what people need

Expectant and new parents have much in common and have similar hopes and anxieties about pregnancy, birth and their babies. But parents are also individuals with different needs. Every woman who comes for maternity care is likely to be influenced by many things, including her family heritage and culture, and her spiritual beliefs. Where these are different from our own it is easy to feel uncertain and inadequate. It may be tempting to collect 'facts' about her particular community or religion and to care for her on the basis of these. But every woman is primarily an individual rather than a member of a group. General information about different cultures and religions tells us little about the person in front of us. What we need is an open, respectful, well-informed, pluralistic approach which enables us to identify the needs and wishes of each individual and to respond to them flexibly and without fuss (Alladin, 1992).

Asking questions

The only person who can tell you what will or will not be appropriate for her is the woman herself. It is necessary, therefore, to give up the role of professional expert and to ask each client what she wants and needs. This can be surprisingly hard, especially for those of us trained in the tradition of the 'all-knowing professional' who always knows what to do and has all the answers. Although we may have accepted intellectually the idea of client-centred care, in which we have to ask about and respond to individual needs and wishes, the remnants of old messages can exert a powerful influence. Having to ask may feel like an admission of failure, of not being a 'good enough' health professional. It also affects the balance of power between professional and client.

> The view that it is enough . . . to go armed with details of people's culture also suggests a top-down approach . . . This approach assumes that the health professional has knowledge (including knowledge about people's way of life) and that this knowledge allows the health professional to meet clients' needs. A different approach, starting with the client, would place the professional in the humbler position of learning from the client. (From Foster, 1988, by permission)

What messages did you absorb during your training or education about asking clients about their needs and wishes?

- How do you really feel about asking clients what they want and need?
- How does asking a client change the relationship between you? How do you feel about this?
- How readily do you ask?
- If you tend not to ask, what gets in the way?
- How easy do you find it to listen to and act on the answers you get?
- How do you manage your feelings and the client's feelings when you get it wrong?

Asking does not always give us the answer, occasionally we are bound to get it wrong. Sometimes we misunderstand the importance of an issue to a client, sometimes it is hard to frame appropriate questions. Our most tactful and respectful questions may be misunderstood, cause offence, or not elicit the answers we need. Asking questions requires courage, but unless we take the risk we will never find out what our clients really need.

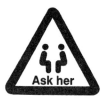

Helping clients identify the key issues

- If someone asks you what your cultural needs are, what do you say?
- Imagine that you are about to go into hospital to have a baby in Bangladesh. In the antenatal clinic a midwife asks you if you have any special cultural or practical wishes during labour and birth, or in the postnatal ward. What would you want to tell her?

To give a useful answer to this question, you need to know quite a lot about the system of maternity care in Bangladesh: what the facilities are, what practices are routine, what options are available, and what the pros and cons of each are. Only then can you select, out of all the possibilities, what is important to you.

'They asked me in the antenatal clinic what I wanted them to do when I was having the baby but I didn't really know what to say. I didn't know anything about what happens or what it was going to be like. I could tell them now.'   English mother

When clients are making decisions or choices in an unfamiliar situation, it is helpful to ask specific questions, to give additional information about the context, and to highlight areas that you think **may** be important to them or may present particular problems.

Table 15.1   Some factors that may be influenced by culture and religion

Daily life	Childbearing
Personal history and heritage	Attitudes to medical care
Religious beliefs and practices	Pregnancy
Religious festivals	Antenatal care
Family structure	Screening
Family relationships	Termination of pregnancy
Attitudes to motherhood	Labour and birth
Naming systems, forms of address	expectations
Diet	support during labour
Fasting	attitudes to pain, pain relief
Clothing	The placenta
Modesty	Welcoming the baby
Jewellery	Postnatal period
Make-up	Naming the baby
Washing	Infant feeding
Menstruation	Circumcision
Body space, politeness	Contraception
Expression of emotion	Premature or very sick babies
Expression of sexuality	Childbearing losses
	infertility
	miscarriage, stillbirth
	neonatal death
	Deaths and funerals
	Post mortem
	Specific health issues

Table 15.1 gives areas of care that may be influenced by culture and religion and which you may find helpful to bear in mind when talking to clients. It is not intended as a checklist to be routinely plodded through, but as a framework to help your own thinking. The areas may be relevant to anyone, whatever their situation, background, or spiritual beliefs, and are not only to do with formal religions or minority cultures. Each client will vary in the importance she attaches to them. With her agreement, record things that are especially important to her, so that everyone caring for her and her family can be aware of their needs.

Explaining your purpose

Some people of minority groups have learned to be cautious about discussing their culture or religion with outsiders or people in authority. They may have past experiences of being judged or criticised, or of having their beliefs and practices misunderstood or distorted. They may feel threatened by your questions and react defensively, especially if they know that your ways are probably different from theirs. Some people may be irritated or sceptical because they have been asked about their needs many times but nothing has ever been done to meet them.

It is important therefore to build up a respectful, trusting and equal relationship before you start asking questions. You may need to explain why you are asking so that the woman can be confident that you are genuinely interested in her and in providing appropriate care.

Managing our own reactions

Gaining insights into other people's lifestyles, beliefs and value systems can be enriching and satisfying. But occasionally people's choices and practices arouse strong negative reactions. It is hard to accept other people's values when they are completely contrary to our own. It can also be difficult when people's lifestyles and decisions conflict with what is considered to be healthy or safe or even within the law. How do we continue to provide responsive and responsible care and at the same time deal with our own views and feelings?

Each of us has certain things that we find particularly hard to deal with. It can be difficult to be sympathetic and supportive to women who persist in smoking or taking street drugs during pregnancy. It may be upsetting to witness family relationships in which women are subservient and all decisions are taken by men. The idea that women are traditionally considered unclean during menstruation may be abhorrent to some health professionals. Others may feel horrified and angry at the possibility of a woman refusing interventions such as a blood transfusion or a caesarean section when her life or the life of her baby is in jeopardy.

> *'The idea that I might have to stand by and watch a woman die unnecessarily from a haemorrhage because she refused a blood transfusion is horrific. I don't know how I'd cope. I just hope it never happens.'*   Student midwife

We are all entitled to hold personal views, but not to impose them on clients. The indiscriminate expression of feelings such as anger, distress, shock, disapproval or horror, even if justified, usually makes things worse. But keeping such strong feelings bottled up blocks our ability to think objectively and makes it hard to provide non-judgemental care. It can also damage our own health and well-being.

Health professionals are responsible for providing respectful care, for meeting cultural and religious needs, for informing and educating on health issues, and for enabling people to make their own choices. They also have a duty to respect the choices people make. Occasionally this may conflict with their responsibilities in relation to child protection, in which case the professional's responsibility to ensure the safety and well-being of the child must take priority.

Separating out professional responsibility and personal beliefs is hard, especially when one's thinking is clouded by strong emotion. It is therefore essential to develop strategies for expressing and releasing feelings constructively and safely, and to choose carefully where, when and with whom you do this.

- It is inappropriate and always unhelpful to do this anywhere near the person or people involved.
- It is unwise to let off steam with someone who shares the client's heritage or values since this can generate anger and conflict and ruin relationships.

> *'I get fed up when colleagues complain to me about Jewish patients. They seem to think that because I am Jewish I am a good person to talk to. But all that happens is that I feel embarrassed, helpless, defensive and resentful. Sometimes they are just prejudiced and stereotyping but even when their complaints are justified, nobody benefits.'*
> Jewish nurse

- In general, avoid letting off steam to other people who are caring for the same client. You risk generating additional negativity against the client.

● Avoid also people whom you know to be prejudiced and negative. Your story is likely to increase their prejudices and is unlikely to help you deal constructively with your feelings. Later on, you may feel that you have made things worse.

The best listener

The best listener is someone who understands that:

● all they need to do is to listen and to remain calm, supportive and objective;
● their own opinions and experiences are not necessarily helpful;
● you need to have your feelings acknowledged and that you need to let off steam;
● what you say and how you say it is not necessarily rational, and that afterwards you may take a different view; and
● everything you say must remain completely confidential.

Once you have had a chance to express your feelings you are more likely to be able to think clearly and to sort out your professional role and responsibilities. You can then work out how to handle the situation and whether action, advice or information is appropriate. In doing so it may be helpful to reflect on the following.

● Your own accepted practice and belief, and the validity of established routines and advice. Can you be sure that you are right and the client is not?

   'When I worked in the East End we put a lot of time and energy into trying to persuade Bengali women to put their babies on their tummies to sleep but to no avail. They persisted in lying them on their backs. The Back to Sleep campaign made a nonsense of our advice. I wonder how much else that we think is sacrosanct will also turn out to be wrong.'   Midwife lecturer

● The fact that people are unlikely to change their values and beliefs, especially if they feel criticised or under pressure.
● The possibility that your cultural or medical values are also causing conflict and distress to clients. We may be unaware of the profound effects that our 'normal' practice in maternity care has on other people.

In the end, unless there is good reason to think that the child may be at risk, health professionals have to accept and accommodate other people's beliefs and decisions, however hard this may sometimes be. Often it helps to understand the context and origins of other people's beliefs and practices. Occasionally nothing helps. All that can be done is to support one another through the pain, and, in the future, to try not to stereotype or to react negatively to people who hold similar beliefs.

16

Personal heritage and religious belief

Our personal history and heritage shapes who we are, what we believe and how we live. We are influenced by the circumstances in which we were brought up, by our parents' way of life, their values, and their beliefs about the meaning and purpose of life. Although the greatest influences for most of us are our immediate family and the society in which we live, we are also likely to have been affected by the origins and beliefs of our grandparents and our great-grandparents.

Take a moment to reflect on your own family history and its influence on you:

- How have your birthplace and upbringing shaped your current attitudes and beliefs?
- How much of your parents' value systems and beliefs do you share?
- What have you rejected or adapted?
- If you or your parents were born outside the UK, how has this influenced you?
- If your grandparents were born and live(d) outside the UK, how has this influenced you?
- If your lifestyle is different from that of your parents, have you noticed times when you have reverted to old familiar patterns of thought and belief?

RELIGIOUS BELIEFS, PRACTICES AND FESTIVALS

When people enter the health care system they are usually asked their religion. The reasons for asking are often unclear and more often than not the answer is merely recorded and an opportunity to find out more about the client's needs is lost. Occasionally the answers may be used in unintended ways, as the following apocryphal story shows.

> At a hospital that recorded Roman Catholics as RC and Protestants as P, and in the days when student nurses served meals, a ward sister challenged a student nurse about the way she was giving out breakfasts. She replied, ' I look at their notes. If they are P I give them porridge and the RCs get rice crispies.'

A client's answer to a question about religious affiliation may seem straightforward, but in reality it tells you little. For example, if a woman says 'Church of England', what does this mean? She may be deeply religious and want to see the chaplain and receive communion. She may have been christened but not have attended church since she was a child. A secular Jew who is not at all religious may reply 'Jewish' purely in order not to be identified as a Christian. A person who says they have no specific religion may have strong spiritual beliefs.

Religious beliefs and values

If religion is discussed at all in relation to maternity care, it is usually in terms of a list of awkward practical requirements and prohibitions which require tolerance and flexibility from health professionals. However there is far more to religion than outward and visible practice. Most people with a strong religious faith have a set of beliefs and values which are woven into the fabric of their being. These beliefs and values influence people's perceptions and reactions, and the meaning that they ascribe to what happens to them. They also determine their priorities and underlie their decisions.

> *'They think we don't understand that they are worried about us fasting. We do, but our ways are different.'*   Pregnant Muslim woman fasting during Ramadan

Think about the following statements of belief:

- This life is a preparation and a test, however hard it may sometimes be, for eternal life in heaven or in the next world.
- Everything that happens is God's will and part of His plan. It is our duty to accept it and to trust Him.
- You've only got one life and there's nothing more. When you die that's the end of you.
- This is just one life in a cycle of many during which we work through the consequences of our past and determine our future. As you sow, so shall you reap.
- There are evil spiritual influences in the world from which we need to take steps to protect ourselves and those we love. There are also good spiritual influences whose power and protection we can call on.

- How might each of these beliefs affect your attitude to life in general?
- How might each of them affect your attitude to:
  - antenatal screening?
  - intervention during pregnancy and labour?
  - termination of pregnancy?
  - a stillbirth?
  - serious illness and disability?
  - death?

Variations in religious belief

For some people their religious or spiritual beliefs are a central part of their lives and affect everything. Others have discarded the formal religious beliefs and practices of their childhood but may still adhere to the ethical system and may celebrate some religious festivals. Yet others do not have any religious or spiritual beliefs but may uphold strong ethical and moral values.

The experience of emigration or of being part of a religious minority leads some people to become less religious and observant; it leads others to rediscover the meaning and importance of their religious roots. Some people also find that important life events, such as a birth, a marriage or a death, lead them back to their religion, and that they have strong feelings about how things should be done. For example, a secular Jew may never attend synagogue or celebrate Jewish festivals, but may want to have her son circumcised. A Christian who never goes to church may feel strongly about having a religious funeral for her stillborn baby.

A strong religious faith can be a source of comfort and strength when life is hard. It may give meaning to tragedies such as the death of a baby. It may give people the purpose and hope they need to carry on. But religious beliefs do not always help and people's feelings about them may be complicated. Women who make choices that are against the precepts of their religion may suffer guilt later or may feel that they have brought punishment on themselves. Sometimes parents may feel guilty if they cannot accept what has happened to them, when their religion tells them that they should. Although tragedy turns some people towards religion, it may lead others to question their beliefs and to lose their conviction that life has any meaning.

It may sometimes be important to help clients talk through their religious or spiritual beliefs and conflicts by listening non-judgementally and supportively.

Understanding and discussing different religions

Many of the fundamental values of the different world religions are similar: belief in the sanctity of life and that life has a spiritual dimension and a greater purpose; belief in the soul and the value of prayer or meditation; the importance of truth and honesty, of doing right, and of fulfilling one's family responsibilities. All religions have their own festivals, times for celebration, reflection and prayer. Historical events are remembered and stories re-told. In most religions there are ceremonies for births, marriages and deaths.

People of different religions may do similar things for similar reasons. For example, a Catholic woman may make a novena of masses to help achieve a successful pregnancy. A Hindu woman might make a special fast.

> 'My mother-in-law has given up eating rice which she especially likes because she has an unmarried daughter and she hopes that her sacrifice will make it more likely that her daughter will marry.'   Indian mother

But there are also many differences in beliefs, values and practices as well as in formal structures. Some religions, for example Christianity, Judaism and Islam, base their beliefs and practices on historical texts and on authoritative statements and interpretations given by religious leaders. Some provide detailed rules covering aspects of daily life such as diet, behaviour between men and women, inheritance law, marriage, divorce, modesty, dress, sexual behaviour, abortion and contraception. Some set out a framework of religious practices and prayer that people must follow. Others have a looser framework of values and principles on the basis of which people make their own decisions and decide their own practice. Some religions stress the importance of public observance; others regard people's religion as their own private affair. Some have a living leader; others may rely on the writings and teachings of past leaders.

There are also variations in practice and belief within each religion. For example, all religions contain certain groups or sects that are stricter and more prescriptive than others. Often there is conflict or suspicion between different groups or sects. People of the same faith whose families originated in different parts of the world may also have different practices and preferences, influenced by their local cultures. For example, although a woman from Bosnia and a woman from Somalia may both be Muslims, their religious attitudes and experiences may vary a good deal. In addition, however clear the authority and laws of some religious faiths, for each person the details of their faith are individual. People may value different things, though their underlying beliefs and practices may be the same. Although it is possible, therefore, to describe in a general way the beliefs, codes of behaviour, festivals, traditions and rituals of a particular religion, there are also always tremendous variations in individual beliefs and practices.

Pastoral care and leadership

The roles of religious leaders vary. In Christianity most leaders have both spiritual authority and a pastoral role. In other religions, emotional and spiritual support may be offered by community members instead. In some religions, formal rituals, prayers and services are led by appointed ministers. In others, they are led by different community members in turn. A person who is employed to lead prayers and care for the place of worship does not necessarily also have a leadership role and authority to pronounce on religious issues. Accepted practice in different communities also changes with changing circumstances. For example, many Jewish rabbis in the UK have taken on pastoral work even though this is not their traditional role.

In some cases health professionals and managers have tried, with the best of intentions, to make contact with leaders or ministers of the different local religious groups and to involve them in decisions on health service provision and practice. This has met with varying success because of the different roles and duties of 'leaders' in the different faiths. In some cases, the official religious leaders, who are generally men, may also understand little about issues such as pregnancy, childbirth and women's health issues and may feel embarrassed at the detailed discussion of such subjects. Sometimes they may take a very conservative line on certain issues, possibly at odds with the views and wishes of many women in the community. It is important to be sensitive to matters such as these and to work out the most appropriate ways of contacting members of different religions and eliciting their views on provision.

Religious festivals

In a multiracial community it is necessary to know the dates and significance of the major religious festivals celebrated locally. It is also helpful to know which festivals are joyful and which solemn so that you can acknowledge the festival appropriately. Major religious celebrations may cause women, in particular, extra work and pressure. Some festivals involve fasting.

Just as women are not given antenatal appointments on Christmas Day, routine appointments should not be made for members of minority religions on their festivals. Most women in hospital would also like to be able to go home to celebrate major festivals, in the same way as many people are allowed home over Christmas. Non-urgent tests, operations or investigations should be avoided as far as possible and routine home visits should also normally wait till the festival is over. At joyful festivals women in hospital may receive cards and presents and are likely to be grateful for recognition that this is a special day for them. Visitors may bring in special festive dishes and any restrictions should be lifted as far as possible.

Some festivals occur on the same dates every year. The dates of Easter and of Hindu, Sikh and Jewish festivals vary slightly each year. The Muslim lunar year is shorter than the Western solar year so the dates of Muslim festivals fall roughly ten days earlier each year.

One person in each unit should be responsible for finding out the dates of the key festivals each year, for circulating this information and for reminding colleagues when an important festival is imminent. In this way clients are more likely to feel that their religious beliefs are valued and respected and appointments are less likely to be missed or resented. (For more on the dates of festivals see Walshe and Warrier, 1993.)

Religion and ritual

Rituals are actions that have no practical benefit but have important social, emotional or symbolic meaning. They offer a way of managing special events. Rituals can provide stability, familiarity and comfort in times of crisis. Having a prescribed way of doing things can help people deal with the uncertainty and anxiety that always accompany new situations, both positive and negative.

Most people are familiar with the concept of rituals in relation to religion; for example, the Jewish tradition of lighting two candles just before the Sabbath, the Muslim requirement to wash in a specific and prescribed way before prayer, the Roman Catholic and Orthodox ritual of making the sign of the cross on entering a church. Different cultures and religions also have rituals associated with events such as greeting and parting, the cycle of the seasons, and important life events.

'Every culture "organises" pregnancy and birth and gives them meaning through ritual' (Hansen, 1990). Many people feel very strongly about the religious and other rituals that surround pregnancy, birth, marriage and death in their family. Even those people whose daily life takes little account of culture or religion may find such rituals important and strengthening.

Identifying individual needs

Asking a client's religion and knowing something about the beliefs and practices of the different religions is a good foundation for identifying potential needs, but these are merely starting points. It is still impossible to predict anything about how devout the client is or what practices she follows. The only way to find out what is important to any individual and what religious needs or preferences a client has in relation to maternity care is to ask, bearing in mind that for many people their religion is a sensitive and personal matter.

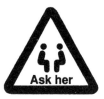

Many of us have grown up with prejudices against different religions, often arising from centuries of mutual dislike, misunderstanding and gross mis-interpretation. Religious differences continue to be a source of suspicion and conflict, even hatred, murder and war. Members of minority religions, in particular, may feel that their faith is often portrayed only in terms of negative stereotypes and distortions. For most people their religion is a sensitive issue. It deals with sacred matters and must not be abused or ridiculed in any way. Many people are reluctant to open themselves and their beliefs to possible criticism or ridicule.

'After Rushdie, the Gulf War, and now Bosnia, I have been forced to describe myself in terms of my religion, to proclaim something that was given and understood before. For 20 years I never thought that being a Muslim was a problem. Then it changed. People would say "but you're so educated and reasonable", as if all Muslims are maniacs.' British Muslim academic and consultant (from the *Independent*, 5.7.93, by permission)

Enabling clients to talk about religious issues and their implications may involve tackling our own prejudices so that we can demonstrate genuine respect and a willingness to listen and learn about the client's perceptions and point of view. We may also need to set aside our own beliefs temporarily. This can be hard when clients express views or make decisions that we find difficult to understand or accept. We may need to make a conscious effort to separate our professional responsibilities from our own feelings (see also Chapter 15).

GOOD AND BAD LUCK

Western scientific 'rationalism' tends to dismiss the concepts of good and bad luck as mere primitive superstition. In reality the belief in good and bad luck is alive and well in the West though it may take different forms from those found in other societies. Superstitions are woven into Western culture so much so that they often go unnoticed. Many hotels do not have a Room 13 and many people are nervous about Friday 13th. Horoscopes abound in magazines and newspapers and have an increasing following. People wish each other luck, have lucky charms or mascots, touch wood, avoid walking under ladders and throw spilt salt over their shoulders.

What people believe can have a profound effect on their lives. Many health professionals have seen patients with reasonable prognoses give up and die for no apparent clinical reason, whilst others with appalling prognoses have recovered against all the odds. An American study found that amongst a group of adult Chinese Americans who were seriously ill, those whose birth year was considered to be ill-fated died significantly earlier than those whose birth year was considered auspicious. Seriously-ill Chinese women with ill-fated birth years died earlier than the men who had ill-fated birth years. This was thought by the researchers to be due to that fact that the men had more exposure to Western culture and therefore did not adhere so strongly to traditional Chinese beliefs (Phillips *et al.*, 1993). Such beliefs die hard. A modern Italian woman may not believe, as her mother and grandmother probably did, that washing her hair after having a baby or during a period will make her more vulnerable to infection. But if she washes her hair and then gets ill, she may regret that she did not follow the old traditions. Many pregnant women in all cultures are reluctant to make preparations for their baby before birth in case something goes wrong. In the UK, department stores accommodate these feelings by reserving cots and buggies to be delivered after the child is safely born.

> *'When I went into a London hospital for my first baby they told me to bring in disposable nappies. I was horrified, not because I felt they should have supplied them, but because I felt it was tempting fate. How could they be so sure that my baby would be all right?'* English mother

It is not possible to predict what any individual will consider lucky or unlucky, or to get it right every time. However it is important to increase your awareness of possible differences and to be sensitive to any verbal and non-verbal clues you get from the mother and other family members about what is and is not acceptable. Where appropriate, ask clients if they have any worries about particular practices.

● Some people believe that it is important to think positively during pregnancy to help ensure that everything goes well. Discussion during antenatal care or in parent education classes of problems, or what might go wrong, should be approached with caution and sensitivity.
● Some parents may be reluctant to make any practical preparation for the baby before the birth.
● Some parents may not be willing to disclose the names they have chosen for their baby until the baby is born or until the formal naming ceremony. In some families a name is not discussed until then.
● Some parents may consider certain days, dates or astrological combinations auspicious or inauspicious. This should be taken into account, if possible, when, for example, an elective caesarean section or induction is planned.
● In most Western cultures, it is considered rude not to admire a baby. In some other cultures there is a strong belief in the dangers of tempting fate and that commenting on people's good fortune or beauty will attract jealousy or the 'evil eye'. Some people may also not show their pleasure or excitement about their own baby in case this is dangerous and attracts bad luck.

17 Families, relationships and roles

Take some time to reflect on the following questions.

- How important is your family to you? Every day? When major life events occur?
- What do you think of as a family? How many people? How many generations?
- What is a family for?
- Which do you think is the most important relationship in the family?
- In your family do men and women have different roles and responsibilities?
- In your family who decides how children should be brought up? Who has the primary responsibility for caring for them?
- Who do you feel has the right to give advice to whom in a family?
- Who do you turn to when you need advice or practical help?
- Do you feel closer to your family or to some of your friends?
- Who would you turn to if your marriage or relationship was in difficulties?
- At what age or stage in their lives do you feel that people should stand on their own feet and be independent of their families?
- Until what age do you feel that parents should have authority over their children?
- Whom should a person involve in decisions about their marriage or relationship?
- Who has ultimate authority over you?
- Does your reputation affect your family? Does this influence your behaviour?
- When you are old do you expect to live with your children?
- What in your life is most important to your self-respect and to the way you would like others to see you?

In the UK, ideas and beliefs about the family and marriage have changed dramatically over the past fifty years. The number of single-parent families is increasing. As more people re-marry or form second long-term relationships more complex families are forming.

'When I came here from Ireland I found the strangest thing was all the divorce. My husband's parents had split up and both re-married and had more children of their own. And they were all part of his family and they all seemed to get on quite well. I was astonished!'   Mother of three

The roles of men and women in the UK are generally less defined and differentiated than they were. Many women are more autonomous and independent. Long-term unemployment has taken the traditional role of breadwinner away from many men. In some families women are now the main earners.

Despite these changes many people in the UK still view the nuclear family – a married couple with children – as the norm, expecting the man to earn and the woman to take the main responsibility for childcare. Most people feel that a married couple should be financially and emotionally independent of their parents and other relatives. Many people have little contact with anyone in their extended family. In English culture marriage does not usually create an alliance between two families; the husband's and wife's parents may never really know each other. Old people often live alone, a fact which shocks many people of other cultures.

Different families

Definitions of what constitutes a family, and ideas about how families should function vary from culture to culture. For example, in South Asian culture (see also Chapter 34) a marriage is traditionally an alliance between two families. A household frequently contains three generations. Men and women usually have clearly differentiated roles and in some communities lead largely segregated lives.

Patterns of authority and decision-making vary. In some families it is traditional for men to make all decisions that relate to the public domain. In many cultures great respect and deference are shown to older people. Older family members may have authority over other adults and children and may make major decisions for them. Some women may not wish to decide about aspects of care such as screening and contraception, without consulting their husbands or older family members. Some may be unwilling to attend appointments or antenatal classes without family approval. Older women may sometimes have a strong influence over how women care for themselves during pregnancy and postnatally, and how the baby is fed and cared for. Providing the client agrees, it may be useful to involve other family members in discussions.

In many cultures people prefer to turn to family members for help and advice; some consider it strange or disloyal to ask outsiders. But families with these values that are geographically divided may have no access to support when it is needed; different pressures in the UK may also mean that other members who live closer cannot help. A study in Bradford found that South Asian mothers who wanted and needed help from social services were less likely to get it than English mothers. 'It was felt by the nurses in antenatal clinics that Asians needed less social services support because of extended family relationships and they indicated (wrongly) that these women . . . were less likely to want help' (Gatrad, 1994).

In cultures where the behaviour of any one person affects the reputation and prospects of his or her whole extended family, there are often strictly enforced codes of conduct. Modesty and discretion may be particularly expected of women. In order to protect them and to preserve their reputations, women in some conservative families only leave the house with permission from their elders. For many people the extended family system provides life-long support. Nevertheless, as in all family systems, there can be tensions and disagreements, particularly where younger people are influenced by a majority culture which has very different values.

Marriage

In the West, monogamy is generally regarded as the only acceptable form of marriage. Polygamy is often seen as licentious and degrading to women. However, in the Muslim religion, for example, men are allowed to take up to four wives under certain conditions (see also Chapter 37). Some Muslims regard this as preferable to the situation they observe in the West where men may father children outside marriage and take little or no responsibility for them, or where families split up and mothers are left to carry the burden of providing for themselves and the children. In certain areas of Africa, including Ghana, polygamy is common and is also practised by some Christians.

For women in a culture where polygamy is accepted as normal there are recognised advantages. The first wife is regarded as the senior and existing wives must agree before their husband can marry again. Wives can support each other. Problems are normally shared and there is someone to offer help and to care for the children when a women is sick or has just given birth. New mothers have the practical help, support and advice of experienced women and are freed from other responsibilities and from pressure to resume sexual relations before they are ready. (It is not legal to make a polygamous marriage in Britain, but a polygamous marriage made in a country that permits polygamy by a resident of that country is valid in British law.)

ATTITUDES TO MOTHERHOOD

A woman's social and economic circumstances, her culture, values and religion are likely to affect the way she adapts to pregnancy and to the massive changes that the baby's arrival brings.

Attitudes to motherhood vary. In the West, for example, there are often sharply contrasting attitudes to motherhood. It may be seen 'as the only thing women are designed by nature to do, or . . . as something that career and professional women should do in the background and on the run' (Kline, 1993). Motherhood is the only role that people are expected to take on 24 hours a day, seven days a week, and 52 weeks a year for a minimum of 16 years without any training or realistic preparation. In the UK the status of mothers is generally low in comparison to some other cultures and countries. Mothers are often poorly supported both emotionally and practically. Nevertheless, they are frequently blamed for the general ills of society and when their children have problems.

The second half of the twentieth century has seen radical changes in Western women's attitudes towards motherhood. For many, motherhood is no longer the absolute fulfilment it was for former generations.

'I went back to work as soon as I could because going to work means you become a person in your own right again.'   English mother of two

Contraception and the legalisation of abortion have given women choices about their fertility, and the feminist movement has raised awareness of inequalities between the sexes. As a result women's expectations are changing and for many motherhood is no longer their main goal. Work outside the home, which is also a financial necessity for many women, may be an important source of fulfilment, self-respect, independence and status. Becoming a mother and giving up work, even temporarily, can mean a loss of status as well as a worrying loss of income. Staying at home and focusing entirely on motherhood can be demoralizing (Bates, 1993).

'My husband tells me I am doing a good job but I do worry that people will think I am just a thick, stupid housewife.'   First-time mother

In contrast, in communities that adhere to more traditional values and gender roles, motherhood may sometimes bring status and identity and a sense of purpose and fulfilment. Women in such communities may be more likely to view marriage and motherhood as their main goal. Becoming a mother may bring a major increase in status and respect. Although mothers in these communities may work outside the home as well, some may depend less on work for their sense of identity and purpose. At the same time, some women in all communities may feel restricted by traditional expectations and may feel negative or ambivalent about the changes that confront them when they are pregnant.

SINGLE PARENTS

In recent years attitudes to single pregnant women have changed enormously. While debates about the potential financial burden on the state and the importance of a stable family unit continue, the social stigma of being an unmarried mother has all but disappeared and increasing numbers of babies are born to single women.

In conservative cultural or religious communities where morality is highly valued, a single woman who becomes pregnant may be viewed very differently. An unmarried, pregnant woman brings shame and disgrace and may ruin the reputation of her whole family and may ruin the marriage prospects of other family members. Such a family may consider secret termination or adoption to be the only options, and any woman who wants to keep her baby risks being isolated and unsupported. This is particularly harsh for women who may be unused to living independently without the support and protection of their own family and culture (Ahmed and Watt, 1986). Women in this situation need supportive and sensitive care.

NAMES AND FORMS OF ADDRESS

Whether we like our name or not, most of us feel strongly about it. It forms part of our identity and can reflect our family history, origins or religion. It is important for most of us that people get our name right and that they pronounce and use it correctly.

The way people address each other reflects their relationship. In English culture calling a person by their personal name implies a degree of friendship, informality and intimacy. Using a title and family name is more formal. Attitudes to formality or informality in the use of names vary between age groups and cultures, and a younger person (including a health professional) who addresses an older person by their personal name may be perceived as disrespectful rather than friendly.

Beatrice Matthews waited for some time in a packed Outpatients Department. At last a young nurse called out 'Beatrice'. Mrs Matthews was so affronted by being addressed in this way by a complete stranger barely out of her teens that she did not reply and the nurse went away. Hours later she was the only person left in the waiting room and someone asked her what she was doing there. By this time the doctors had gone so she left without being seen.

- How do you feel about your personal name(s) and your family name?
- Who chose your personal name(s) and why?
- Does your name reflect your origins or religion?
- How do you feel when people pronounce your name incorrectly or change or shorten it?
- How do you feel when someone you do not know addresses you by your personal name?

In the UK people commonly talk about Christian names and surnames. This assumes that everyone is Christian, an assumption reflected on many forms. This is clearly inappropriate in a multicultural society. (See Chapter 14 for more about recording names and addressing people correctly.)

FOOD AND DIET

Food is not simply a matter of nutrition; it often has profound personal significance. It can symbolise love, security, moral and religious values, attitudes to health, and our beliefs about ourselves and about the world.

Local diets reflect climates, seasons and agricultural patterns. There may be special foods for different occasions and in many cultures it is traditional to prepare special foods for major family events such as births, marriages and deaths and for religious ceremonies and festivals. Familiar food is also comforting and reassuring, especially at times of stress.

In most cultures and families women are responsible for preparing food and pass their knowledge informally to their daughters and, sometimes, to their sons. Most women cook and eat what they like and are used to, and know how to prepare. People are unlikely to change their eating habits and tastes when they migrate, or the cooking methods they are familiar with.

> *'My children go to school and get Western food to eat. I try to cook Nigerian food at home so they are accustomed to it and like it and won't find it strange when they visit the family back home.'*   Nigerian woman

Meal times can be important social occasions when friends and family spend time together. The concept of good table manners may be universal but how they are defined varies. In some cultures great importance is attached to who eats with whom, who serves whom, and the order in which people are served. In some cultures making a noise while eating indicates that you are enjoying and grateful for your food; in others it is considered rude. In many cultures it is polite always to offer visitors food and drink, and polite for the visitors to accept.

Different cultures also have different ways of eating. For example a Chinese woman who normally eats with chopsticks may find a knife and fork difficult to manage in hospital. Even if she brings in her own chopsticks, the food she is presented with may not be cut small enough. Many South Asian people prefer to eat with their fingers; sometimes this has given rise to offensive comments from staff and other people on the ward.

Think about your attitudes towards food:

- How important were/are meal times in your family?
- What do you like to have for breakfast?
- Which foods do you eat with a knife, fork or spoon and which do you eat using your fingers?
- How do you react when you are given something unfamiliar to eat?
- What sorts of foods do you feel like eating when you are feeling ill or vulnerable?
- If you have been abroad, how did you feel when confronted with a menu in a language you do not understand?
- How did you make a choice and how did you feel when the dish arrived?

Attitudes and beliefs about food

The importance assigned to food varies in different cultures. In French culture food is a major topic of interest and pleasure. Food also plays a crucial role in Jewish culture. In British culture it is not usually regarded as particularly important. This is reflected in the lack of attention often paid to feeding clients in hospital. In 1994 a survey in a British hospital found that 200 out of 500 patients admitted were undernourished. Nevertheless, there was no nutritional information in most patients' case notes. While the patients were in hospital, the nutritional status of most of them worsened. One third of those who were admitted moderately undernourished became severely undernourished during their stay. In such a climate, meeting the nutritional needs of clients whose diet is different from that of the majority may have even less priority.

Many cultures have strong beliefs about what people should eat or avoid to keep healthy. Each culture has its own view of what constitutes a good diet. In the West this is usually based on the nutritional values of different foods, in traditional Chinese and South Asian cultures it is based on the idea of contrasting food types which should be balanced to achieve maximum health. Beliefs about diet may be particularly important during pregnancy. In many cultures it is also considered important for women to eat a very nourishing diet after the birth and while breast feeding so that they regain their strength and are not vulnerable to illness.

Food and religion

For some people food also has a religious and spiritual significance. There may be religious requirements about the way food is prepared. For observant Jews meat must be specially slaughtered and prepared in order to be acceptable. Meat and milk products must be kept strictly separate (see also Chapter 39). Islam also lays down rules for the slaughter and preparation of meat (see also Chapter 37).

When preparing or serving food for people who are vegetarian or who eat only halal or kosher meat, it is very important to ensure that:

- No prohibited food comes into contact with the food that is being served. A salad from which a slice of ham has been removed has already been contaminated and cannot be eaten.
- Separate utensils and dishes are used for prohibited food. The same spoon must not be used, for example, to serve minced meat to other people and then potatoes to a Hindu, a Sikh or a Muslim who follows food restrictions.

If people cannot be sure that foods have been kept completely separate they may feel that it is best to refuse all food.

Fasting

Fasting is an important component of religious practice for people of many different religions, though its significance and implications vary. Many Muslims and Jews observe set annual fasts while some Hindus fast or restrict their food intake on certain days. Most observant Jewish women will not attend antenatal clinics or classes during fasts as these are also religious festivals. Muslim women who are fasting during Ramadan may find it difficult to keep early appointments and may also be reluctant to give blood. (For more about fasting and different religions see Part Five.)

Most women are exempted from stringent fasts if there are genuine medical contra-indications. However, fasts have an important spiritual and personal significance for many people and some may be reluctant to miss them. In most cases fasting is not contra-indicated during pregnancy though adjustments may be necessary for women on medication.

Dietary advice

People are unlikely to follow advice that does not take their real situation into account or that does not make sense to them. They may also be worried or alienated by inappropriate advice. Advice about diet is therefore only worth giving if it is based on a thorough understanding of the client's existing diet, and of the beliefs, traditions and financial and other factors that may affect or limit her choices. Often these constraints are practical. For example, most women living in bed and breakfast hostels have very limited access to cooking facilities and may find it impossible to cook meals, especially if they have children to care for at the same time (Schott and Henley, 1992).

It is also important not to assume that people who eat an unfamiliar diet are malnourished and need dietary advice. Dietary changes should only be recommended if they are really necessary, and the reasons and benefits to the client must be made very clear (Holmes, 1993).

'Just because we follow vegetarian or vegan diets, don't assume that we are anaemic or that we don't know how to eat a balanced diet.'   Rastafarian mother of two

Food in hospital

In hospital, it is clearly important that women get food that they find appetizing, healthy and, where relevant, acceptable in religious terms. Menus need to offer a good range of choices in order to meet the needs of all clients.

This means finding out in detail what is appropriate to different groups and working out a range of acceptable menus with women from the local community. It is important to be very specific; an African, South Asian or Indian diet does not exist. People's diet varies according to their religion, culture and area of family origin. For example, some people of South Asian heritage are vegetarian. Some eat no eggs. Some eat no onions, garlic or root vegetables. Others eat meat but only if it is halal. Others eat all meat however slaughtered; some refuse beef and pork. Some usually eat chapatis with their meals, some usually eat rice, and some eat both. People whose families originated in different areas use different ingredients, spices and cooking methods. What suits the members of one community is unlikely to suit others.

'Our local maternity hospital serves different vegetable curries which most of the Indian, Pakistani and Bangladeshi women are happy to eat. Many of the Somali women find them too hot but there isn't anything else really suitable as they are Muslims and most only eat meat if it's halal.'   Community worker

Women who follow religious food restrictions and are unfamiliar with English cooking and ingredients may find it impossible to select from hospital menus. If they do not know what has gone into a dish, for example what cooking fat has been used, they may be unable to eat it. Hospital kitchens and menus should indicate which foods are suitable for people who follow the different religious food restrictions. If this is not done it may be necessary for ward staff to find out.

Bringing in food

Some families try to solve the problem of inappropriate hospital food by bringing in food from home, though this is not always easy. It is important not to assume that all ethnic minority women are being satisfactorily looked after by large families. Torkington (1987) describes an incident where a South Asian woman was left for two days without food. Apparently the ward staff knew she was not eating hospital food but presumed that her family was providing something. In fact her husband was abroad and she had no visitors.

Bringing in food does not always solve problems. If food is brought in between mealtimes some women may feel conspicuous eating it. Although it is possible to draw the curtains round the bed, this is often perceived as an unfriendly act by other people on the ward. Storing and heating food can cause problems, not only for women on wards but also for parents of babies in neonatal units and people accompanying women in labour. Since the lifting of Crown Immunity from health service premises, local authority Health and Safety officers interpret the relevant guidelines. In some cases inflexible interpretations make it difficult to respond to people's needs.

'I have been trying in vain to get our local Health and Safety officers to change their minds and allow us to give soft boiled eggs to elderly people in long-stay care. Many of them cannot eat protein in any other form. We don't want to have to rely on protein drinks and anyway they like soft boiled eggs. But the officers insist that all eggs should be hard boiled.' Consultant physician in public health

Clearly some precautions are necessary. Food should not be stored in hospital fridges without careful regulation. Re-heating must be thorough. But rules that prevent people eating properly are not helpful. If hospital food is unacceptable to clients for whatever reason, provision must be made, in conjunction with Health and Safety staff, for food to be brought in, and stored and heated as necessary.

As hospital stays become shorter it can be tempting to ignore the importance of food. But it is both damaging and inhospitable to keep women hungry at a time of physical stress when nourishing and acceptable food is essential for their well-being.

CLOTHING

International fashion has changed the way people dress; tee-shirts and blue jeans have become almost a world-wide uniform for young people. However, clothing is much more than passing fashion. What we wear and how we wear it can reflect our personality, lifestyle, age, the community in which we live, the work we do or even our politics. Clothes also reflect our cultural or religious values and ideas about modesty.

We tend to judge and categorize people, correctly or incorrectly, by the way they dress. Looking a little different may gain approval and admiration; looking very different often attracts criticism. Some people hold the view that everyone living in the UK should wear Western clothes. However, clothes are an important part of identity and security. When the British colonized other countries they rarely adopted the local style of dress. Instead they continued to wear what they were used to and comfortable in, sometimes adapted to the local climate.

Modesty

People's feelings about modesty in relation to dress vary enormously. What is acceptable to some, shocks others deeply. Some women are happy to sunbathe topless or nude, others may never have seen themselves, let alone anyone else, without any clothes on. Some people have different standards of modesty for different situations, others maintain the same standards all the time.

- When you were growing up, what messages did you receive about modesty?
- Do you have different standards of modesty:
  - at work?
  - in your doctor's surgery?
  - on the beach?
  - at a social event?
- How do you feel when your standards of personal modesty have been violated?

Many religions and traditional cultures require people to dress and behave modestly. Women may be required to dress in certain prescribed ways, especially in the presence of men and in public. Orthodox Jewish women and some Muslim and other South Asian women are likely to cover their upper arms and their legs to below the knee and to wear high necklines. Some women traditionally cover themselves from head to toe when they leave their homes. Modesty in dress and behaviour are likely to be particularly important when the reputation of a whole family depends on the behaviour and reputation of each of its members.

- What sort of clothes do you like to wear? What do you feel most comfortable and at ease in?
- Do you dress differently for different situations?
- How do you feel if you are expected to wear clothes, say for a wedding or interview, that you would not normally choose to wear?
- What do you wear to sleep in?
- What do you prefer to wear if you are feeling vulnerable or unwell?
- If you were in hospital and could wear what you feel most comfortable in, what would you choose?
- Have you ever worn a hospital theatre gown? How did you feel? (If you haven't, try it.)
- Have you ever felt uncomfortable because you were wearing the 'wrong' clothes for a situation?
- Has anyone ever made incorrect assumptions about you, based on the clothes you were wearing? How did you feel?

Hair

The way we care for and wear our hair is also important in terms of our well-being and self-expression. For some people there are also cultural and religious considerations. For example, many Muslim and Orthodox Jewish women keep their hair covered. In some cultures long hair is regarded as a symbol of holiness. Some devout Sikh men and women, particularly those who have taken amrit (see Chapter 41), never cut their hair. Married women normally keep it tied up in a bun. Some Rastafarian women and men keep their hair covered at all times and do not to cut it. Orthodox Jewish men may wear side locks and keep their heads covered.

Clothing in hospital

Information booklets about coming into hospital often assume that women coming into a maternity unit will wear night-dresses and dressing gowns. But not everyone wears or owns such garments. For example, some Chinese women may feel more comfortable in pyjamas. Many South Asian women wear shalwar kameez (a loose tunic top and trousers) at night as well as during the day but may feel that they have to buy night-dresses and a dressing gown for hospital. Some women may also feel embarrassed wearing a night-dress in a public ward where men go in and out. Verbal and written information about what to bring into hospital should invite women to wear whatever they find most comfortable.

Ideally, long-sleeved, high-necked, full-length coloured night-gowns should be available for women who for some reason need to wear hospital clothing. Theatre gowns, especially those that tie up at the back, are unacceptable to many women. Some may also find white gowns unacceptable since white is the colour of mourning in parts of South Asia and China.

Visiting clients at home

It is important for professionals to consider the way they dress and the impression they give when visiting clients at home so as not to cause unnecessary offence. In conservative families or with older family members, tight clothing, short skirts, bare arms and low necklines, for example, may prevent mutually respectful relationships. They may also be seen as unprofessional.

> 'I once stayed with a friend to keep her company while her baby son was being circumcised and to help afterwards. After he had performed the ceremony the mohel came up with the baby and told me what to do and what not to do. Or rather he told my feet. He didn't take his eyes off them and would not look at any other part of me, I assume because I was wearing trousers and my hair was uncovered.' Secular Jewish mother of two

In many cultures people take off their shoes when entering a home or a place of worship. If you see a row of shoes by the door, it is polite to take your own off.

JEWELLERY AND MAKE-UP

In most cultures a woman is given a piece of special jewellery with a symbolic meaning when she marries. This may be, for example, a ring, bracelets, a necklace or nose jewels. Just like a wedding ring, most other wedding jewellery is never removed. Some women may fear that removing wedding jewellery will bring bad fortune to themselves or their families. In some cases it is anyway impossible to remove wedding jewellery without breaking it. Many women would regard this as disastrous.

Much jewellery has religious significance. This may include, for example, special threads around the body, amulets containing holy texts, medals, crucifixes and other blessed items. Sometimes these have been blessed or come from a place with special spiritual significance. Many devout Sikhs wear a steel bangle and other religious items which must never be removed (see Chapter 41).

Sometimes religious jewellery is specially put on to protect the wearer against illness and danger, or to help ensure a successful pregnancy or an easy birth. Parents may also put religious items on or near their babies especially if the baby is unwell. Such items are clearly tremendously important and should never be removed without the parents' agreement.

Certain types of make-up may have also special religious or cultural significance (see, for example, Chapters 33 and 36).

All wedding jewellery and all items of religious significance should be treated with respect. They should never be removed without permission. In most cases there is no need to ask a woman to remove jewellery, threads or amulets. If there are genuine medical reasons it is important to find out first what significance the item(s) have for her. Where necessary, wedding jewellery and religious items should be taped.

WASHING

Beliefs and practices in relation to washing and cleanliness are linked to health, social acceptability and to personal comfort and well-being. Cultural patterns of washing have developed in response to local climates, terrains and circumstances.

Most people whose families originated in hot countries place a greater importance on washing than is generally found in traditional English culture. Some people may feel dirty and uncomfortable, for example, if they cannot wash or shower and change their clothes at least twice a day. In most hot countries people do not sit in a bath; they shower or pour water over themselves with a bowl. Some people feel that only running water gets them clean and may find the idea of sitting in a bath of water in which they have washed extremely distasteful. They may also prefer to use water rather than paper to clean themselves after using the lavatory. In many countries running water or a jug for carrying water are routinely provided in lavatories.

Washing may also be symbolic and rituals involving washing are part of several religions. Most Muslims wash in a prescribed manner before each of the five daily prayer sessions. Many Orthodox Jews wash their hands before eating bread. Many Sikhs and Hindus wash before praying. Some cultures also have restrictions on bathing at certain vulnerable times, for example, after childbirth and while menstruating.

In South Asian and some other cultures the right hand is used where possible for touching food and other clean things. It may be important to consider this and to ask the client when, for example, siting drips, or positioning food trays.

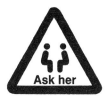

- When you were a child what were you taught about:
  - how often you should bath or shower?
  - washing before meals
  - washing after going to the lavatory
  - washing after touching certain things?
  - how often you should change your clothes?
- Do you prefer a bath, a shower or a strip wash?
- Do you bath or shower in the morning, at night, or both?
- Do you oil your skin after washing?
- If you are go to the doctor's knowing you might be examined, do you wash and put on clean underwear first?
- Do you wash before having sex? After having sex?
- After going to the lavatory, do you clean yourself with paper or with water?
- Do you shave some or all of your body hair?
- If you are a woman, do you alter your washing habits during and at the end of a period?
- What assumptions do you make about the cleanliness and washing habits of people whose skin colour, culture or religion is different from yours?

Since an individual's personal hygiene habits are linked to their comfort and self respect, it is important to respect and accommodate the needs and wishes of each client.

Ideally, baths, bidets and showers should be all available so that women can use whichever they prefer. If no showers are available, some women may prefer to have a jug in the bathroom so that they can stand in the bath and pour water over themselves. Some may also appreciate being offered a jug in which to take water into the lavatory for washing. As it is not possible to predict who will want what, it is better to make a gentle tentative offer which might be refused, than to leave a woman feeling uncomfortable because it is difficult to maintain her usual washing routines in hospital.

It may be helpful to keep a mop available in bathrooms and lavatories so that women can mop up spilt water.

Pregnancy and antenatal care

Women's attitudes and expectations

Women in the UK and elsewhere have a wide range of attitudes towards what kind of care is needed during pregnancy and childbirth. Some regard them as potentially problematic, necessitating frequent and careful medical supervision. Others regard them as normal healthy processes that do not usually require medical intervention. The attitudes and expectations of women who grew up in, for example, places where medical care is in short supply, or in countries with private, insurance-based health care systems, may differ widely.

In many Third World countries, pregnancy and birth are traditionally the concern of women. They are generally considered to be normal and natural events, though higher rates of perinatal, infant and maternal mortality and morbidity may mean that they are also regarded as dangerous. Most women expect to maintain their usual work and routines during pregnancy. There may be little formal care, especially in rural areas. Hospital antenatal care and births are often reserved for serious problem cases. Although women living in towns and cities are more likely to have access to hospital maternity care, lack of resources in many countries means that most hospital facilities are severely overstretched, overcrowded and under-equipped, and many staff inadequately trained and supported.

Women who are unfamiliar with Western attitudes and patterns of care may sometimes be surprised by the amount of energy and time devoted to clinical care and by the lack of attention paid to the more spiritual and emotional aspects of pregnancy. In many parts of the world it is traditional for women to do everything they can to avoid stress and negative thoughts during pregnancy and to concentrate on positive images. Peace of mind is highly valued and thought to have beneficial effects on the baby. The advantages of this tradition are supported by research on the physiological effects of stress. It appears that stress during pregnancy can affect the well-being of the fetus and also increases the incidence of pre-term delivery (Hedegaard *et al.*, 1993; Niven, 1992).

Health professionals' attitudes and expectations

Each medical system defines what health and illness are and how people should behave when they are in need of care. Each has its own definition of 'good' and 'bad' patients. This is also true of maternity care. There is a strong tendency for health professionals everywhere to regard the way they organise antenatal care as the best and only way. Other ways of doing things may be considered inferior. But we need to be cautious about assuming that what we do, and what we expect of clients, is always best especially as 'the changing fashions in obstetric medicine constantly redefine the boundaries of acceptable maternity behaviour' (Ahmad, 1993).

It is always important to respect and accommodate differing beliefs and customs in relation to pregnancy. There are very few cases where different practices genuinely jeopardise the well-being of the mother or the baby. And it is only too easy to damage people's confidence and ability to cope well and so, perhaps, to create rather than solve problems.

> *'We have to ask ourselves what is really important to tackle and what is not. How willing are we as health professionals to look at alternatives and variations? Is it really essential or just the way we do it?'*   Director of midwifery education

> *'Having been born and brought up here I tend to think that the Western, scientific approach to pregnancy and birth is better than the traditional ways my mother would like me to follow. But some of the traditional ways of doing things do work very well.'*   Indian mother of twins

CHOOSING THE STYLE AND PLACE OF CARE

The right of each woman to choose the style and place of her antenatal care and of the birth is enshrined in *Changing Childbirth* (Department of Health, 1993): every woman should 'be able to feel that she is in control of what is happening to her and . . . able to make decisions about her care'.

These important decisions are usually made very early in pregnancy, often during the woman's first interview with her GP or midwife. In order to make a meaningful choice, the woman needs first to know what the options for antenatal care and labour are, and then the pros and cons of each option. Increasingly, women are given time to discuss and consider all the possibilities before deciding. However, in some cases they are automatically channelled into the predominant local pattern of care, or into the type of care that it is thought will be best for them. For example, in some parts of the country, even articulate, well-informed women are still having to fight hard for their right to choose the place of birth although there is no justification for encouraging everyone to give birth in hospital (Campbell and Macfarlane, 1994; House of Commons, 1992).

Exercising the right to informed choice is likely be particularly difficult for some women of minority groups. Some may not know that they have a right to choose or may not be aware of the choices available to them. Others may feel obliged to comply with whatever they are offered, or may lack the confidence to say what they want and to negotiate with health professionals. Language barriers make it harder to exercise choice, as do the assumptions that some health professionals make about what is most appropriate. Women of minority groups who do voice their needs and preferences may be perceived as difficult and demanding.

> *'When a white woman says what she wants she is called assertive, when a black woman does the same, she is labelled aggressive.'*   African-Caribbean woman

For many women of minority groups, community-based care from a small team, care from a midwife with her own caseload, domino schemes or home births may be the best choices: such schemes normally provide greater flexibility and attention to individual needs, more continuity of care and better caring relationships. They may also cut down the need for women to travel; this may be especially important for women who are not used to going out alone, for those who find public transport hard to manage or fear racist attacks, and for those who speak little or no English.

For women who have practical support from their families or close friends, home birth may be most suitable. They are more likely to feel in control and less likely to feel lonely and isolated.

'Many of the Vietnamese women we look after really appreciate having their babies at home. They are more relaxed because they are in familiar surroundings and have come to know us and trust us even though there are often language difficulties. They are well supported by their families, can have their own familiar food which they consider to be extremely important. They can maintain the tradition of remaining secluded and protected at home for the first month after the birth. If they went into hospital, they would have problems with diet and be stressed by trying to communicate with strangers across language barriers and by having to make the transition from hospital to home.

'We also look after many African-Caribbean women at home. They prefer it because they feel more in control and in charge. Some have said that their husbands and partners participated much more at home than they would have in hospital as many find hospitals intimidating or threatening so it is just easier not to be there.'
Community midwives

ANTENATAL CARE

A great deal of time, money and energy are invested in antenatal care in the West. Most women have been socialized and educated into regular clinic attendance, which is considered to be extremely important despite the fact that many components of routine antenatal care have no proven benefits (Enkin *et al.*, 1990; Steer, 1993).

It has been known for some time that many women find antenatal clinics tiresome and unrewarding and that they do not meet their needs (Gladman, 1994). Too often women have been passive targets, expected to turn up, wait for hours and then accept 'care' which does not always address their concerns (Thorley and Rouse, 1993). The social, emotional and spiritual aspects of pregnancy important to many may be ignored (Vincent Priya, 1992). Some women are subjected to unexplained procedures and investigations (Smith and Marteau, 1995). Childcare facilities are rare, and mothers are often distracted and stressed by the demands of their other children, both in the waiting area and during the consultation. Journeys may be long and difficult. Nevertheless, most women spend large amounts of time, energy and money travelling to and attending clinics.

Women of minority groups may encounter a range of additional disincentives to antenatal attendance. For example:

- Being in an alien environment, feeling conspicuous and out of place.
- Unwelcoming or racist attitudes and behaviour.

- Appointment times that disregard religious festivals or family commitments.
- Health professionals who do not understand or respect their needs and preferences.
- Being addressed incorrectly because staff do not understand their naming systems.
- Language barriers (Narang and Murphy, 1994).

For some women the whole concept of antenatal care as organised in the West is new and they have to adapt to unfamiliar systems and values. Medicalised antenatal care, blood tests, ultrasound, urine tests and amniocentesis may be completely new concepts. Women who do not understand the purpose of antenatal care and the various checks, or who feel threatened and uncomfortable at clinics may see little point in attending.

'We had a lot of trouble persuading some women from rural areas of Africa to bring urine samples to the clinic. They always smiled but said they had forgotten. Eventually I realized that they could not see the point and what is more they thought we were extremely odd to ask for their urine. To them it seemed as crazy as we would think a request to bring in our toe-nail clippings. Once we explained, there was no problem.'   Obstetric registrar

'Bangladeshi women who have had several babies back home may not see the relevance of antenatal care. They managed quite well without it before. They may also be wary of having investigations or treatment imposed on them.'   Midwife teacher

Women who live completely within their own communities may not have had direct contact with the majority culture before using the maternity services. The wider the cultural gap, the more bewildering and difficult the experience is likely to be.

'I felt grateful for so much attention from the doctors. But I was afraid that some of the tests would harm my baby. And often I did not understand why they were doing them. I had two babies in Bangladesh without all these tests and everything was OK. I did not worry so much there.'   Mother of three

In addition, some women worry about the 'policing' and monitoring role of health professionals, and fear that they may get into trouble if they do not conform or if they inadvertently reveal some practice or aspect of behaviour that health professionals might disapprove of.

The impact of reputation

Once they are in the system many women feel powerless. Women of minority groups may have reason to feel even more so. Reports of poor care, abuse or rudeness travel fast. Women who book late or 'default' on appointments are usually seen as irresponsible and unco-operative, but some may have good reasons. Those who have experienced or fear unsympathetic or inappropriate treatment may vote with their feet.

'In the late 1980s, Asian women who were going to have their babies at the local district general hospital started to delay booking until they were 24 weeks pregnant. They had heard through the community grapevine that a consultant obstetrician there had decided that all women over forty should have amniocentesis.

'No consent was obtained, nor were the procedure, the risks, or the decisions that might have to be made afterwards explained. Amniocentesis was forcibly carried out on

women, some of whom were held down during the procedure, regardless of lack of consent and the fact that many would not have contemplated termination on religious grounds. Not surprisingly, women who heard what had happened to sisters and friends took the only action they felt able to. Avoidance.'   Midwife teacher

'In the clinic where I worked, women undergoing pre-natal diagnosis came in expecting abdominal ultrasound. Many of the Asian women, who had less explanation than the others, and were not asked for their consent, were particularly horrified and humiliated to find they were expected to submit to trans-vaginal ultrasound performed by a male doctor using a transducer covered with a condom. One woman who spoke little English became extremely distressed when the doctor continued against her obvious resistance.'   Student midwife

What kind of care does your antenatal clinic offer?

Take a fresh look at your antenatal clinic. One way of reviewing some aspects of your service is to sit quietly and unobtrusively in the reception or waiting area and watch.

Consider the following questions:

- What is going well? What concrete evidence do I have for my conclusions?
- What needs improving? How can these improvements be achieved?
- Is everyone, including clerks and receptionists, friendly, respectful and welcoming?
- Is bureaucracy kept to a minimum?
- Are people addressed correctly? Are there mechanisms for recording names of women and their partners or husbands correctly (see Chapter 14).
- Are women put at ease? Do they know what to do next at each stage and where to go?
- Are appointment procedures sufficiently flexible to take account of different religious festivals and of each woman's work, family and childcare commitments?
- Do the posters and leaflets reflect the variety of cultures and groups in your community?
- Are there crèche facilities?
- Are interpreters readily available for all the main local languages? Is there a system for getting hold of an interpreter for a client who speaks a language that is not normally catered for?
- Whose agenda is being met? Are women's concerns being addressed?

MODESTY

Modesty may seem an old-fashioned concept to many people, hardly compatible with a liberated woman. In reality, most women still carry strong messages about keeping their skirts down, their knickers up and their knees together. Pregnancy changes all that. Women suddenly find that they are expected to shed years of conditioning, to respond readily to questions about the most intimate aspects of their lives, to undress and to accept, without question, physical examinations from a succession of complete strangers, often men. Women who are pregnant often say that they feel their body is no longer their own, not because they are carrying another human being, but because other people suddenly act in a proprietary way towards them.

Physical and vaginal examinations during antenatal, intra-partum and postnatal care are a source of embarrassment and emotional distress for many women regardless of culture or religion. When a group of English women were asked how they felt about vaginal examinations, they initially responded that such things just had to be done and women should just accept them quietly. When asked how they really felt, all the women said they found the vaginal examination distressing but that they had to hide their feelings.

> 'Well I grit my teeth and put up with it. I smile and try to look calm because that's what they expect of me, I mean it's important not to make a fuss. But now that you ask me what I really feel, I hate it, it's embarrassing, humiliating and degrading. Sometimes I feel I'm not a person any more.'

Several women said that their husbands had been upset at seeing them examined internally by a male doctor but had not been able to say so at the time. Several older women also said that the memory of their humiliation and distress had remained with them all their lives.

In a recent survey of 500 women volunteers in the UK, over 100 reported that their experience of gynaecological or obstetric procedures was 'very distressing' or 'terrifying'. Thirty women fulfilled the criteria for a diagnosis of post traumatic stress syndrome (Menage, 1993).

Women of minority groups

If women who have been brought up to accept internal examinations as part of medical care find them difficult to cope with, it is not surprising that many women with a different upbringing find it especially hard to overcome their reticence. Women whose culture or religion requires strict modesty are likely to find such examinations especially traumatic. They may be deeply disturbed about the humiliation, shame and wrong-doing associated with exposing themselves in any way. These concerns may even discourage some women from seeking care, especially if they see little benefit in it.

> 'When I worked in an area where there were many South Asians it was common for the women coming to clinic to be very frightened of internal examinations. I was frequently asked 'How long are the doctor's fingers?'   Midwife

In traditional South Asian culture and in Islam, many women keep their bodies completely covered. Some women have never seen another woman partly naked and consider that exposing any part of their body, especially to a man, would be profoundly shocking and humiliating. For some it is unacceptable to expose even their back for an anaesthetist to insert an epidural. Internal examination, especially by a male doctor, is traumatic. Women may feel violated and polluted as a result. They may also feel that what they have done is deeply shameful and may be very concerned that family members and others do not hear of it.

> 'We don't tell our mothers that we see male doctors.'   Pathan woman (from Currer, 1986)

It is important to do everything possible to protect women's modesty and self-respect and their requirements for privacy during physical examinations. This can be achieved by:

- Reducing physical examinations of any kind, and vaginal examinations in particular, to a minimum.
- Reviewing routine practice in order to re-define what is essential (Clements, 1994).
- Offering total midwifery care to women who are particularly concerned about being examined by men.
- If examination by a doctor is essential, respecting a woman's request for a female doctor if at all possible. If this is not possible, many women will accept examination by a male doctor provided the medical reasons are fully explained to them and they are supported throughout by their midwife. Some women may prefer a male doctor who does not share their culture or religion since he may also not share her embarrassment as he is less aware of the cultural or religious prohibitions.
- Obtaining informed consent beforehand; this means ensuring that the woman understands why examination is being suggested, how it will benefit her and what disadvantages there may be.
- Finding out about each woman's concerns about modesty and agreeing with her what can be done to minimise her exposure and embarrassment. For example, it may be important to ensure that only the part of the body to be examined is exposed and that the rest, including the legs, is kept completely covered.

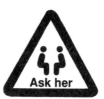

- Discussing with women the most suitable clothes for clinics and for labour. For example abdominal and breast examinations can be performed with minimal exposure if the woman wears a separate top and long skirt. Vaginal examinations can often be done under a skirt or sari as in many cases the examiners rely on what they feel, not on what they see.
- Keeping the number of people present to the minimum, always shutting the door and placing additional screens around the examination couch.
- Only using the lithotomy position when it is absolutely essential, and ensuring that the woman's legs are completely covered.

Discussing intimate matters

People's sense of modesty and self-respect can be damaged not only by physical examinations but also by questions about and discussion of intimate matters. In some cultures pregnancy is a matter of pride and is generally seen as a public event to be discussed and celebrated. Pregnant women may feel happy to talk about intimate physical changes and behaviour with strangers, especially in a clinical context. In other cultures pregnancy is largely a private event, not discussed openly and perhaps not even publicly acknowledged for several months. Attention is not drawn to the physical changes a women is experiencing and it is regarded as immodest to do so, particularly when men are present.

People also have very different views about what is appropriate to discuss with whom. For example in ultra-Orthodox Jewish communities women might discuss intimate matters such as their menstrual cycle and vaginal discharge with their rabbi, since these have a bearing on religious observance. Many people also accept the need to talk to both male and female health professionals about topics that they would never discuss with anybody else. However in some cultures, any discussion of intimate subjects, especially between men and women, even health professionals, is out of the question.

ANTENATAL SCREENING, DIAGNOSTIC TESTING AND TERMINATION FOR FETAL ABNORMALITY

Screening and the detection of fetal abnormality has become a major component of routine antenatal care, despite the fact that the vast majority of women who reach the second trimester have healthy babies (Green and Statham, 1993). As the technical scope of antenatal screening and diagnosis widens, the associated practical issues and dilemmas become increasingly complex, while strategies for managing the social, emotional and ethical implications of screening and diagnosis lag behind.

Underlying the acclaim that greets each new 'breakthrough' in screening for fetal abnormality, are the assumptions that it is good to have as much information as possible about a baby before birth, and that a high uptake of screening programmes is desirable. On a personal level the reality can be less straightforward. Antenatal screening and diagnosis do not offer solutions. Instead they may precipitate women and families into a series of agonizing choices and dilemmas, including, ultimately, a decision about terminating a pregnancy that is often welcome and wanted.

> '*It's mind-boggling. In a generation abortion has gone from something that was illegal, unobtainable and shameful, to being an underlying and acceptable part of antenatal care.*'   Gynaecology nurse

The way a woman reacts to antenatal screening and the decisions she makes will be influenced by her attitude to her pregnancy and her feelings about becoming a mother. She will also be influenced by her own and her community's attitudes towards normality and disability, by economic factors and by religious and moral beliefs.

Many parents want screening and see it as a positive advance which widens their choices. However they may be unclear about what these choices involve. They may not understand the purpose and scope of the tests that are offered, or that the potential end result of many tests is the termination of a pregnancy.

> '*I had no idea during my first two pregnancies what the tests I had might lead to. I assumed that if they found something wrong they could put it right. I was horrified to discover during my third pregnancy, that the only option I would have had was a decision to get rid of the baby.*'   Professional woman

Some parents may feel that it would be irresponsible to refuse the tests they are offered. Others may accept certain tests and refuse others for 'non-medical' reasons.

'Well, they offered me a blood test and a scan to see if the baby was alright, so I had the scan because I can't stand needles.'   Mother of three

Some parents may be confused about the distinction between screening, which assesses **how likely** they are to be carrying a baby with a specific condition, and diagnostic tests, which can tell 'with reasonable certainty' **whether or not** the baby is affected. (Green and Statham, 1993). They may accept testing without realizing the psychological risks and benefits and that their anxiety may in fact be increased rather than diminished (Van den Akker, 1993). They may also assume that if the results of all the tests are negative, their baby will definitely be healthy.

Ultrasound is generally considered a positive psychological experience for pregnant women and many parents welcome a routine scan as an opportunity to see their baby. But because women are often given far less information about the purpose of scans than about serum screening tests they may be unaware that their baby is being screened for anomalies (Smith and Marteau, 1995). If even a minor problem is found, anxieties are raised and their relationship and attitude to their baby during the rest of the pregnancy is likely to be altered (Boyle, 1994).

'My sister-in-law had a scan and they told her they'd found placental lakes and she was to come back in a month for another scan. At that scan they found them again, so they sent her away for another month. She was worried sick. When she went back the third time they told her cheerfully that the lakes had disappeared. She plucked up the courage to ask what it all meant and they told her they didn't really know, but placental lakes were quite common and usually went away. Her pregnancy had been ruined by three months' worry.'   Postnatal support worker

Women who accept screening such as the 'triple test' may not realize that dealing with the results and deciding what action to take is sometimes far from simple.

'There's a lot more anguish about. Every week I listen to women trying to make decisions on the basis of numerical probabilities. Probabilities aren't tremendously helpful when you are trying to decide whether or not to accept diagnostic procedures which carry their own risks and may lead to a decision about whether or not to abort a baby.'   NCT teacher/tutor

Some professionals assume that women make a positive choice to undergo screening and diagnostic testing in order to abort the fetus if it is abnormal, but this is not necessarily so (Van den Akker, 1993). They are far more likely to be seeking reassurance that their baby is all right (Gladman, 1994). For some women, termination, however distressing, may be preferable to giving birth to a child with a disability or life-threatening disease. But for others, termination is unacceptable on personal, moral or religious grounds. Some parents who, before testing, thought they would have a termination if the result was positive, may change their minds when faced with the decision. Others may never consider a termination but may want to know if their baby is abnormal so that they can begin the process of adaptation and acceptance before he or she is born.

Pregnant women now have to search their own souls and make a positive moral decision whether they would want to continue with the pregnancy or have a termination ... And that day that they take the decision will have changed them. (From Nicolaides, 1994, by permission)

Pre-test counselling

Women need reliable, consistent, impartial information about the choices they have to make (Baldwin, 1994). Otherwise they may find that they have, without knowing it, embarked on a course of action from which there is no turning back. But the practicalities of offering comprehensive and effective pre-test counselling are considerable, and there is a tendency to introduce screening programmes with insufficient resources for counselling (Green, 1994). Effective counselling is time-consuming and complex. It also needs to be done earlier and earlier in pregnancy.

'We can sometimes spend up to an hour in the booking visit explaining the various tests, what they might show and what the potential next steps would be. It's not what they expect when they come and it's a lot for people to cope with when they are only just getting used to the idea of having a baby.'   Community midwives

Tests are becoming increasingly complex and difficult to explain (Green, 1994; Vyas, 1994). One book written for parents takes 94 pages to explain the various tests and their implications (Godsen *et al.*, 1994). If highly educated parents find it hard to understand and decide about screening, women with less understanding of medical issues may find it even more difficult to make informed choices. Nevertheless, they are just as likely to want to make their own decisions rather than hand over control to staff (Green *et al.*, 1990).

The content, quality and consistency of counselling varies, as do the knowledge and skills of those expected to fulfil this role. 'There is an urgent need to consider what counselling should consist of and who should undertake it' (Green, 1994). It has been suggested that pre-test discussions should include:

- a description of the test
- what it involves and when it is done
- the condition it could identify
- the chances of it occurring
- when the results will be available
- the meaning of a positive and a negative result
- the options if the result is positive, and how parents can get more information (Smith *et al.*, 1995).

Health professionals need considerable knowledge and skill to help and support parents. They need opportunities to develop their knowledge base, to improve their communication and counselling skills and to increase their confidence. There are therefore important cost implications in terms of time, staffing levels, training and updating (Whittle, 1993).

Accepting parents' decisions

Offering people choices must include accepting and supporting their decisions. Women who do not want certain screening tests also need respect and acceptance, and the normal care given to all pregnant women.

'I decided not to have any antenatal screening even though I know I carry a genetic disorder, because I would not consider a termination. Throughout my pregnancy I had to deal with other people's reactions. Of course it was hard to deal with comments such as 'you ought to be sterilised', but even neutral responses were difficult to cope with since I tended to interpret them as negative. The people who really helped were those that treated me as normal. One midwife asked me if I would breast feed my baby and I thought, at last, someone who thinks that things could go well rather than badly. She got it right. My baby was born strong, healthy and unaffected.' Mother of four

Because the issues surrounding screening are so emotive it is important for health professionals to be aware of their own beliefs and attitudes:

■ How do you feel about antenatal screening and diagnosis of fetal abnormality?
■ How do you feel about termination for fetal abnormality?
■ What do you think you would choose if you yourself were faced with these choices?
■ How do you feel when people make decisions that you would not make? How do you behave towards them?
■ How do you manage uncertainty in yourself? In others?

Religious and cultural issues

The amount of screening offered during a normal pregnancy may particularly surprise or worry women who have strong religious views on interventions and/ or on the termination of pregnancy, or who are unfamiliar with British antenatal care. Some may feel threatened, frightened, confused or assaulted. Some may not have the confidence to ask questions or to challenge routine practice. As always, language barriers increase any difficulties.

● It is important not to assume that quiet acceptance equals consent and to ensure that all women, whatever their background, are informed of the purpose, scope, risks and benefits and limitations of the various tests, and that they understand that they have choices.
● The cultural, religious, spiritual, social and emotional implications of testing should be taken into account. At the same time it is important not to assume, for example, on the basis of a client's religion, what she is going to decide. Women who make decisions contrary to the teaching of their religion may be in particular need of understanding and comfort. Scrupulous confidentiality must be maintained.
● Some women may have concerns in relation to specific procedures. Some may be unwilling to have blood taken during pregnancy in case it weakens them. Muslim women who are fasting during Ramadan may be unwilling to give blood and may refuse glucose tolerance tests. Some Orthodox Jewish women, who are usually certain about the date of their last period, may see no point in having a scan to date their pregnancy. The physical exposure required to carry out a scan may present problems for some women.

- Women who normally make major decisions jointly, or whose husbands or older female relatives normally make such decisions, may want the consent and support of other family members before deciding whether to accept screening or diagnostic tests. Information and counselling about screening and diagnostic testing should therefore be available to husbands or partners and other family members. However, care should always be taken to ensure that the woman gives consent or refuses on her own behalf.
- Appropriate counselling and screening should be offered to people known to be possible carriers of genetic diseases such as the haemoglobinopathies and Tay–Sachs disease (see Chapters 25 and 29). However questions about people's origins and family histories should be broached sensitively and with clear explanations of the reasons for asking.
- In some parts of the world there are enormous cultural, social and economic pressure to have sons, especially if a couple only has daughters (Booth *et al.*, 1994; Imam, 1994). Health professionals may be concerned about telling some parents the sex of their unborn child in case they decide to terminate the pregnancy if the baby is a girl. Termination on these grounds is illegal and is abhorrent to most people. But before making judgements about others, it may be useful to remember that many parents' decision to abort an 'abnormal' fetus in the UK is influenced by the knowledge that our society does not provide adequate resources for the disabled, and that able-bodied people are ignorant and prejudiced about disability. Similar social and economic constraints are at work when women in India choose to abort girl fetuses (Grant, 1993).

ANTENATAL EDUCATION

Although the aims and effectiveness of antenatal education have always been unclear, in most areas antenatal classes are an integral part of maternity services (Nolan, 1994). The style and content of antenatal education has changed over the years and has tended to reflect prevailing social attitudes and medical practice (Combes and Schonveld, 1992).

Recently, antenatal education has moved towards group-centred learning and identifying and meeting parents' needs, based on knowledge of how adults learn and the philosophy of woman-centred care and informed choice (Braun and Schonveld, 1993; Priest and Schott, 1991). Many health professionals are developing group skills and innovative interactive teaching techniques. However, some classes are still mainly 'chalk and talk' with parents as passive recipients. Too often the content is still based on the health professionals' agenda rather than the parents' needs, and some classes cover issues that should be part of routine clinical care.

Antenatal classes may be unattractive to people for a variety of reasons. Women whose experience of education has been negative, those who for a variety of reasons are wary of authority figures, and those who are worried about making a fool of themselves or appearing ignorant are particularly likely to avoid classes. The words 'classes' and 'education' imply formality, while 'groups' may sound trendy or threatening. Parentcraft is a misleading title and is especially unlikely to appeal to people who do not want to be 'taught' or who expect to learn about childcare from their family.

Some women may be anxious about being in a minority because of their social situation, their skin colour, or their religious or cultural background.

'Classes are for hoity-toity people'   African-Caribbean mother of three

In some cultures the idea of turning to outsiders for help and information about pregnancy and childbirth is extraordinary. Women expect to learn all they need to know from older female relatives, informally and as and when they need it. Some women may not understand the function of antenatal classes or may assume that they deal only with the practical care of the baby after the birth. Some may be discouraged from coming by conservative family members.

Organisation and content that ignores the variety of beliefs and lifestyles among expectant mothers is alienating. For example the timing and location of classes may not be suitable. Modesty may be an issue for some women and their families. They may be shocked by the idea of discussing intimate matters in public, sitting on the floor, practising positions and exercises, or seeing anatomical charts or videos of a birth, especially if men are likely to be present. If classes are mixed some women may be totally inhibited and silent.

Some people do not make any preparations for the baby or announce the child's name before the birth for fear of attracting bad luck. Classes that focus on what to prepare and what to buy may be off-putting.

Some women consider it very important for their baby's well-being to think positively during pregnancy and may be distressed by discussions about what can go wrong during pregnancy and birth. People who believe that discussing problems is actively harmful may not want to come to classes when certain topics are covered or if they arise spontaneously, may want to opt out at the particular point. If the content of the course is negotiated with participants at the first class it may be possible to identify reservations such as these and to work out a way of balancing different needs.

The biggest barrier of all is language. Even English speakers have to learn the language of labour and birth, to add words such as 'cervix', 'effaced' and 'dilatation' to their vocabulary, and to get used to talking about topics and body parts not usually mentioned in public. When women speak limited English, classes can be confusing, increase feelings of isolation, and decrease their self-confidence. Unless there is an interpreter, classes are obviously useless to those who speak little or no English.

Consider how to meet the needs of those who do not normally come to classes and take a moment to step into the shoes of the people you want to reach.

■ What might their concerns and needs be? How could you find out more?
■ How could you meet their needs and deal with their concerns?
■ How do you feel about changing your content and approach to meet their needs?
■ What information and support would you need?

Finding ways to meet differing needs

The fact that some women to do not attend classes does not mean that they do not need or want support, information and opportunities to ask questions and to talk about their hopes and fears. In many cases their needs are greater than the needs of those who come to classes. For women, for example, who are not supported by older female relatives, classes may be particularly important.

Identifying and finding ways to meet differing needs requires time, sensitivity and innovative thinking. It may be necessary to scrap some or all of the existing content, or to abandon the idea of classes altogether and to try completely different approaches. What is needed will vary depending on local needs. This might mean:

- Befriending key women in the community and finding out what the issues are.
- Choosing times and venues to suit the participants. For example, it may be more appropriate to hold sessions in local community centres, or to hold them immediately after antenatal appointments so that women only have to make one journey.
- Offering informal drop-in sessions.
- Offering both women-only and couples sessions.
- Offering expectant fathers opportunities to meet without women, if possible with a male health professional.
- Finding out and responding to what participants want to know even if it means abandoning existing course plans.
- Running courses for particular groups.
- Teaching with professional interpreters who can act as a bridge between the cultures and advise on input and approaches.
- Finding a more appealing name for classes.
- Finding out about and accommodating women's concerns about modesty. This means taking care when choosing videos and other visual material, and ensuring that participants have a choice about what they see. It means thinking afresh about topics, activities and the language you use.
- Including mothers and sisters, mothers-in-law and sisters-in-law in classes, especially if they will be present during labour and birth. Older women who had their own babies outside the UK can find current practices strange and worrying. They need to know what to expect in the delivery suite and what choices are available to women.
- Where relevant, including discussion in classes of relevant cultural or religious issues, for example, the way parents may want to welcome babies at birth, circumcision, ways in which parents can maintain cultural and religious preferences in relation to diet, washing, dress and prayer while in hospital.
- Training women who are already taking a lead within their community to run their own pregnancy and postnatal sessions.

Finding different and acceptable ways of offering support and information to people who do not attend traditional antenatal classes is time-consuming. It requires flexibility and commitment not only from staff but also from management. It also requires staying power. Word of mouth is the most effective form of advertising, but it can take months or even years for the message to spread throughout the community and for people to feel sure that what is on offer is relevant, accessible and rewarding.

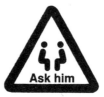 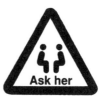

Labour, however straightforward, is not 'usual' to women experiencing
it.

Ralph and Alexander, 1994

Throughout history women all over the world have been giving birth and
successfully handing down skills, traditions and expectations from generation to
generation. Different societies have developed different approaches. Many
Westerners consider their methods superior, but current practice has both
advantages and disadvantages. Just as the West is beginning to re-appreciate the
benefits of supporting rather than managing the process of labour, and of enabling
women to move around and to give birth in whatever position they choose, the
medicalised approach is being adopted in the Third World where women are now
often encouraged to labour and deliver on their backs (Vincent Priya, 1992).

In the UK, most women labour and give birth in hospital. Although policies
and practices vary, most are still heavily influenced by the medical model.
Labour and birth are generally viewed as risky until proven otherwise. Practices
such as regular vaginal examinations throughout labour, amniotomy, continuous
electronic fetal monitoring and exhorting women to hold their breath and push in
second stage persist, despite lack of evidence for their benefits when used
routinely (Enkin *et al.*, 1990; UK Amniotomy Group, 1994).

Most women in the UK have come to expect a certain amount of technology
during labour. Some are reassured by practices such as electronic fetal
monitoring and many welcome pharmacological pain relief. However, others
dislike the clinical environment, the focus on technology and the 'chemistry of
fear and doubt which is often felt in the atmosphere of a modern hospital'
(Vincent Priya, 1992). Having to give birth in hospital may distress women who
strongly dislike being away from the comfort and safety of their home and from
their families at such an important time. Some women also associate hospitals
with serious illness, fear and death.

Many women assume that health professionals know what is best for them and
are happy to comply. Others may feel under pressure to conform and to do as they
are told or to do what they believe is expected of them. For example, if a woman
is shown into a room with a bed, she may assume that she is supposed to lie down
in labour even if she would prefer to be upright and mobile. Some women,
especially those from certain minority groups, may not feel able to say no or even
ask questions in case they cause offence and alienate their carers.

Women's experiences during labour matter, both at the time and much later. There is growing recognition that most women have vivid recall of their labours, remembering what was said and how they were cared for. Many carry lasting memories of pain, anger and exhaustion (Bates, 1993). Ralph and Alexander (1994) suggest that some women suffer from post-traumatic stress disorder following childbirth.

Women who have been well supported and listened to, and who have understood what was happening and why, are likely to feel more positive about their experience afterwards even when their labour was difficult. One study showed that women who felt that staff had given them enough information during labour were more likely to say that they were happy with the way their labour was managed than women who had wanted more information (Fleissig, 1993). Nevertheless hospital delivery suites and birth technology can be terrifying, especially, perhaps, for women who grew up expecting to give birth at home, supported by people they knew and trusted (Ahmed and Watt, 1986). Stresses of which their carers may be unaware, such as being cared for by a succession of strangers, worries about preserving modesty, and inability to communicate their needs and fears may all add to their fear and distress.

A survey carried out in 1990 found that women want a positive welcome when they arrive in the labour suite, and that during labour they want individual and continuous care from their carer, honest information, empathy, support and encouragement (Hutton, 1994). In response to these and other concerns, many health professionals have worked to humanise care during labour. They are giving women more information, choice and greater continuity of carer, and are taking steps to preserve their privacy and autonomy. Many labour suites are more home-like and in many places equipment is kept out of sight unless or until it is needed.

IDENTIFYING WOMEN'S NEEDS

Since attitudes, needs, beliefs and practices concerning labour vary widely, the only way to be sure of providing appropriate care is to find out from each woman what is important to her. This is best done antenatally, when the woman is likely to feel less pressured and stressed than she will at the onset of labour. One way of helping a woman to decide what she would like and ensuring that her wishes are followed as far as possible is through the use of a birth plan.

On occasions labour does not progress as expected. Women may change their minds about what they want or intervention may be needed. Writing a birth plan is therefore rather like planning the route for a journey. Often the journey is uneventful but sometimes there are unexpected hold-ups which make diversions necessary. Birth plans need, therefore, to be viewed flexibly by both women and their carers: women should know that they can change their minds; when intervention is indicated, health professionals should ensure that they are given good information and clear explanations.

Birth plans have received a mixed response from health professionals, but they can be particularly useful for women with special religious or cultural needs. They act as a focus for helping women to formulate their ideas, to identify their preferences and needs, and to discuss how these could best be met. The process of working with a woman on her birth plan increases the professional's understanding of what she and her supporter(s) want and expect during labour and birth, and highlights those issues about which they need more information. A written birth plan also enables everyone involved in a woman's care to identify and respect her particular needs. It can be included in her notes or given to her to bring in when she is in labour.

If a woman brings in a birth plan that appears abrupt, negative or dictatorial it is prudent to reflect on why this might be before reacting. This is especially important if the birth plan was written by someone whose first language is not English.

Cultural and religious factors

In addition to a woman's personal preferences about how her labour and birth will be managed, cultural or religious issues should be addressed. These might influence:

- who and how many people she wants with her
- the degree of involvement the father wants and any needs he may have
- concerns about modesty
- religious observance including prayer and diet
- attitudes to pain, pain relief and intervention
- how the baby is to be received and welcomed to the world
- whether the mother wants the baby placed on her tummy or washed beforehand
- whether the mother has any preferences about disposing of the placenta.

Although people's beliefs and practices in relation to labour and birth vary enormously, certain themes are found in widely differing cultures. The labouring woman's vulnerability and need for protection are often recognised. Women in labour may keep special prayer cards or religious items with them, recite prayers, or wear special amulets, threads or girdles to protect them during labour.

> 'Siobhan wore a red cord around her tummy throughout her labour to protect her and her baby and ensure an easy birth. It was the same cord that her mother had worn 30 years ago in Ireland during Siobhan's birth.'   Community midwife

In many cultures mobility during labour is the norm, and the importance of letting go and opening up in order to give birth are understood. This recognition maybe symbolized, for example, by opening doors and releasing knots, particularly if the labour is slow or difficult.

EXPECTATIONS OF SUPPORT DURING LABOUR

Traditionally, labouring women throughout the world have been cared for and supported by one or more older women who have themselves had babies. These may be family members or women of the local community, often with a tremendous range of skills and experience in the care of women during labour and birth. 'Even in the most patriarchal societies ... pregnancy and birth are the primary arenas in which women have status and prestige' (Vincent Priya, 1992).

Women who are well supported in labour benefit both physically and psychologically. Continuous psychological support during labour appears to reduce the need for analgesia, make caesarean sections less likely, and improve the outcome of labour for both mother and baby (Thornton and Lilford, 1994). Studies have shown that women who have the companionship and undivided attention of a supportive lay woman have shorter labours, require less intervention and have more confidence and self-esteem (Hofmeyr *et al.*, 1991; Sosa *et al.*, 1980).

Nowadays, at least in the West, it is more common for women to labour and give birth with help from health professionals and their husbands or partners, From a historical perspective, the involvement of men in childbirth is relatively recent. Almost within one generation fathers in the West have moved from pacing the floor outside the labour ward or retreating to the nearest pub, to being in the delivery suite actively supporting their partner throughout labour and birth. The pendulum has swung so far that it is now generally assumed that a father will be present, though it has also been suggested that some men feel unduly pressurised and that, for some, being there may not be a good thing (Seel, 1994). However, a recent survey in the UK indicates that many men choose to be with their partners for labour and birth and afterwards are pleased to have been there (RCM, 1994).

Supporting labour supporters

Being a labour supporter is not always easy. Some men may be unprepared for the range of powerful emotions that they experience. They may feel helpless in the face of their partner's pain, inadequate, stressed and on alien ground (Hall, 1993). Because the involvement of men is relatively recent there are few helpful role models for them to learn from. Providing care and support for fathers and other supporters during labour helps them in their key role of supporting the mother (Niven, 1992).

> *'We expect a total role reversal when couples are having their babies. Men, who have been conditioned not to show their feelings, to be the ones in charge, the ones who know, the ones who lead, are expected to take a supportive secondary role, to provide tender, sensitive and responsive care and to intuitively know what the woman needs. Women, who are generally conditioned to be more accepting and to take a secondary role, are expected to make decisions, stand up for their rights and be assertive.'* Antenatal teacher

It is important not to make assumptions about whom and how many people a woman will want to support her in labour, or about who is willing and able to come. Some women prefer female family members to support them if possible. Where there is none available, a mother may be forced to call on her partner, especially if she speaks little English and there is no interpreter. This may not be what either of them would have chosen and may be difficult for both of them to handle. In such a situation the kinds of support the man can give may be limited.

Increasingly younger couples from conservative communities are deciding to be together during labour and birth. Some may stay throughout, others leave during internal examinations and sometimes for the birth. Some may wish to be present but may not, sometimes for religious or cultural reasons, touch the woman during the labour or birth (see Chapter 39). Some women may wish to have both their husband and another woman to support them, especially if the husband will not be present the whole time or cannot help physically. Men who decide to come need to feel welcomed and accepted regardless of their degree of involvement.

Some men may be under pressure from older family members not to attend. Others are concerned and supportive but are reluctant to be there because they are frightened or squeamish or do not know how they can help (Niven, 1992). They may be unsure about entering a traditionally female arena and feel intimidated by hospitals and health professionals.

'I'm glad I had my baby at home, for one thing it meant my partner stayed with me. If I'd been in hospital he would have found any excuse to be somewhere else. He feels very uncomfortable and like a fish out of water in those places.'   African-Caribbean woman

'I find some midwives hostile towards the Asian men. They criticise the men if they don't stay with their wives during labour, and accuse them of wanting to control their wives if they do. Most of the men are concerned and want to help. But we do need a male link worker. We have no one to communicate with them if they don't speak English.' Director of midwifery services

Couples and families who are making the decision about who will be there during the labour need information about the options and about what to expect. Possible supporters need opportunities to think about what the experience might be like, what their role could be and to reflect on how they might feel before a decision is reached. A male health professional may be needed to talk to a man who feels unable to discuss intimate matters with an unrelated woman.

Labour supporters of either sex may observe cultural or religious practices which should be respected and accommodated. Female supporters who had their own babies outside the UK may also find much of what happens in the delivery suite strange and alarming. They too are likely to need support and explanations. Their methods of providing encouragement and support to the labouring woman should be respected and accommodated unless actively harmful.

'Recently I cared for a young Bengali woman who was having her first child and was being supported by her mother. Neither of the women spoke any English. All went well, the baby was born and I was just waiting for the placenta when I looked up and was astonished to see the mother stuffing her daughter's hair into her mouth. Presumably this was to make her gag and bear down to push the placenta out. There is no syntometrine in rural Bangladesh.'   Midwife

■ Where do you think a father should be during labour and why?

If he is present:

■ What do you think his role should be?
■ How do you react to men who do not fit in with your expectations?
■ What kinds of needs and feelings might fathers experience during labour?
■ How do you feel about respecting the different reactions and meeting the variety of needs that fathers have?

ATTITUDES TO PAIN AND PAIN RELIEF

> When compared with the pain associated with a number of illnesses and traumatic conditions, the intensity of pain in labour is severe.
>
> Niven, 1992

A woman's behaviour when she is in pain is likely to be influenced by her personal and cultural values, her individual situation and the context in which she is experiencing the pain (Melzack, 1973). Exactly the same factors are likely to influence health professionals' assessment of the appropriateness or inappropriateness of the woman's behaviour, their responses to her and the care they give her. Caring well for a woman in labour is always demanding. It requires sensitivity, concentration and empathy. Where there are cultural and other barriers the task of assessing what will best meet her needs becomes even more complex.

Within any cultural group individual women manage their pain in different ways. Some worry about 'making a fool of themselves' in labour and afterwards may apologise for 'making a fuss'. Some feel that it is best to express their pain and let their feelings go. Others may see labour as an opportunity to demonstrate their strength and stoicism in a particularly female way. Some women feel that it is important to remain quiet; others find that it helps to make a noise. They may, for example, moan, scream, rock, sway, click their fingers or tap rhythmically, shake their hands, chant, pray or call on God.

> *'I'm quite a self-controlled person but at the end I found myself moaning loudly and rhythmically. I needed to hear that it was still there and hadn't drowned in the pain.'* English woman

Some women may also be influenced by what they perceive as locally acceptable pain behaviour.

> *'I had my fifth baby in Egypt. In Somalia I was brought up to accept pain stoically but in Cairo everyone else was screaming in the labour ward so I did too.'* Somali mother of five

Some women react strongly to labour pain and behave in ways that are completely alien to their normal behaviour. Many are shocked and surprised both by the intensity of the pain and by how they respond. A woman who is noisy in labour may be coping well. Alternatively, she may be communicating her fear and isolation, or her urgent need for pain relief. A woman who cannot communicate her needs or feelings, who cannot benefit from her midwife's verbal support, reassurance and encouragement, or who does not know enough about the available methods of pain relief to ask for one, may have no other way of expressing what she is feeling.

Health professionals

Health professionals' attitudes to pain behaviour are affected not only by their upbringing, culture and personal values but also by the culture in which they work. It can be hard to witness the expression of pain or strong emotion in others, especially if we are not allowed to express our own pain and emotion. Some professionals find it hard to understand why some women, particularly those who make a lot of noise, do not accept pain relief (Wilson, 1994).

'I wish people would realize that some women prefer to shout rather than have pain relief. We want to move freely and don't want to be restricted by monitors, belts and drips.'   Rastafarian mother of four

Many health professionals think of pain control in labour mainly in terms of pharmacological methods (Rajan, 1993). However, women and their helpers have traditionally used a variety of techniques including massage, hot or cold compresses, being active and mobile, and changing position in response to what they are feeling at the time. Emotional support and the undivided attention of another person can be one of the most effective ways of helping women manage their labour.

'I stayed with a woman during her labour, just holding her hand and giving her my complete attention and discovered that I could be even more effective than 100 mg of pethidine.'   Student midwife

If the ability to keep labouring women quiet is considered, officially or unofficially, to be a sign of professional competence, caring for a woman who expresses her pain and refuses pain relief can be both personally and professionally threatening. Some health professionals may also need to deal with their own discomfort at witnessing the expression of pain.

'Some years ago I was taken round a labour ward by the sister in charge. She stopped in the corridor and said "Listen". I could hear nothing and said so. "I know", she said, "aren't epidurals wonderful things?"'   NCT teacher

Some health professionals find it hard to listen to women and accept the reality of what they are describing. One study showed that health professionals were significantly more likely to agree with each other than with the woman they were caring for about the effectiveness of the pain relief she had received during labour! They were also unlikely to agree with women who thought that the pain relief they had been given was poor (Rajan, 1993). It is important to avoid personal and institutional assumptions about different women's reactions to pain and their need for pain relief, and instead to assess each woman individually. It is also important not to criticise labouring women for expressing pain, for being 'weak' or for 'making too much fuss', and at the same time not to press analgesia on women who do not want it.

Certain minority groups, including South Asian women, are often stereotyped as making 'too much' noise in labour, having 'low pain thresholds' and 'attention seeking'. Sometimes this behaviour is explained as 'cultural'. However, in the Indian subcontinent, especially in rural areas, most women have their babies at home within earshot of the rest of the family and of other children, a situation in which they are anxious not to make a noise. Bowler in her observations of the care given to a small group of white and South Asian women on a labour ward, found that although the midwives shared the common stereotypes, they offered the South Asian women less pain control than the white women. She concluded that this might have been because the language barrier prevented them from explaining what was available, or 'maybe the midwives thought that the [South Asian] women did not need (or deserve) pain control because of their known "low pain" thresholds' (Bowler, 1993).

What 'messages' did you get as a child about expressing pain?

■ How do you manage your own pain?
■ What do you find helpful and unhelpful?
■ What choices did you or would you make for yourself about managing pain in labour?
■ How do you feel about witnessing pain?
■ How do you react?
■ How do you feel when someone chooses to manage their pain in ways that you would not choose?
■ How are women who make a noise during labour regarded where you work?

Pain relief: information and individual assessment

None of the major religions proscribes the use of pharmacological pain relief in labour. Nevertheless, for some women in all communities giving birth without pain relief may be important to their self-esteem. Others may be grateful for and happy to use whatever help is available. Some women may be concerned about the effects of certain drugs on the baby and on their own awareness. Women for whom physical modesty is very important may reject the idea of an epidural, particularly if the anaesthetist is male.

Because there is such a wide variation in the way women experience, manage and express pain in labour it is essential to find out from each individual what support and/or pain relief she would like. This involves making sure that each woman comes to labour with information about available methods of pain relief and the advantages, disadvantages and limitations of each. Preparation for labour and information about what is likely to happen as the labour progresses also help reduce anxiety and the need for pharmacological pain relief (Enkin *et al.*, 1990). Anxiety has been shown to increase pain, and high levels of pain both heighten the mother's anxiety and can have adverse effects on the baby (Niven, 1992). It is also important that each woman knows that she has the freedom to do what she wants, to make choices and to change her mind. Women should be actively encouraged to use their own self-help techniques and not to be inhibited by the unfamiliar environment of the hospital.

The intensity of pain and the desire for pain relief can only be gauged by the person who is experiencing them. Because cultural, personal and other factors affect the way a woman expresses her pain, and because of the influence of their own preconceptions, professionals cannot rely simply on their own assessments. Crying and moaning may be a culturally appropriate way of managing pain. So may silence. Neither is a reliable indicator of whether a woman wants or does not want pain relief (Cheung, 1994). If a woman regards her experience as pain it should be accepted as pain (Merskey, 1986). She should be supported and offered whatever pain relief is possible and appropriate.

In situations where it is difficult to assess the level of pain or the effect of the pain relief you have given it may be helpful to ask a woman to describe her pain using a colloquial analogy (Salim, 1993). For example, if the most extreme pain imaginable is a pound, how many pennies' worth is she experiencing at present? Once pain relief has been administered, has the amount gone down and by how much?

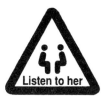

INTERVENTIONS DURING LABOUR AND BIRTH

Intervention is sometimes essential for medical reasons. However, some women view all intervention with suspicion and worry that doctors and midwives may intervene routinely and without good reason. Although this occasionally happens, more often problems arise because interventions have been carried out without sufficient explanation and without sufficient trust between a woman and her carers. In some cases, fathers have been persuaded to put pressure on their partners to accept intervention, especially when the women speak little or no English

If a woman needs or is likely to need intervention it is important to discuss with her (and, where appropriate, with her partner or supporter) the reasons, risks and benefits, and to discuss any questions or worries. Detailed discussions are clearly not possible in emergencies, but a pre-existing respectful and trusting relationship between parents and their carers can make it easier to manage decisions well even then.

Unnecessary intervention may be more likely if women's progress is considered slow in relation to arbitrarily defined 'normal' rates. Some women of African descent, for example, have a more pronounced tilt to the pelvis; this increases the angle of inclination which delays the engagement of the head and is associated with longer labours (Enkin, *et al.*, 1990). Women in this situation may be compromised if they are in a recumbent or semi-recumbent position; activity and mobility can change pelvic angles and internal dimensions quite dramatically (Sutton and Scott, 1994). Slower than 'average' progress during labour should not by itself be an indication for intervention when the mother and baby are in good condition (Enkin, *et al.*, 1990).

Caesarean section   Although some women may welcome a caesarean section in certain situations, others, for personal or cultural reasons, may strongly wish to avoid them. For women whose primary role, sense of purpose and self-esteem comes from giving birth and being a mother, a caesarean section can have serious emotional and social consequences. Some women may feel that they have failed if they have not given birth normally. A few may be criticised by their husbands or communities for 'not being a proper woman'. Some women fear that a caesarean section will jeopardise future births and limit the number of children they can have. This may be a serious concern for women who want large families.

Induction and acceleration   Parents for whom the precise time of a baby's birth is of great importance may be reluctant to accept induction or acceleration as this influences the time and date of birth. Other parents may not object to induction itself but may be concerned that their baby is born on a day or date that is considered to be auspicious.

WELCOMING THE BABY

In the 1970s Frederick Leboyer's work on the way babies are treated at birth prompted people to think about the unique sensitivity of a new-born baby and what it might be like to be precipitated into bright light, hung by the feet, slapped and then separated from the mother (Leboyer, 1975).

Some of the measures that Leboyer advocated are still practised, for example placing the baby on the mother's tummy at birth. However, parents who regard secretions and fluids associated with birth as polluting may want the baby washed first.

Some parents may want to perform a ceremony at or shortly after the birth. Except for Islam (see Chapter 28), the major religions do not have a formal ceremony at this time. Some Christian parents may want to baptise their baby immediately if he or she is severely ill (see Chapter 35).

THE SEX OF THE BABY

Great importance is attached to the sex of a new baby in all cultures. One of the first questions everyone asks is whether a baby is a boy or girl. Having at least one son is important in most cultures and very important in some. It is generally most important in those societies where men and women have very different roles, where men are dominant and women are regarded as inferior, and/or where important practical matters such as the family name and status, and the family wealth and business are handed down through the male line. For some people, preferring a son is a personal issue.

> '*I was very glad I had two sons. I didn't want to bring a girl into the world because girls have such a bad deal. I wouldn't want to be responsible for putting anyone through what I have been through.*'   English woman

In some societies there are major practical and religious implications for couples who do not have a son. In traditional South Asian culture, for example, sons and their wives are responsible for looking after parents when they get older (see also Chapter 34). For some Hindu fathers it may be very important to have a son who can light the funeral pyre when he dies and help ensure religious merit and righteous passage into heaven (Ahmed and Watt, 1986). It is, however, important never to assume that parents of certain communities will place a higher value on boys, or will not welcome a daughter.

Until the biological facts were discovered, women were always considered responsible for the gender of their children. Attitudes are changing as people become better informed. However, occasionally women are still blamed and may blame themselves for not having a son. This can be very distressing to witness, not only because it is unfair, but also because it is hard to see baby girls and their mothers devalued. In a few cases a woman may be devastated at the birth of another daughter, sometimes expressing her distress through physical symptoms (Ahmed and Watt, 1986). Women in these circumstances need sensitive support.

THE PLACENTA

In Western obstetric and midwifery practice, the placenta has generally been regarded either as clinical waste to be disposed of safely, or, until the advent of HIV and AIDS, as a source of income to the unit. In certain other cultures there are strong traditions concerning the handling and disposal of the placenta and cord. Some parents may worry that if the placenta and cord are not dealt with properly the baby could become ill or have bad luck in life. Parents who wish to take the placenta and cord home with them should be allowed to do so.

In some cultures it is traditional to bury the placenta. In farming communities this may be done in the place where the child will grow up and work so that the child knows where he or she belongs. Sometimes a tree is planted over the placenta. In some Jewish communities when a child was about to marry, the tree under which their placenta was buried was cut down to form one of the posts of their wedding canopy. A few people advocate eating the placenta. Some dry and preserve the cord. In some cultures and religions, for example, Islam, the placenta and cord are regarded as polluted (see Chapter 37). They should be removed quickly and disposed of.

It is important to find out from each woman what, if any, significance she attaches to the placenta and if she has any preferences about how it should be disposed of.

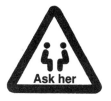

The postnatal period

Most women give birth in hospital and afterwards have to adjust to life in the postnatal ward. Many adapt fairly readily, but women of minority cultures and religions may have special concerns about how their needs can be accommodated and managed in relation to such things as religious observances, washing, diet and clothing.

The importance of the postnatal period

Despite the fact that the postnatal period is recognised as a time of immense physical and psychological adjustment, current Western practice places far more emphasis on caring for mothers antenatally. The 'lying-in period' has become a thing of the past and women are expected to be up and taking care of their babies from the beginning. Increasingly women are sent home, where most have little or no support or help, within a few hours or days of the birth.

Many women prefer to care for their babies right from the start. However in order to care for and cherish their babies, women need to be cared for and cherished themselves. In most parts of the world, rest and care during the postnatal period are considered essential for a mother's health and well-being. Women who have recently given birth are believed to be especially vulnerable and in need of protection, warmth and seclusion, and nourishing foods to help them regain their energy and strength. They have a duty to rest and recuperate. In many communities it is traditional for the other women of the family to take charge of the household and of older children, and to care for the baby. In parts of the Indian subcontinent an expectant mother may go home to her parents' house for the birth and remain there for several weeks afterwards as a treasured guest. Little is required of her but to recover from the birth.

There are now known to be sound medical reasons for encouraging women to be mobile as soon as possible after the birth. However, women who have been brought up with deeply held beliefs about the importance of several weeks of rest after giving birth are often shocked when hospital staff expect them to be up and about immediately, taking complete responsibility for their baby. They are also likely to be worried and upset by the lack of sleep common in postnatal wards. Many women in such a situation feel neglected and frightened, especially if they believe that their long-term health may be affected, and even more so if they have had difficult deliveries or a caesarean section. The reasons for postnatal mobility should be discussed antenatally to avoid unnecessary distress and resentment on both sides (Bowler, 1993). Women who wish to rest and who require help with the care of their baby during their time in hospital should be supported as far as possible.

The common tradition of seclusion for mother and new baby for about six weeks may also mean that women are reluctant or may be unable to attend postnatal check-ups or other appointments during this time. In some cases, older women of the family feel strongly that women should remain at home until the period of rest and seclusion is over. In addition, for those women who are unaccustomed to transporting babies anywhere, let alone on public transport and in urban areas, simply getting to clinics may be difficult.

Cultural traditions

Cultural traditions after giving birth vary. Some women may consider it very important to dress warmly and avoid draughts, chills and cold drinks. Some may also refuse baths or showers, preferring to sponge themselves down. Diet is often important and women may avoid certain foods. In many cultures new mothers are given particularly nourishing food; families may want to bring in special traditional dishes.

> 'My friends used to sneak in real food after I had my baby.'   Nigerian woman

For women of all cultures it may be very important at this vulnerable time to do things the right way, the way they were taught as young girls. This may be especially true if they are away from home and missing their families. Women who cannot look after themselves and their baby as they know they should, may worry about the long-term effects. A Ghanaian woman having her first baby in Switzerland wrote:

> After we got married and during my pregnancy I began to get a bit worried that we couldn't afford to bring my mother here to take care of me after my giving birth just as it is done at home. I also worried that both the baby and I would not get the herbal baths for strength and energy. How could I get my pepper soup with dried smoked meat and dried okra to heal the wounds of the womb? And what of the millet flour water to produce milk for the baby? I was in constant fear that I could get ill if I didn't get all the matnaa attention. Matnaa means after [the] birth. (From Bieri, 1993, by permission)

Many of the problems that women experience in hospital postnatally can be reduced or eliminated if carers take steps to understand their needs, expectations and perceptions. It is important to ask each woman, both antenatally and after the birth, about her likely needs, and to take steps to accommodate them as far as possible. In some cases this may mean re-assessing the clinical necessity for routine practices. Sensitive discussion of possible problems beforehand may also help. For example, if women know that they will be expected to care for their own babies in the postnatal ward, they have time to adjust, to discuss their concerns with midwives, and perhaps to reach an acceptable compromise.

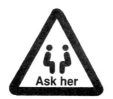

Modesty

For some women, modesty and the need for privacy may be particularly important issues in an environment where strangers, including men, come and go. Some may wish to draw their curtains during visiting times so that they are not seen in bed by other male visitors, especially of their own community (Currer, 1986).

Washing, especially of the vulval area, is generally considered personal and private. Women should be asked if they want help or if they would prefer privacy so that they can wash themselves after the birth.

Some women may be distressed and humiliated by perineal examinations or requests to see soiled sanitary pads. Some women consider that lochia is dirty and polluting. Others may worry if their flow is light because the discharge of lochia is considered cleansing after the birth.

Visitors

Birth is a family event and in many cultures it is customary for members of the extended family and friends to visit the new mother and baby. Not to do so may be considered an insult and some women will have many visitors who may come in groups. In some communities, however, it is not customary for women to visit a new mother in hospital as this would involve contact with unrelated men. Female relatives and friends may wait till a woman has gone home before they visit.

Where large numbers of people wish to visit it may be necessary to restrict the numbers at the bedside at any one time in order to minimise stress for other women in the ward. However it is important to be sensitive to the obligation many people are under to visit and to try to find ways of accommodating their needs.

Going home

Women who consider rest essential for their health may be upset if they are sent home soon after the birth, especially if there is no one there to look after them, or if they have other small children to care for. The timing of discharge may also be important. Some women very much want to be home for festivals. Some Orthodox Jewish women, for example, may want to be home for Shabbat (see Chapter 39). They may also be unable to travel during Shabbat and other festivals. Concerns about rest and care, and about the timing of discharge, can be identified and addressed if plans are discussed with the women in advance.

Symptoms after childbirth

The current Western focus on antenatal and intra-partum care has resulted in much less research, awareness or discussion of problems in the postnatal period (Trevelyan, 1994). However postnatal symptoms are common. One survey of women's experiences showed that 85 per cent of women experienced at least one health problem in hospital, 87 per cent had at least one health problem in the first eight weeks at home, and 76 per cent continued to experience at least one problem thereafter (Glazener et al., 1993). However, in most cases postnatal symptoms are not recognised or reported (Bick and MacArthur, 1994).

All women, regardless of their religion and culture, are likely to experience similar physical and emotional reactions after giving birth, though the way these are acknowledged, expressed and managed may vary. Women who have been brought up to get on and cope are likely to do just that even if there is something wrong, so it is important to ask each woman specific questions about how she is feeling both physically and emotionally. General questions are unlikely to elicit symptoms or feelings that are precise enough to be discussed and dealt with (Bick and MacArthur, 1994). It is necessary to ask specific questions and to take time to listen and respond to the replies.

Women who regard the postnatal period as a time of vulnerability may be more vocal about their needs and problems. It is important not to assume that women who do not complain are necessarily symptom-free, nor that those who do complain are making an unnecessary fuss. One UK study of long-term health problems following childbirth found that South Asian women were more likely than white women to experience backache, frequent headache, aching shoulders and pains and weakness in their limbs. The researchers suggested that lack of vitamin D might be a contributory factor (MacArthur et al., 1993).

Postnatal depression

The debate over the exact definition of postnatal depression continues. However, as far as women and their families are concerned, the priority is recognising when something is wrong and trying to make it better (Niven, 1992).

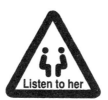

During the postnatal period mothers are adjusting to enormous physiological, psychological and social changes, especially with their first babies. At the same time they are experiencing fluctuating emotions and many have the so-called postnatal blues. Some mothers experience longer-term symptoms such as tearfulness, sleep disturbance, exhaustion, anxiety and irritability which may or may not be identified as postnatal depression.

Language barriers make it particularly difficult for women to communicate psychological distress. However, assumptions about women of minority groups can also create powerful barriers and can interfere with health professionals' ability to recognise symptoms of postnatal depression. The Commission for Racial Equality cites the following 'myths' about South Asians and other minority ethnic communities which make it less likely that depression will be picked up and treated:

> The idea that they 'look after their own' through the extended family structure . . . and therefore do not need help from public services.
>
> The belief that people from non-Western cultures do not experience depression as a psychological condition, and that their religion and community values gives them different understanding of themselves as individuals.

The view that women from 'non-Western cultures' do not fully understand their feelings and that they only talk about physical symptoms. (From CRE, 1993, by permission)

Some women's anxiety and depression after giving birth is exacerbated by additional stresses such as isolation, anxiety about not having the traditional period of rest and seclusion, and fear of racist abuse or attacks. A woman who is living far from the rest of her family may experience renewed grief over separation from loved ones at a time when she would traditionally receive their support, encouragement and advice, and when everyone would be celebrating the arrival of a new family member.

Women who are bereaved during pregnancy tend to delay their grieving (Lewis, 1979). Asylum seekers and refugees are likely to have been bereaved or to have witnessed or been the victims of violence. During pregnancy they may find it impossible to continue the enormous and lengthy psychological task of coming to terms with their experiences and may be distressed by a resurgence of their grief after the baby is born.

THE 'GOOD MOTHER'

Most people have theories about what makes a good mother (Paradice, 1993). The definition of a 'good mother' varies from culture to culture and through history. Health professionals' expectations of women postnatally are based largely on current Western assumptions of 'normality' in relation to the mothering of a new-born baby. Women who are happy to take total care of their babies in hospital, and who therefore meet professionals' expectations, are considered to be behaving normally. Those who are not happy to do so may be seen as difficult or lacking normal maternal instincts (Bowler, 1993; Woollett and Dosanjh-Matwala, 1990).

Current Western views of normality include the importance of bonding; a concept which prompted hospitals to change the routine separation of mothers and babies after birth. Although the change was and is welcomed by many parents, there is no evidence that there is a crucial period for bonding in the early days after birth or that the amount of contact a mother has with her baby at this time affects their long-term relationship. 'It therefore seems sensible to conclude that close, intimate physical contact immediately after birth and in the first few postnatal days is not essential for adequate bonding' (Niven, 1992).

A woman who does not willingly take on full care of her baby is not necessarily uninterested, a poor mother, or rejecting the baby. She may be behaving perfectly normally and in her view prudently. She may also assume that in the absence of her family, the staff will care for her and her baby. Where there are no female relatives to support and advise a woman, the role of midwives as 'surrogate sisters' may become particularly important (Currer, 1986).

A woman who does not look at her baby directly or who pays him or her little attention may also be protecting her baby from bad luck and danger (see Chapter 16). Some people may become distressed if other people admire their babies in case this too increases the risk of harm to the baby.

'I visited an Indian family and said, "What a lovely baby!" Immediately the grandmother rushed out and brought back some black stuff and marked the baby's face with it.'   Health visitor

Alternatively, there may be more practical reasons:

'The midwives are often critical of women who do not pick up their babies in the first few hours after the birth. When we ask the woman why, it is often because the baby has not yet been bathed properly. For us, washing the baby is very important because it removes the pollution of birth. So we bath her baby and everyone is happy.'   Bangladeshi health aide

'I visited a woman who had had her fourth baby two days earlier. The midwives were critical because she did not change the baby's nappy and assumed she was rejecting her. In fact, she didn't know how to use disposable nappies. She hadn't used them at home. Nobody had asked her if she needed help and she did not feel able to ask.'   Interpreter

It is easy to assume that differences are abnormal. Before judging, consider whether there may be good religious, cultural or practical reasons for what people do.

Caring for the baby

New-born babies are universally regarded as vulnerable and in need of care and protection from physical harm and, in some cases, from less tangible influences. However, there are wide variations in how the need for care is translated into practice. For example:

- In some cultures it is considered natural and right for mothers to take their babies into bed with them. In others this is considered dangerous because of the risk of overlaying. Where the marital relationship is considered primary, a new baby in the bed may be seen as an intruder and as setting a dangerous precedent.
- Some women wrap their babies well and stay indoors, taking great care to avoid draughts. Others regularly undress their babies to oil and massage them. Others feel that fresh air, even if cold, is good for babies.

'I was told firmly to wrap my baby up well and put her in a pram at the bottom of the garden all day. I was only to bring her in every four hours for a feed. The fresh air would be good for her lungs and the four-hourly feeds would teach her discipline. When I think about how my daughter looked after her babies it makes me laugh.'   English grandmother

- Some people shave the baby's hair to remove the pollution of birth. Others observe a religious prohibition against cutting hair.
- Some people say special prayers to protect the baby and help ensure a happy life. They may also give the baby religious symbols such as medals, prayer cards, special threads or amulets.

GIVING ADVICE

The confidence of new parents is often very fragile. It is therefore especially important to respect the different ways that parents react to and care for themselves and their babies.

Advice to do things differently should only be given when it is essential or when parents specifically ask for it. Before offering advice or intervening consider if it is essential for the baby's safety and health or whether your way is just a different way. It may also be salutary to reflect on how much Western expectations and assumptions have changed over the past few decades, and how, even within Western Europe, health professionals often hold very strong and opposed views on what is best.

> *'When Mark was born in England 22 years ago I* **had** *to stay in hospital for ten days even though everything went normally. And my husband wasn't allowed to touch the baby till we got home. I was told in no uncertain terms that all this was medically essential.'*   Mother of two

> *'In Britain I was encouraged to have lots of baths after giving birth to help me relax and heal. In Germany I was strictly forbidden to bath for six weeks after the birth in case I got a perineal infection. I had to plant my husband on the front doorstep in case the midwife called while I was in the bath.'*   Mother of three

In some cases putting pressure on parents to do things differently can cause them serious conflict and anxiety, and can lead to a breakdown in trust between clients and health professionals.

> *Susan had her third baby in Switzerland and was told by the doctor and the midwife to feed him fennel tea with sugar in the first few days. This is regarded as essential to avoid hypoglycaemia in the new-born. In the UK she had been strongly advised not to feed her babies anything but breast milk as this could prevent her producing enough milk and affect their willingness to suckle. When Susan refused to give the fennel tea she was told firmly that she was being irresponsible and risking her baby's life. If he became seriously ill it would be all her fault. Susan became confused and very anxious. She believed that what she had been told at home was right but feared that if anything went wrong she would be blamed. She lost faith in Swiss midwives and doctors and worried about the baby's health. She also became extremely careful about what she told health professionals from then on in case she was disapproved of or got into trouble.*

Conflicting advice from different health professionals can also confuse and worry clients. Women who are trying to adapt to new ways of doing things in an unfamiliar environment may be particularly anxious. There may also be conflicts between the advice given by health professionals and that which a woman is receiving from other sources. In families with a strict hierarchy of authority, older women are likely to give a new mother advice and will expect it to be followed. Even if this advice conflicts with that of health professionals, most women will follow it, especially if they live with the older women. Where there are real problems it may be important to offer to talk to everyone involved and not just to the new mother herself.

INFANT FEEDING

> At no stage should the mother be given the impression that bottle-feeding is equivalent to breast feeding or without risk. (RCM, 1991)

Despite the mounting and convincing evidence of the benefits to babies of breast feeding, the number of women in the UK who breast feed for any length of time is disappointingly low. The decision on how to feed a new baby is highly personal. In addition to their own feelings and convictions, women are likely to be affected by practical and commercial pressures. However, social influences appear to have the greatest impact. A UK study found that women who were themselves breast fed and whose friends breast fed their babies, were more likely to breast feed successfully (OPCS, 1992).

The role of health professionals

Most people decide well before the birth whether they will breast or bottle feed and those who have made firm decisions are unlikely to change their minds (Oxby, 1994). Nevertheless, health professionals have a key role to play in raising awareness of the advantages and disadvantages of each method so that all women can make their decisions in the light of research-based information.

Some health professionals are reluctant to 'promote' breast feeding in case they induce guilt in women who decide to bottle feed. Such reluctance appears, however, to be selectively applied. There seems to be less concern about inducing guilt when encouraging women to give up or reduce smoking, discussing the importance of antenatal clinics and classes, or promoting immunisation. It may be useful for health professionals concerned about discussing breast feeding to be clear about the difference between promoting one method over another, and providing the information and evidence to enable women to make their own informed choices. The decision a woman finally takes must of course be respected, and her need for on-going practical help, information and encouragement must be met.

- How do you **feel** about breast feeding?
- Were you and/or your siblings breast fed?
- Before becoming a health professional did you see women breast feeding?
- If you have children, did you breast feed them?
- If so, was it a generally positive or negative experience?
- How might your own views and experiences influence the way you help inform and support women?

Infant feeding and minority groups

Breast feeding is the norm in most Third World countries. In many parts of the world most people cannot afford artificial milks. Advertising and pressure by baby milk manufacturers stress the benefits to the baby of artificial milks (Ahmet, 1990; Price, 1989). Being able to bottle feed is therefore often seen as progressive and as better for the baby. There are no religious constraints on breast feeding. Islam encourages mothers to breast feed.

One study of Bangladeshi women in the UK found an increased tendency to bottle feed: 'the greater exposure to Britain and midwifery services here, the less chance there was that the mother would exclusively breast feed' (Ahmet, 1990). This finding speaks volumes about the subtle but powerful influences that exist within Western society in relation to infant feeding. However, some of the women in the study quoted above were shocked when asked how they planned to feed their babies, seeing this as 'the equivalent of asking if she planned to keep her baby clean'.

Women who are having problems breast feeding need intensive emotional and practical support until the crisis is over. Lack of consistent advice and information, support and encouragement are likely to contribute to low rates of breast feeding. Some women may also not know where to turn for help, and may not see health professionals as a source of information or support (Ashwood, 1994). Stereotypes about the attitudes and language skills of minority ethnic women may also mean that midwives and other professionals do not always provide them with the full range of information and support on important issues (Ahmet, 1990; Bowler, 1993). For women who speak little English, discussion in their own language backed up by written material that deals with their particular concerns is essential.

Cultural and other factors

Some women may be influenced or feel constrained by a range of cultural and personal factors in relation to breast feeding. These need to be acknowledged and respected when feeding is discussed. For example:

- The demands of other children, especially in large families, may make breast feeding impractical. Bottle feeding, with which older children and other people can help, may seem easier.
- In many parts of the world it is traditionally believed that colostrum is dirty or unhealthy. Alternatively, some people may believe that it is not proper milk and therefore of no value to the baby. Women who worry about the effects of colostrum may refuse to breast feed their babies until their milk comes in and may be upset by pressure to do so. Although colostrum is now known to be important it is not essential. The experience of women in the Indian subcontinent and elsewhere clearly shows that delaying the first feed for several days need not prevent successful breast feeding later. Many women who delay breast feeding until their milk comes in then go on to breast feed for many months. If a woman does not want to breast feed her baby straight away it is important not to assume she wants to bottle feed, or to imply that she will be unable to establish breast feeding. When discussing feeding antenatally it may be helpful to discuss the issue of colostrum and to outline its known benefits. Women who have had the benefits of colostrum explained but do not wish to feed their babies immediately should be given any help they need with bottle feeding until their milk comes in. Some women may wish to combine breast and bottle feeding. Providing this is going well there is no reason to intervene.
- Some women may worry that they will pass pain or infection on to their baby through their milk.
- Some women, for personal, cultural or religious reasons may need complete privacy when breast feeding. Postnatal wards are busy places with many people, both male and female, constantly coming and going. Bed curtains offer little guaranteed privacy and some women find this totally inhibiting. Drawing the curtains may also be seen as a hostile act and some women may be reluctant to do it (Currer, 1986). Whenever possible, nursing chairs should be provided in the nursery and women who wish to breastfeed in private should be encouraged to use them. Achieving privacy at home may also be difficult,

especially for women in inadequate accommodation. Bottle feeding may be a more practical and less stressful solution.

- Some women have never looked at or handled their own breasts and may never have allowed anyone else to see or touch them. They may be acutely embarrassed by the idea of having help, for example, with positioning the baby on the breast.
- Women who have to return to work immediately may find breast feeding impossible.
- Women who eat a halal, kosher or vegetarian diet may need advice to enable them to choose baby milks and foods which do not contain animal products.

NAMING THE BABY

In Western culture, most parents choose their baby's name and are happy to announce it straightaway. In some cultures the baby's name may be chosen by the grandparents or other relatives. In some the choice may be influenced by the baby's horoscope. Some parents prefer to delay announcing their baby's name, until the formal naming ceremony. If the relative choosing the name lives abroad, it may take several weeks to hear from them, and the baby may be given a temporary nickname. Occasionally a name does not arrive until after the legal registration date, in which case the family has to register the child under a temporary name. The family may need help and advice later on changing the name legally.

When there is a delay, or when the parents' naming system is different from the Western naming system, it is essential to check with the parents before recording the baby's name in health records, and before notifying the Registrar. Recording the baby's name incorrectly can give deep offence. It can also cause long-term confusion in health records, which can have serious clinical consequences, and can cause difficulties for the parents when they register the birth (see also Chapter 14).

> 'My name is Roshanara Begum. Because we were waiting for my mother-in-law to choose his name, the staff labelled my baby son Baby Begum. My husband and I were upset and we felt very awkward. That name is still on his medical records. When we went to register the birth, the man was unpleasant. He did not want to accept that Begum could not be our little boy's last name.'   Bengali mother

WELCOMING CEREMONIES

The birth of a child is a rite of passage for parents, bringing new purpose and responsibilities. In many cultures there are rituals to welcome the baby into the social or religious community and to enable parents to make a public commitment to the spiritual and physical well-being of their child. This is often the time when the baby's name is formally announced. The timing and content of such ceremonies vary in different cultures and religions. Increasing numbers of people do not have a specific religious affiliation or may not feel able to approach any religious authority. They may organise a non-religious ceremony to mark the birth of their child and to make a formal and public commitment.

Although ceremonies and family gatherings are joyful occasions they are also nearly always stressful. Often there is a great deal of organising, co-ordinating and cooking which falls mainly on the new mother and can be physically and emotionally draining.

CONTRACEPTION

Contraception is a delicate and highly sensitive topic which can touch on people's deepest feelings about their sexuality and self-esteem, their relationships, and their perceptions of themselves and of their families. Contraceptive choices may also be affected by moral, cultural and spiritual values (Prasad, 1994).

People's decisions about the number of children they would like are likely to be based on many factors (Mares *et al.*, 1985), including:

- family and social traditions and pressures
- how they (men and women) see their roles and the purpose of their lives
- income and other economic factors
- the benefits and costs of children, and the degree of material prosperity that people feel that they and their children require
- the space and time available for children as opposed to other priorities
- religious and moral beliefs
- the extent to which parenthood is valued and supported in the community or society
- the extent to which children are valued in the community or society
- who makes the decision
- the availability of suitable and acceptable contraceptive methods and ease of access to them.

In the West, children are expensive and are the focus of strong consumer pressure. They can often be more of a worry and a drain than a pleasure, especially to parents on low incomes with restricted options and poor housing and other facilities. With an increase in working mothers, the problems of organising and paying for childcare have also become a major disincentive to having a large family.

In most Third World countries children are an important economic asset. They can help on the farm, in the home or wherever help is needed. In the absence of a welfare state, they are the only source of income and support when the parents become too old to work or look after themselves (Mares *et al.*, 1985). One study of a failed population control programme in India concluded that 'to practise contraception would have been wilfully to court economic disaster' (Mamdani, 1972). Parents who have grown up in societies that regard children as a blessing and an asset are likely to wish to have a large family in Britain. In cultures where motherhood is women's main or only role, and their chief source of satisfaction, pleasure and self-esteem, women are more likely to want several children. Nevertheless, there is also evidence that attitudes to family size in the UK are changing amongst those groups which traditionally have large families (Daud, 1992).

Contraception can also be a political issue and a means of social control. In China couples are permitted to have only one child and this policy is generally rigorously enforced. In the 1970s under Mrs Gandhi there were forcible sterilisation programmes in India. Experience both in the Caribbean and in Britain has led some African-Caribbean women to regard family planning advice and provision with suspicion. Many people see it as no coincidence that the first ever use of black people in advertising in the West Indies (in the late 1960s) was to promote contraception. At that time the Rastafarians were one of the most politically aware groups and led the resistance to the campaign. In the 1960s a popular slogan in Jamaica was 'Family planning – a plot to kill off the black race' (Mares *et al.*, 1985). In Britain family planning leaflets were the first to be translated into minority languages. Some women may also be concerned about being pressurised to use certain methods such as long-term injectable contraception and suspect that they are not being given the information they need about all the options.

In the UK, many people hold the view that parents who have more than three or four children, unless they are wealthy, are irresponsible and feckless and a drain on the state. There is strong prejudice against larger families, especially if they are black. Some people of minority groups experience negative reactions, open criticism and hostility for having or wanting large families.

'Because I'm Asian too the other midwives get at me. When an Asian women comes in to have her fifth or sixth baby they are so rude to her, especially if she doesn't speak English. They say terrible things right to her face, like, 'I'd do something to your husband if I could' or 'This one should be sterilised' and often she just smiles politely because she doesn't understand. And then they come and tell me to tell her that she mustn't have any more babies. They say, "She's one of yours, tell her it's revolting to have so many children. Somebody should do something to her husband".' South Asian midwife (From Mares *et al.*, 1985, by permission)

In some cases it is assumed that women of minority groups are not interested in contraception and little or no information is given (Bowler, 1993).

Religious and cultural factors

While it is helpful to be aware of factors that might influence choices, it is important not to an make any assumptions about what individual women will decide. Only they can decide what will fit in with their social situation and their cultural and religious values.

Religion   Most religious doctrines support procreation (Daud, 1992). Some see procreation as the only function of sexual activity and prohibit the use of contraceptives entirely. Members of some religions only accept contraception if there are medical or social reasons for avoiding pregnancy. But religious teachings and personal practice are not necessarily the same. Within religious groups that do not sanction contraception there are different degrees of observance and many people make their own decisions. The Catholic church, for example, forbids the use of all artificial means of contraception. However, many Catholics in the UK use contraception and regard this as a question of personal conscience.

Menstruation   Religious and cultural beliefs and traditions in relation to menstruation, and therefore to any vaginal blood loss, may affect the contraceptive choices people make (see below). Throughout the world there are common themes in relation to menstruation, some of which may affect contraceptive and other decisions. In many cultures and in some religions, sexual intercourse during menstruation is regarded as disgusting and is forbidden. For Orthodox Jews intercourse is prohibited during menstruation and for seven days after bleeding stops. In some cultures menstruation is seen as a cleansing process. Women may take a special bath at the end of each period, and some also shave their pubic hair. Some women may be anxious that they are not properly cleansed if their menstrual flow is light. Some women are considered and may feel impure during a period and do not pray formally or enter a holy place. Traditionally some women do not cook or serve food to others whilst they are menstruating, though this is rarely practical in the UK.

Different methods   People who decide to use contraception on a long- or short-term basis may find certain methods more acceptable than others. For example:

- **Female barrier methods** may be unsuitable for women who find the idea of touching their genitals unacceptable. Women who use their left hand to wash with and keep their right hand clean will find it impossible to insert a **cap** using only one hand. **Contraceptive sponges or spermicides** may be unacceptable for similar reasons. Some women may also lack the necessary privacy and washing facilities to use the cap (Urwin, 1994).
- **The coil** may be unacceptable to some people because it is an abortifacient. Side effects such as spotting and irregular bleeding can cause problems for women who observe religious and social restrictions while they have any blood loss. Some women dislike the idea of having a foreign body inside them.
- **Post-coital contraception** may be unacceptable to some people because it acts after conception.
- **The condom** may be unacceptable on religious grounds to some people because it contravenes the biblical prohibition against 'spilling seed'.
- **The pill** may be unacceptable to people who do not wish to take drugs. Breakthrough bleeding may also cause problems for some women. It is important to discuss the necessity of taking the pill regularly, especially with women who are likely to fast.
- **Intra-muscular preparations** may be unacceptable to some women because they can cause spotting and side effects which must be tolerated until they wear off. Some women may be distressed if they experience amenorrhoea, especially if they see menstruation as a way of purifying their system. Some women may regard intra-muscular preparations with suspicion (see above).
- **Sterilization** (male or female) may be unacceptable on religious grounds because it is permanent, or because people see fertility and potency as important aspects of their sexuality and self-esteem.

It is important to check, where appropriate, that a woman's husband or partner also has the information he needs. Where men take responsibility for contraception they may prefer to use a condom or withdrawal. Some men may be unwilling to discuss intimate matters with a female health professional and it may be necessary to find a male health professional.

Offering family planning advice and services

It is essential to make sure that each woman and/or couple are as happy as possible with the method chosen or at least see it as the best option. All clients need full information about what is available and the advantages and disadvantages. All information and advice must, as always, be **seen to be** respectful and sensitive and must take into account the needs of the individual. A woman who decides not to use contraception must also be treated with complete respect.

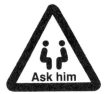 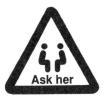

The **timing** of contraceptive information and advice for women who have just had a baby is important. Many women find the routine discussion of contraception shortly after birth and before discharge from hospital offensive (Hutton, undated). Some feel that the implication of such discussions is that they should not have any more babies, or that they should not have had one at all. Some feel that it is being implied that they should resume intercourse soon, when this may be the last thing they feel like. Although some women have intercourse soon after birth, many wait for several weeks or even months. Women whose religion or culture bars sexual relations for several weeks or months after the birth may see the postnatal discussion of contraception as inappropriate or disrespectful.

This presents a dilemma to health professionals. It is important that advice about contraception is available to all couples before they resume sexual intercourse. It is also important not to offend people, or possibly to discourage them from using family planning services, by raising the subject inappropriately.

One solution is to include discussion of contraception in routine antenatal care, for example at the 36-week check-up, when the birth is becoming a reality and when parents need to begin to think about the practicalities of life afterwards. Raising the subject when there is less urgency about reaching a decision is likely to make it easier for health professionals to find out tactfully whether a woman is interested in using contraceptives and, if she is, to identify her needs and concerns.

Needs and preferences vary with regard to the **location** of family planning services. Women who have family commitments, who are reluctant to travel outside their own familiar area, or who fear racist attacks may prefer local clinics. For others, particularly those in tightly knit communities, confidentiality and privacy may be of paramount importance. They may prefer centralized clinics where they are less likely to meet people they know or to be seen entering the clinic. Some women may be unwilling to seek advice from their GP, especially if he is male and is part of the same community. For some women, the preference for seeing a female doctor may outweigh the disadvantages of a language barrier.

Pregnancy and birth are generally assumed to be joyful and happy. However, the outcome is not always positive. Childbearing losses, including infertility, prematurity, or the birth of a disabled baby, can have profound and lasting effects on women, their partners and their families. The ultimate loss is death, either of the baby through a miscarriage, stillbirth or neonatal death, or, very occasionally, of the mother. Culture, religion and traditional customs can become very important around the time of illness, death and bereavement, even for people for whom they are unimportant at other times (BHAN, 1991).

Reactions to loss

Culture and religion are likely to influence people's perceptions of loss and their reactions to it. Some people with a religious faith find strength and comfort and may discover that their religion supports them through their loss; others may gain little help or comfort and may feel that their beliefs seem irrelevant, or they may lose their faith. Some may feel that it is their duty to accept whatever God sends. Some may be expected by others to do so and to behave in a restrained manner. Some may feel that the loss is a punishment for previous wrong-doing.

Different religious and cultural traditions also affect the amount of support parents receive when their baby dies, as do the attitudes of other community members and of religious leaders. Theological and religious teaching often ignore the importance of the life that has been lost. In many religions there is little or no formal religious recognition. There may be no ceremony, for example, when a baby miscarries or is stillborn. For some parents this adds to their distress and isolation.

'Outwardly I was calm and accepting. But I was screaming and furious inside.'
Bereaved mother

Although it is helpful for health professionals to understand the framework of different religious and cultural beliefs so as to be able to provide more sensitive support, it is important never to assume how parents will react or what they will want.

In communities where it is important to have the funeral as soon as possible, some parents may feel deprived of opportunities to hold and spend time with their baby and may feel that their decisions about the funeral and other matters are rushed. They may also feel cut off from the support of health professionals.

> *'My baby was in the neonatal unit for three weeks before he died. The staff were great and really looked after us. But he was buried the day after he died and suddenly I lost all that support. I had no reason to go back to the hospital and I felt desperately alone and deprived.'*   Orthodox Jewish mother

In such cases it is important to find ways of offering continuing care and help to bereaved parents.

Expressing feelings

The way people express or do not express grief varies enormously. In the UK it is generally acceptable for women to display grief as long as it is reasonably restrained. One study showed that women in the UK felt they had to limit their grieving so that they did not increase the distress of those close to them (Rajan, 1994). The expression of emotion is generally less acceptable in English men, who are often conditioned to be strong and to suppress their feelings in order to support their wives or partners and families. As a result men's own needs for support are less likely to be recognised or met. Bereaved parents may misinterpret each other's reactions and may feel misunderstood and out of step with each other.

In some cultures the external expression of grief is considered normal. Bereaved people may be expected to grieve loudly; in some communities it is traditional to hire professional mourners to wail at funerals. Health professionals who have been brought up and trained to control their feelings may find it hard to witness the free expression of grief. In contrast, some religions forbid the loud expression of grief although quiet weeping is acceptable. Official mourning is suspended by Orthodox Jews during the Sabbath and on festivals, and some people may also suspend expression of their personal grief during this period. In some cases both loud and overt grieving, and the suppression of grief have been taken to indicate unhealthy reactions and a need for psychiatric help.

> *'I was phoned at 10 pm one night and asked to come into the Neonatal Unit where I was a volunteer parent supporter. A baby had just died and his mother was yelling and screaming and throwing herself around on the floor. I was surprised they had called a volunteer, but the staff were distraught so I went in. The woman was OK. She was reasonably and understandably devastated and was expressing herself in the way that was normal for her. After a bit she came and sat down and talked and talked about her baby and how she felt. All she needed was to be accepted and listened to. I sometimes think she eventually came to terms with her loss more easily than many of the women I saw who felt unable to express their feelings freely and 'behaved well'.*
>
> *'Another woman I supported was from the Philippines. She had had two previous premature babies and then a third who was very handicapped. She was very demure and quiet while she was in the Unit, but when she got home she threw all the plates at the wall. The staff were horrified when they heard about it but she felt a bit better.'*   Volunteer parent supporter in a neonatal unit

Although it can be difficult, it is important to try to distinguish between changes of behaviour that are the result of accepted religious or cultural patterns, normal individual variations in the timing and pace of grieving, and abnormal reactions that might indicate the need for intervention.

Supporting minority group parents

Each couple needs to be able to grieve in their own way, and to have the privacy and space to be themselves. They also need support, and health professionals are increasingly involved in listening to and comforting distressed and grieving parents. This is generally much appreciated, especially when carers show their own sorrow about the loss (Rajan, 1994). However, many health professionals feel less confident about offering this kind of support to people from other religious or cultural groups. As a result, minority parents may feel deeply hurt and isolated.

> *'When things go wrong for us don't keep your distance. We need your support as much as anyone else. Put your arms around us too'.*   African-Caribbean woman

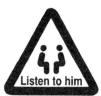 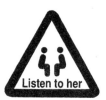

INFERTILITY

Infertility may not generally be regarded as a bereavement. However, couples with fertility problems experience a series of disappointments and losses. For many men and women, the realisation that they have fertility problems is in itself a shock. It can be a blow to their self-esteem and may profoundly affect the way they view themselves and their sexuality.

Couples trying to conceive may experience a loss of spontaneity in their love-making. Those who seek medical help have to discuss and answer questions about a very intimate and private area of their lives. They have to cope with the stresses and humiliations of investigations and treatment.

People who are in the end unable to have children can feel that they have lost their hopes, dreams and purpose in life. Their disappointment may sometimes overshadow their whole lives. They may also have to deal with the disappointment of potential grandparents and other family members as well as other people's insensitivity, since in most communities parenthood is considered the norm.

Cultural attitudes to infertility

The ability to have children is generally regarded by both men and women as an intrinsic part of being an adult. In some cultures proving one's fertility is traditionally more important than marriage. In a family-centred culture, the failure to produce children can be a social as well as a personal tragedy for both women and men. Failure to father or bear a child can have serious social and emotional consequences. In cultures where motherhood is the primary and perhaps the only accepted role for women, infertility can be particularly hard to bear and may lead to rejection and social isolation.

Historically, infertility has been regarded as the woman's fault. Although people are nowadays more aware that the physical problem can lie with either the man or the woman, attitudes are slow to change especially in cultures where men are generally in authority, or where men's self-esteem and masculinity are fundamentally linked with their ability to father children.

'Some women will take great care to protect their partners from any implication that there might be something wrong with them. They will come to the clinic secretly and alone and some are prepared to have invasive investigations without our having had an opportunity to check their partner's sperm sample first.'   Registrar in obstetrics and gynaecology

In some cases women who come for infertility investigations and treatment may have good reasons to be particularly concerned about confidentiality and privacy.

'I didn't even want my partner to know I was seeking help. If he thought for a moment that I might be infertile, he'd walk out.'   African-Caribbean woman

When the causes of infertility are poorly understood, people may fear that it is catching, that it is caused by the evil eye, or that it is a punishment for past misdeeds. In some communities a married woman with no children may be barred from family and religious celebrations. In some communities infertility is acceptable grounds for a husband divorcing his wife.

Religious and ethical issues

Religious beliefs and personal philosophy may influence people's attitude to infertility and the decisions they make about investigation and treatment. However, the desire for children may lead deeply religious people to make decisions contrary to religious teachings. It is therefore essential not to assume what individuals will or will not find acceptable, but to listen to and respect each person's needs and concerns.

Some people may find any treatment unacceptable, perhaps believing that they must accept God's will. Others may find particular methods of investigation or treatment unacceptable on moral or religious grounds. For example, some men may not be willing to produce sperm samples because of religious prohibitions against masturbation. Treatment that involves donor eggs or sperm, or that might lead to the selective reduction of implanted embryos, may also be unacceptable to some people on religious or ethical grounds.

Barriers to care

Some people with fertility problems do not seek help, either because they feel too embarrassed and ashamed, or because they do not know how to get access to services, what to expect or what investigations and treatments are available. Some may be reluctant because of worries about confidentiality. Some may fear the physical examinations and other processes involved. It is extremely important to respect people's modesty and to avoid in any way further diminishing their self-esteem. It may also be more appropriate for discussions about investigations and treatments to be conducted by men for men, and by women for women. Interpreters should always be of the same sex as the client. (For more about developing flexible, culturally sensitive services see also the sections on Antenatal Care in Chapter 19.

The highly charged nature of infertility means that when people come for a consultation it is especially important to set aside personal feelings and reactions, to take into account the cultural and social pressures and the emotional turmoil that they may be enduring, and to understand and accept the range of possible sensitivities and concerns that they may have.

TERMINATION OF PREGNANCY

Of all childbearing losses, termination is potentially the most emotionally complicated and can, therefore, be the most difficult for professionals to handle well. Furthermore, it is a loss not always recognised or understood. Most professionals inevitably have personal feelings about termination which are likely to influence the care they give.

Deciding to terminate a pregnancy at any stage can be harrowing. People's reasons for having a termination may be complicated and may give rise to feelings whose depth and complexity even they cannot fully comprehend. There may be particular distress if the termination is of a wanted pregnancy carried out because of fetal abnormality or social pressures. Parents have to come to terms with the loss of a baby for whom they have usually begun to make emotional space. They may also need to grieve for lost hopes and dreams. They may feel failure and guilt. Parents whose baby was abnormal may lose faith in themselves and their bodies. They may also find themselves grieving for the normal baby they wanted but did not have (see also the section on Antenatal Screening in Chapter 19).

Parents who have decided to terminate a pregnancy, for whatever reason, often receive little understanding and emotional support from others. It is often assumed that termination is easier to cope with than other childbearing losses because the parents 'chose' it. For some people this is true, and the termination brings relief from intolerable pressures. For others, the fact that they 'chose' it merely adds to their distress. They may find it particularly hard to get understanding and support if their decision was contrary to the teachings of their religion. In some communities people who are 'unable' to produce a healthy child may be stigmatized. Some parents may decide not to tell family and friends that they decided to terminate the pregnancy, or that their child had a disability. For some it may be vital that nobody knows they were pregnant. Confidentiality is of paramount importance.

Preparation for termination   Whatever the reason for the termination, or the stage of pregnancy at which it takes place, parents should always be fully informed about what will happen. They need to know how the termination will be carried out, what is likely to happen during and after the termination, and what support and help will be available to them. Some people may wish to see and hold their baby after the birth. At a later gestation, women for whom this is important may therefore prefer to have their labour induced rather than to have a dilatation and evacuation. Induction may also be the best choice if it is important to carry out a post mortem (SANDS, 1995).

All these issues should be discussed with parents beforehand. They should be asked, sensitively, if there is anything they feel strongly about and what they would like (see also Managing Death in Maternity Care below). Some parents may wish to bury the baby or to carry out a religious ceremony. For many it is important to know that their baby's body, or the products of conception, will be handled and disposed of respectfully.

THE SICK OR PRE-TERM INFANT

Parents whose baby is ill or born prematurely are also likely to experience a range of losses. Pregnancy may have been unexpectedly short and labour difficult and often terrifying. The anticipated joy of the baby's arrival is marred by fear. The mother is separated from her baby and usually goes home long before her baby is ready to leave hospital.

Being the parent of a baby in a neonatal unit is often extremely stressful. Parents have to adapt to a bewildering, noisy and highly technical environment. They are likely to experience a roller coaster of emotions in response to the unpredictable and rapid changes that can occur in premature and sick babies.

'I used to stand outside the ward door, plucking up courage to go in and dreading what I might see and hear.'   Mother of premature twins

Parents can often feel confused, isolated and exhausted by long-term anxiety, by travelling to visit their baby, and by the mixture of tedium and stress involved in sitting in the unit. When babies are transferred to other hospitals or to regional centres, parents may face long and often expensive journeys which some can ill afford. Some parents are torn between caring for older children at home and visiting their new infant. All these stresses are increased where there are cultural and language barriers.

Parents who spend time in the unit may also have particular religious or cultural needs. For example, those who observe special diets will probably need to bring in, store and heat their own food (see also Chapter 18). Some people may need privacy for prayer, possibly at certain set times every day. Modesty may be an important factor for women who are trying to establish breast feeding. Orthodox Jewish parents may observe prohibitions against travel or using the telephone or other electrical equipment on the Sabbath and other festivals (see Chapter 39). Some parents or other family members may want their baby to wear religious items such as amulets or threads to protect them. Others may want prayer cards, prayer books, rosaries or other religious items to be kept in or near the baby's incubator.

Some parents welcome the support and prayers of the chaplain or their own religious leader. Some Christian parents may want their baby baptised. Parents of other faiths may also want a religious ceremony to welcome and protect their baby. In communities where religious leaders do not have a pastoral role, family members may wish to recite prayers and carry out religious rituals themselves, possibly with members of the extended family and community present. Wherever possible, space and privacy should be made available for this and people should be welcomed.

Disability

In many cultures, disabled or sick children are traditionally cared for by their families, particularly by the women of the family. However the practical problems of caring for a disabled child in urban Britain without the support of the extended family may be far greater than many parents can manage. Those who are unfamiliar with statutory provision and who speak little or no English may need special help in gaining access to services and also to suitable informal support networks.

Many people in all cultures feel a sense of shame and failure if they have a disabled child. These feelings may be more severe if people know little about heredity or the causes of disability, or feel that they are to blame. Parents of disabled children may also be very isolated. In some communities the presence of a disabled child may make it difficult to arrange good marriages for other members of the extended family, though attitudes are changing with greater understanding and more external support. Counselling and support should always be offered and, where appropriate, parents should be referred to specialist genetic counsellors.

MANAGING DEATH IN MATERNITY CARE

Cultural and religious traditions

In the West, rituals and traditions surrounding death and mourning have tended to lapse. Death is almost a taboo subject. Many English people, for example, are embarrassed and discomforted in the presence of people who have lost a spouse, a child or someone close to them. Many are afraid to see a dead body, even of someone they loved very much. Once the funeral is over even close relatives of the person who has died are often expected to carry on as before, although it can take many months or years for people to work through the normal grieving process and to reach the stage when they can begin to take an interest in life again (Ainsworth-Smith and Speck, 1982; Worden, 1991). The loss of a baby is generally still seen as less severe than that of a child or an adult relative. Parents whose baby has died during pregnancy or at birth often receive even less public acknowledgement and support.

In many cultures there are formal ceremonies and traditions which provide some structure for managing the practicalities of an adult death, though childbearing losses are often handled differently. The importance of grieving may be more widely understood and in some traditions there are specific ways of acknowledging and meeting the needs of the bereaved. The length of the necessary grieving period is also recognised. In some religions there is a formal ceremony to mark the first anniversary of the death and an annual remembrance ceremony thereafter.

> *'My mother and aunts wore black for a year when any close relative died. I hardly remember my mother ever out of black. But it meant that everyone knew and I think people were more supportive.'* Austrian woman

When a death occurs in maternity care it is always a shock. Much of what follows refers to the death of a baby during pregnancy or around the time of birth. Cultural and religious requirements in the case of an adult death are sometimes different.

When a baby dies

It is now well recognised that the death of a baby during the second half of pregnancy and around the time of birth is deeply traumatic, and that earlier loss is often equally so. Any childbearing loss, at any stage can have severe long-term effects for parents. These are likely to be worse if the care parents receive at the time of the loss is inappropriate and insensitive to their needs. Although practice has improved dramatically in most places over the past few years, health professionals may still feel less confident about how to respond flexibly and sensitively to the needs and wishes of individual parents of minority groups.

Care around the time of death

Some relatives may need privacy and time for prayer around the time of death. Some may want a religious leader to be present. Others may wish to say prayers and perform any religious rituals themselves. Some Christians may want their baby baptised (see Chapter 35).

In some cultures it is customary for the whole extended family to gather at the bedside, sometimes to pray together. This may be particularly important if the death is that of a baby, since it is the only chance for most family members to see and remember him or her. Whenever possible, arrangements should be made to accommodate all family members and to respect their privacy. Since many parents whose baby dies have never experienced a death before, they may be frightened and unsure and need support. Their need for privacy should be balanced by regular and sensitive offers of support and reassurance (SANDS, 1995).

After a death, stillbirth or miscarriage: finding out what parents want

The needs and wishes of parents following the death of a baby are likely to vary tremendously. What is now accepted as standard good practice in the UK may not suit everyone, whatever their background. It is also important not to assume that parents of a particular religious or cultural community will or will not want certain things. The views and feelings of each individual must be ascertained, respected and met. Where there are decisions to be made, parents must be given unhurried explanations of what is involved so that they can decide what is right for them in their own time.

Childbearing losses are rarely talked about until they happen. Few expectant parents know or have thought much about the traditions, beliefs and practices of their own religion or culture in dealing with miscarriage, stillbirth or neonatal death. Most parents are completely unprepared for the physical and emotional impact of their loss. They are unlikely to know immediately what arrangements they want to make, or to be aware of the choices they can make and their implications. Some may want to consult their families, and community members or religious leaders before making any decisions.

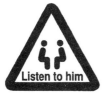 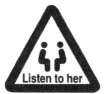

Stress and grief affect people's fluency in a second language. Parents whose first language is not English may need an interpreter even if they normally speak it well (see also Chapter 11).

Creating memories

Grieving is a normal and necessary process which is harder when there are few or no memories of the person that has been lost (Lewis, 1976). Helping parents and families to create memories is now recognised as an important step towards enabling them to begin this long and difficult process. However, this is a new idea to many parents. Parents of different cultural or religious groups may also find different things helpful or acceptable. In some cases religious rulings or traditions may affect their decisions.

Health professionals caring for bereaved parents need to give careful and gentle explanations of what parents can choose and the possible benefits later on. If parents refuse what is offered, tactful and sensitive questioning may be needed to establish the reasons. If there are specific cultural or religious prohibitions, further encouragement is clearly inappropriate. It is always important to ask and listen.

- Some parents may prefer not to see or hold their baby after death. For a few it may be important to avoid seeing or touching a dead body. Some parents may want their baby to be washed before they hold him or her because the fluids associated with the process of birth are traditionally regarded as polluted.
- For some parents it may be very important to give the baby a name, however early the loss. Others may not wish to name a baby who died before birth.
- Many parents are grateful for photographs of their baby. Some may refuse or be unsure because the idea is new and strange to them. However, a few parents may strongly object to the idea of photographs, possibly on religious grounds. Since many parents who refuse photographs later regret their decision, health professionals need to try to find out sensitively the reasons for parents' reluctance before deciding whether to discuss the matter further. This requires tact and time.
- Similarly, many parents are grateful for mementoes of their baby such as hand and foot prints, or a lock of hair. Again it is important, especially if parents are initially reluctant, to take time to discuss the options with them and to explain the possible benefits of having concrete things to remember the baby by. Nevertheless, a few parents may find some or all physical mementoes unacceptable on personal, cultural and religious grounds. In some communities, for example, birth hair is traditionally regarded as polluted and is usually shaved and discarded after the birth. Cutting a lock of the baby's hair may also be unacceptable to people who observe a prohibition against cutting hair.

Preparing the body

When an adult or an infant dies the parents or relatives should always be asked if they have any wishes about how they want the body to be prepared. Some may want to wash and dress the body themselves, or to be present while this is done by hospital staff. In some communities it is traditional for certain members of the community to wash and prepare the body and this should be accommodated.

If the body is to be washed by the family or other community members, find out what, if anything, the relatives want hospital staff to do first. It is usually acceptable to remove intravenous lines and other equipment, to straighten limbs and to wrap the body in a plain sheet or blanket. Some people, for example, Orthodox Jews and some Hindus and Muslims, may want staff to wear gloves before touching the body.

If the relatives want hospital staff to wash and prepare the body, find out how they would like this to be done. Ask how they would like the body dressed. It is important to ensure that any clothing such as shrouds is non-denominational and to ask before placing flowers on or near the body. Also check with the relatives before removing any jewellery or religious items such as threads, bracelets, rings, amulets or crucifixes.

Find out how the relatives would like the body positioned. Non-Christians for instance may be distressed if the arms are crossed. The head of a Muslim should be turned to the right so that he or she can be buried facing Mecca. Traditionally the body of a Jew is placed on the floor wrapped in a shroud and is never left alone.

Seeing the body

Personal views and beliefs, cultural and religious traditions all influence people's attitudes to the body of someone who has died. For some people seeing the body is unimportant. For others it may be actively discouraged or even forbidden. For many people, however, seeing, touching or holding the body is very important. Some families will wish to take the body home, possibly so that people can come and pay their respects before the funeral. Others may not want to take the body home but large numbers of family members may wish to see the body in order to pray and pay their last respects. In some cultures this is a binding duty; if the body is in the hospital it is very important to understand and respect people's obligation to come, and to accommodate large numbers of people when the need arises.

The chapel of rest

Some people may make a brief visit to the chapel of rest, others may want to stay and mourn and may want to touch and hold the body. Great distress may be caused when, as in some hospitals, relatives are separated from the body by a glass screen or wall. The justification for this separation is unclear and probably has more to do with the cultural attitudes to death of the planners and managers concerned than with any rational or objective reasons. Where such barriers exist, steps should be taken to have them removed as soon as possible. In the meantime relatives should be forewarned and, if they wish, arrangements should be made for them to spend time with the body elsewhere. When a baby has died parents should have complete access and as much time as they wish with their baby.

Before non-Christians visit the chapel of rest, it is important to check that all Christian religious symbols, such as a crucifix have been removed, and, when appropriate, replaced by symbols of the family's own religion. Community leaders of the different local religious groups could be asked about appropriate symbols for the chapel of rest and about where they should be placed. Care should also be taken about positioning the body. For example the body of a Muslim should be placed with the face towards Mecca. Religious symbols should always be placed near the head, not near the feet.

Burials and cremations

For many people the choice between burial or cremation is a personal one. For some the decision may be influenced by religious rulings. When hospital staff are asked to organise the funeral or disposal of the body of a baby who has died or miscarried **at any gestation** it is important to find out if the parents have any religious or other objections to the hospital's normal arrangements (SANDS, 1995). For example, Jewish law requires all bodies or remains, of whatever gestation, to be buried. Islam also requires burial rather than cremation. In the Hindu and Sikh traditions adults are cremated but babies and children are buried. For many parents it is simply important to know that their baby's body, at whatever stage of gestation, will be handled and treated respectfully.

Funerals and ceremonies

Cultural and religious traditions, requirements and prohibitions are likely to have a major influence on parents' decisions about funerals and other ceremonies. Both parents with strong religious beliefs and those with none may find it important and helpful to organise and attend a funeral or other ceremony to mark their baby's life and death. However this may not be right or possible for everyone. It is important to avoid assuming that all parents will want, be able to have or benefit from the same kinds of arrangements.

In some communities, women traditionally do not attend funerals. In others they may attend the funeral but do not go to the graveside. Some women do not enter a place of worship or pray formally when they are bleeding after a birth. In some religions only a simple ceremony is carried out for a baby who is stillborn or died shortly after birth.

Because current thinking in the UK stresses the importance of funerals and other events in helping parents and other family members to accept and deal with the reality of their loss, it can be hard for health professionals to accept that other people may view things differently.

'A Nigerian woman gave birth to full-term twins, one of whom died suddenly and unexpectedly just before they were due to go home. The mother was deeply shocked and so the father was asked about funeral arrangements. He was quite definite that there should be no funeral ceremony and that the baby's body should just be got rid of as it would have been back home.

'The staff found this extremely disturbing and distressing but eventually concluded that they had to respect the father's wishes and could not impose their own cultural expectations on this family.'   Psychotherapist attached to a neonatal unit

It can sometimes be even harder for parents who feel caught between two cultures with very different beliefs:

'When I was back home on holiday I went into premature labour and lost my twins. They were taken away and buried and when I asked where they were, they would not tell me because they said it would be unlucky and they wanted to protect me. Having

lived and worked in the UK I had different ideas and expectations and found this extremely distressing. It made me very angry.' British midwife originally from Nigeria

Post mortems

Many people find the idea of a post mortem distasteful. To some people post mortems are also unacceptable on religious grounds. According to Jewish law the body must be complete and whole when it is buried; a post mortem is considered a desecration of the body. Many Muslims also refuse post mortems on religious grounds. For members of those religions that require burial as soon as possible, a post mortem may mean an unacceptable delay.

In the UK, consent for a post mortem has to be obtained under the Human Tissue Act (1961) for all stillborn babies (i.e., those babies born dead after 24 weeks' gestation) as well as for all babies born alive. Although permission to perform a post mortem on a pre-viable baby born dead is not officially required, the parent's consent should always be sought as a matter of good practice.

If parents do not want a post mortem but the coroner requires one, they are likely to be extremely distressed and to need sensitive support. Where possible, a partial post mortem should be performed, all organs should be replaced, and the body carefully stitched and restored.

Some parents give consent to a complete or partial post mortem in the hope that an explanation can be found for their baby's death, even though they may find the idea of a post mortem very distressing. Parents should always know in advance if such an explanation is likely to be forthcoming, and if they will be able to see their baby's body after the post mortem. They should be forewarned about the position of stitches and the baby should be dressed so that stitch-lines are covered as far as possible.

Certificates and registration

Many people need guidance and help with the legal requirements concerning the registration of deaths. Parents faced with the distressing task of simultaneously registering their baby's birth and death may need extra practical help and emotional support, especially if they are unfamiliar with British bureaucratic systems or speak little or no English. In some cases hospital staff may need to accompany parents to the Register Office.

Some religions require funerals to be held as soon as possible, usually within 24 hours. Parents and relatives may need help both from hospital staff and from staff at the Register Office to get paperwork completed as soon as possible. In some areas the Register Office makes special provision to issue certificates out of normal office hours.

Parents of babies born dead before the legal age of viability are often distressed by the lack of official recognition that their baby existed. In some hospitals, special certificates are offered to parents giving their names, the baby's date and time of birth and death, the baby's name if one was given, and the name of a member of staff involved in their care. This formal acknowledgement can be extremely important to parents, validating the fact of their baby's existence, confirming their status as parents, and acknowledging their loss. It is extremely important to take care to get the baby's and the parents' names right on the certificate, especially if the family's naming system is unfamiliar.

Remembrance books, cards and services

Many hospitals keep a remembrance book, send out sympathy cards to parents and invite parents to memorial services. These should all be non-denominational so that nobody feels excluded. In areas where there are different cultural and religious communities it may be more appropriate to hold services in a local community hall or centre rather than in a church or chapel.

STAFF SUPPORT

Childbearing losses of any kind are distressing and hard to bear. Health professionals and other staff also need good support systems so that they can acknowledge and deal with their own feelings. This is especially necessary when they are looking after people who may express themselves in ways that professionals find unfamiliar or disturbing, and who may make choices and decisions that health professionals may find hard to accept (see also Chapter 15).

USEFUL ADDRESSES

SANDS – Stillbirth and Neonatal Death Society
28 Portland Place
London W1N 4DE

SATFA – Support for Termination for Fetal Abnormality
29–30 Soho Square
London W1V 6JB

The Miscarriage Association
c/o Clayton Hospital
Northgate
Wakefield
West Yorkshire WF1 3JS

23 Implications for purchasers, service managers and educators

In order for maternity services to be truly accessible to everyone, the needs of cultural and religious minorities must run as a continuous thread through all health planning, policy making, management and practice. This is the only way to ensure that the Charter Standards for maternity care are met for all women, regardless of their culture, religion or ethnic group. Minority needs should not be seen as 'different' or 'separate', or only considered in relation to certain issues or services. Practitioners need the active support and encouragement of well-informed purchasers, managers and educators so that they can deliver sensitive, flexible, high-quality care.

A commitment to equality

The basic foundation for tackling discrimination, improving care and redressing inequalities is a policy that commits the organisation to providing **equal access to services** for all who need them. The policy should outline the requirements of the Race Relations Act 1976 and its implications for health care provision (CRE, 1994) (see also Chapters 4, 5 and 6). It should include the needs of people of cultural, ethnic and religious minorities, of people who have a disability, and of people who experience social deprivation and homelessness.

The organisation's commitment to equality should also be reflected in a policy on **equal opportunities in employment** and in the active implementation of such a policy in all areas. The policy must include strategies for identifying and dealing with harassment, discrimination and victimisation within the workplace (CRE, 1991; RCN, undated) (see also Chapters 4, 5 and 6). It is inconsistent to expect staff to be committed to equal access to care if they do not see the principles of equality working within their own organisation.

Identifying local needs and issues

Purchasers and providers must identify all the different cultural, linguistic and religious groups in their locality in order to consult on and plan to meet their needs. This includes groups that are small, isolated or less obvious (Li, 1992). Members of small and isolated minority groups often face greater barriers to services than members of larger minority communities precisely because their needs are not recognised.

Ethnic monitoring is an important first step towards identifying different groups within the local population, but it will not give the whole picture. The categories are crude, and individuals have a choice about whether and how they identify themselves. People belonging to the same 'racial group', such as Indian or Black-Caribbean, may be culturally very different (Senior and Bhopal, 1994). They are also likely to have differing religious needs. People who do not use the health service will not be identified at all.

To get a full picture of the diversity within the local community and of the groups to be involved in consultation about services, it is therefore necessary to compare ethnic monitoring data with local census data. It is also important to consult community midwives, health visitors and others whose work might bring them into contact with people who are not using the service, such as asylum seekers, refugees and homeless people.

Consultation

The people for whom maternity services exist must be central to the whole process of identifying needs and working out ways of meeting them. If the different minority groups are not consulted, services will remain biased towards white, middle-class norms. Failure to consult minority service users should provoke as many objections as if a group of men were to devise and implement policies and practices specifically for the care of women (Alladin, 1992).

Consultation should take place from the beginning. It is unacceptable, insulting and pointless to call in people of minority groups simply to 'rubber stamp' the final documents. They must have continuous opportunities to influence the whole process. A clear distinction should also be made between consultation and information-giving. Meetings which are publicised as part of a positive consultation process, but which are really forums for managers to announce firm decisions cause lasting anger, resentment and suspicion and may lead to breakdowns in communication. It is also important not to begin a process of consultation without a firm and genuine commitment to making as many of the changes that are needed as possible.

> *'People keep asking us what we want from the health service and we keep telling them. But nothing ever changes.'*   African-Caribbean women's group

Effective consultation in maternity services involves building links with women of different communities and inviting them to participate in planning, evaluating and monitoring the quality of services. Care should be taken to consult a broad section of each community. Religious leaders are a starting point for identifying religious teachings and practices, but do not necessarily provide an insight into how people actually live their lives (see also Chapter 16). Ethnic minority health professionals often have a good understanding of the range of possible needs and of the problems people face in getting care. Community workers who are in close contact with people of minority groups, and other professionals, may also have useful information and insights into varying needs. However, it is also important to seek the views of people who may be less assimilated and more traditional. Interpreters may be needed so that those who face the greatest obstacles in communicating can participate in the consultation process (SHARE, 1992).

The consultation process should be carefully organised. Arrangements should to be made to accommodate people who are not used to voicing their views in public, or who feel uncomfortable talking publicly about sensitive and delicate issues. Meetings in small groups are likely to be more effective, especially if service users outnumber policy-makers, and if the same group meets several times so that trust and mutual respect can develop. Policy-makers must listen actively and with empathy, and must be genuinely and visibly flexible and responsive.

Reviewing existing services

Maternity satisfaction surveys usually yield positive responses. However, apparently high levels of satisfaction often conceal important problems. Research indicates that when asked if they were satisfied most people said 'yes'. This may be because:

- they had a healthy baby
- on the whole they were helped and many are incredibly grateful
- they don't speak the language well
- they know the staff are under pressure
- they prefer to forget about their experiences
- most people have little basis for comparison and do not know how things should be.

People may also be reluctant to criticise or complain because:

- they are dependent on the health service and on health professionals
- they fear the possibility of cuts, closures and privatisation
- they feel vulnerable and fear reprisal and racism
- they do not understand their rights.

To find out about people's real views and experiences it is necessary to ask very concrete questions. A general question such as 'Are you happy with the choices your GP gave you?' almost always elicits a 'yes'. A specific question such as 'Did your GP tell you that you could have a home birth or a Domino?' is much more likely to elicit an accurate reply and also provides more useful pointers as to what needs remedying.

Questions must also address those issues that are important to users. These can be identified through the consumer representatives on Maternity Service Liaison Committees and through the complaints procedure, as well as through the consultation process outlined above. Issues raised by health professionals should also be included; they are often aware of service problems and shortcomings because of their direct contact with clients. Involving professionals from an early stage is also an important way of gaining their commitment to changes and improvements.

SETTING AND MONITORING QUALITY STANDARDS

A range of issues should be considered when purchasing maternity services. With a few exceptions (such as counselling and screening programmes for the haemoglobinopathies or Tay–Sachs disease), separate or special services are not needed. Instead, all services should be broad-based and flexible, so that varying needs can be easily accommodated as they arise.

The quality standards below cover some of the key issues in providing services that will enable women and families of all communities to benefit equally from them. Achieving some of the standards will require additional resources in terms of time, training, support and facilities. Some may not immediately be achievable, but all should be regarded as important goals. The process of working out how to achieve and monitor the implementation of each standard will help purchasers and providers assess the resources that will be required and decide on a time scale.

Several of the quality standards listed below can be audited as part of regular quality-monitoring visits. Others can be monitored by checking levels of service use. However, some of the factors that are most important in ensuring that services are acceptable and accessible are the hardest to measure. This should not be a reason for ignoring them.

- The unit will have a policy on equal access to services, and steps will be taken to ensure that all staff, including clerks and receptionists, understand the policy and its implications for their work. The rest of the standards outlined below could be incorporated in this equal access policy (see Chapter 6).
- There will be a policy on equal opportunities in employment, and steps will be taken to ensure that it is implemented at every level (see Chapter 4).
- Procedures for tackling discrimination, harassment and abuse will be in place and will be well publicised (see Chapter 4).
- Antenatal appointments will be made at times and locations to suit clients and will be responsive to cultural and religious needs (see Chapter 19)..
- Procedures will be implemented to ensure that clients' names are accurately recorded and used, and can be retrieved correctly. Computer systems and all charts, forms, and labels will accommodate differing naming systems (see Chapter 14).
- Screening and counselling programmes will be flexible, will respect different religious beliefs, and will take into account the genetic conditions that are relevant to local minority groups (see Chapters 19, 25 and 29).
- Antenatal education sessions will be held at times and places to suit clients and will be culturally sensitive and responsive to minority needs (see Chapter 19).
- Care plans and birth plans will be used as vehicles for discussing and recording specific cultural and religious needs (see Chapter 20).
- Privacy will be provided in all clinical areas (see Chapter 19).
- Women for whom modesty is a particular issue will have access to women doctors (see Chapter 19).
- Men for whom modesty is a particular issue will have access to male staff when intimate matters are discussed (see Chapter 19).
- Written information will accommodate differing religious and cultural issues and will be available in languages appropriate to local community

needs, as a back-up to verbal information (see Chapter 13). This will include:
- letters and appointment cards
- hospital and clinic direction signs
- health education material
- information leaflets on what to bring into hospital, on screening and on diagnostic tests
  - a standard letter explaining the significance of client-held notes and offering the services of an interpreter if the client would like help in understanding her notes.
- Posters and visual aids will be culturally inclusive (see Chapter 19).
- A range of foods will be offered so that all clients can choose foods to suit their religious or cultural needs (see Chapter 18). Menus will include details of ingredients.
- Relatives will be free to bring in food from home. Adequate storage and heating facilities (within appropriate health and safety guidelines) for such food will be provided (see Chapter 18).
- Privacy and space for families to pray or spend time together or to perform religious ceremonies will be provided (see Chapter 16).
- Both showers and baths will be provided in all wards (see Chapter 18).
- Women will be able to have more than one person to support them during investigations such as ultrasound, and during labour (see Chapters 19 and 20).
- Discharge procedures will be planned jointly with women and will take account of religious constraints and festivals (see Chapter 21).
- Professional interpreters who speak the main local languages will be available for clinics and routine appointments, and will be on call for the labour ward on a 24-hour basis (see Chapter 11).
- Arrangements will be in place for contacting interpreters who speak languages that are less frequently needed (see Chapter 11).
- Interpreters will receive training on the psychological as well as the practical aspects of optimum care (see Chapter 11).
- The religious and cultural needs of parents with babies in the neonatal unit will be identified and met (see Chapter 21).
- Family planning information will respect and be responsive to cultural and religious differences (see Chapter 21).
- All staff will adopt a flexible and responsive approach to procedures after miscarriage, stillbirth and neonatal death and will accommodate differing religious and cultural needs (see Chapter 22).
- Relatives will have complete access to the body of an adult or infant in the chapel of rest (see Chapter 22).
- Religious symbols appropriate to the main local religious communities will be available in the chapel of rest and, when relevant, will be put in place before the relatives arrive (see Chapter 22).
- There will be an accessible, responsive and well-publicised complaints procedure.
- Information about complaints procedures will be available in all languages relevant to the local community.

IMPLICATIONS FOR SERVICE MANAGERS

Our own cultural assumptions and beliefs influence our views and actions. Managers too need to reflect on their own attitudes in order to manage a service that is flexible and responsive to everyone regardless of culture, religion or need.

Service managers also need to take into account the fact that providing culturally sensitive care:

- **takes longer**, and it is unreasonable to expect staff to do it well without extra time.
- **requires appropriate resources**, such as well-trained interpreters.
- **takes thought and self-awareness** and people cannot be expected to do it well without training. Such training needs to be skilfully designed and sensitively run so that participants can examine their own beliefs and attitudes as a foundation for understanding those of other people. It should not consist of 'facts' about different groups (see Chapters 1 and 2). Training should be available to all grades and to anyone who has contact with clients, including all front line staff. One rude or insensitive person can easily nullify the efforts of everyone else.
- **requires flexibility**. Once people understand the principles and aims of equal access they should be encouraged to use their imagination and common sense in devising care that really meets the needs of different clients. Innovations that do not work should be treated as part of the learning process and those responsible for them should not be blamed (Cheung-Judge and Henley, 1994).
- **is demanding**. Staff should have easy access to support systems. They should have time with their managers to evaluate their workload and identify their training needs.

IMPLICATIONS FOR EDUCATION AND TRAINING

In a multiracial, multicultural society it is essential that all health professionals are able to understand, respect and meet a diversity of needs. The necessary information, skills and awareness should be woven into the initial and continuing education of all health professionals.

It is important that issues such as the cultural and religious needs of minorities are not simply tacked onto the end of the curriculum. This reinforces the idea that such needs are extraordinary and abnormal, and that meeting them is optional, whereas everything learned in the main body of the curriculum is the norm. It helps to perpetuate inequalities in provision.

All health professionals and students need training in the subtle skills required to provide health care in a multiracial, multicultural society, sensitively and without stereotyping. Training should include opportunities for professionals and students to develop awareness of their own culture and culture-based assumptions. Inequalities in health, the effects of racial discrimination and poverty, and the implications for maternity services of the 1976 Race Relations Act (CRE, 1994) also need to be addressed. Different cultural and religious issues and the knowledge and skills needed to provide flexible, sensitive care should be considered in relation to each aspect of physical and emotional care as it arises in the curriculum.

Awareness of racism and inequality should be a strand throughout the educational curriculum, with positive attempts made to expose learners to all aspects of caring for women from a wide variety of ethnic backgrounds. (Kroll, 1990)

Such training requires knowledge, skill and sensitivity on the part of educators and trainers. It must be carried out in an atmosphere of trust, respect and safety. Subjects such as inequality and racial discrimination are emotive and difficult to discuss without arousing defensiveness, anger, guilt and resentment. Feelings can run high, especially as the students and health professionals involved are themselves likely to be of different cultures, religions and ethnic groups and may bring their own, often painful, experiences to the discussion. Health professionals and students can learn a great deal about such issues from each other, but they must first learn to value each other more positively (McGee, 1994) and there must be enough safety within the group to make learning possible. Potential difficulties such as these should not be reasons for inaction. Educators who lack the necessary knowledge, confidence and appropriate skills need training and support.

References and further reading

Ahmad, W.I.U. (1993) Making black people sick: 'race', ideology and health research. In *'Race' and Health in Contemporary Britain* (ed. W.I.U. Ahmad), Open University Press, Buckingham

Ahmed, G. and Watt, S. (1986) Understanding Asian women in pregnancy and confinement. *Midwives Chronicle and Nursing Notes*, **99**, May, 98–101

Ahmet, L. (1990) A model for midwives – support for ethnic breastfeeding mothers. *Midwives Chronicle*, 103 (January), 5–7

Ainsworth-Smith, I. and Speck, P. (1982) *Letting Go: Caring for the Dying and Bereaved Patient*, SPCK, London

Alladin, W.J. (1992) Clinical psychology provision: models, policies and prospects. In *The Politics of Race and Health* (ed. W.I.U. Ahmad), Race Relations Research Unit, Bradford University

Ashwood, C. (1994) Cultural differences in breastfeeding. *Nursing Times*, **90**, 10–11

Baldwin, J. (1994) Obstetricians: safety and quality. *Modern Midwife*, **4**(12), 4

Bates, C. (1993) *A Feminist Perspective of Motherhood* (unpublished). MA dissertation, London University

BHAN (1991) *AIDS and the Black Communities,* Black HIV and AIDS Network, London WC1N 3XX

Bick, D. and MacArthur, C. (1994) Identifying morbidity in postpartum women. *Modern Midwife*, **4**(12), 10–14

Bieri, A. (1993) Does anybody speak Bimoba? In *Cupid's Wild Arrows* (ed. D. Dicks), Bergli Books, Weggis, Switzerland

Booth, B., Verma, M. and Singh Beri, R. (1994) Fetal sex determination in infants in Punjab, India: correlations and implications. *British Medical Journal*, **309**, 1259–61

Bowler, I. (1993) Stereotypes of women of Asian descent in midwifery: some evidence. *Midwifery*, **9**, 7-16

Boyle, M. (1994) *Antenatal Investigations*, Books for Midwives Press, Haigh and Hochland Publications, Cheshire

Braun, D. and Schonveld, A. (1993) *Approaching Parenthood*, Health Education Authority, London

Campbell, R. and Macfarlane, A. (1994) *Where to be Born? The Debate and the Evidence*, National Perinatal Epidemiology Unit, Oxford

Carlson, E. and de Wet, M. (1991) *Bangladeshi Food and Food Habits*, Nutrition and Dietetic Department, Bloomsbury Health Authority, London

Cheung, N. (1994) Pain in normal labour: a comparison of experiences in southern China and Scotland. *Midwives Chronicle*, **107**(1,277), 212–16

Cheung-Judge, M. Y. and Henley, A. (1994) *Equality in Action: Introducing Equal Opportunities in Voluntary Organisations*, NCVO Publications, London

Clements, S. (1994) Unwanted vaginal examinations. *British Journal of Midwifery*, **2**(8), 368–70

Combes, G. and Schonveld, A. (1992) *Life will Never be the Same Again*, Health Education Authority, London

CRE (1991) *Race Relations Code of Practice in Employment*, Commission for Racial Equality, London

CRE (1993) *The Sorrow in My Heart: Sixteen Asian Women Speak about Depression*, Commission for Racial Equality, London

CRE (1994) *Race Relations Code of Practice in Maternity Services*, Commission for Racial Equality, London

Currer, C. (1986) *The Mental Health of Pathan Mothers in Bradford: a Study of Migrant Asian Women* (unpublished thesis). Department of Sociology, University of Warwick

Daud, S. (1992) Abortion, contraception and ethnic minorities in the UK. *Planned Parenthood in Europe*, **21**(3), 9–12

Department of Health (1993) *Changing Childbirth*. Report of the Expert Maternity Group, HMSO, London

Enkin, M., Keirse, J. and Chalmers, I. (1990) *A Guide to Effective Care in Pregnancy and Childbirth*. Oxford University Press, Oxford

Fleissig, A. (1993) Are women given enough information by staff during labour and delivery? *Midwifery*, **9**, 70–5

Foster, M.-C. (1988) Health visitors' perspectives on working in a multiethnic society. *Health Visitor*, **61**, 275–8

Gatrad, A. R. (1994) Attitudes and beliefs of Muslim mothers towards pregnancy and infancy. *Archives of Disease in Childhood*, **71**, 170–4

Gladman, J. (1994) Antenatal care in the 90s. *British Journal of Midwifery*, **2**(10), 449–503

Glazener, C., Abdalla, M., Russell, I. and Templeton, A. (1993) Postnatal care: a survey of patients' experiences. *British Journal of Midwifery*, **1**(2), 67–74

Godsen, C., Nicoliades, K. and Whitting, V. (1994) *Is my Baby Alright? A Guide for Expectant Parents*, Oxford University Press, Oxford

Grant, J. (1993) *Midwives and Prenatal Screening* (Unpublished). MSc (Sociology) dissertation, South Bank University, London

Green, J. (1994) Serum screening for Down's syndrome: experiences of obstetricians in England and Wales. *Student British Journal of Medicine*, **2**, 423–5

Green, J., Kitzinger, J. and Coupland, V. (1990) Stereotypes of childbearing women: a look at some evidence. *Midwifery*, **6**, 125–32

Green, J. and Statham, H. (1993) Testing for fetal abnormality in routine antenatal care. *Midwifery*, **9**, 134–5

Hall, J. (1993) Attendance not compulsory. *Nursing Times*, **89**(46), 69–71

Hansen, H.P. (1990) Ritual understanding of pregnancy and delivery. *Nursing Times*, **86**(17), 57

Hedegaard, M., Henrikson, T., Sabroe, S. and Secher, N. (1993) Psychological distress in pregnancy and preterm delivery. *British Medical Journal*, **307**, 234–9

Hill, S. E. (ed.) (1990) *More than Rice and Peas: Guidelines to Improving Food Provision for Black and Ethnic Minorities in Britain*. The Food Commission, London

Hofmeyr, G., Nikodem, V., Wolman, W. *et al.* (1991) Companionship to modify the clinical birth environment: effects on progress and perceptions of labour and breastfeeding. *British Journal of Obstetrics and Gynaecology*, **98**, 756–63

Holmes, S. (1993) Force of habits. *Nursing Times*, **89**(35), 48–50

House of Commons (1992) *Health Committee 2nd Report: Maternity Services*, HMSO, London

Hutton, E. (1994) What women want from midwives, *British Journal of Midwifery*, **2**(12), 608–11

Hutton, E. (undated) *What Women Want from Midwives, Obstetricians, General Practitioners and Health Visitors*, The National Childbirth Trust, London

Imam, Z. (1994) India bans female feticide. *British Medical Journal*, **309**, 428

Kline, N. (1993) Motherhood, consider it leadership. In *Women and Power: How Far Can We Go?*, BBC Books, London

Kroll, D. (1990) Equal access to care? *Nursing Times*, **86**(23), 72–3

Lamblia, J. (1980) The image of the fetus in the first trimester. *Birth and the Family Journal*, **7**(1), 5–14

Langford, J. (1994) Forward planning. *New Generation*, **13**(4), 22–3

Leboyer, F. (1975) *Birth without Violence*, Fontana/Collins, London

Lewis, E. (1979) Inhibition of mourning by pregnancy: psychopathology and management. *British Medical Journal*, **ii**, 27–8

Lewis, E. (1976) The management of stillbirth: coping with an unreality. *Lancet*, **ii**, 619–20

Li, P.-L. (1992) Health needs of the Chinese population. In *The Politics of 'Race' and Health* (ed. W. I. U. Ahmad), University of Bradford

Lumley, J. (1980) The image of the fetus in the first trimester. *Birth and the Family Journal*, **7**(1), 5–14

MacArthur, C., Lewis, M. and Knox, E. (1993) Comparison of long-term health problems following childbirth among Asian and Caucasian mothers. *British Journal of General Practice*, **43**, 519–22

McGee, P. (1994) Educational issues in transcultural nursing. *British Journal of Nursing*, **3**(21), 111–15

Mamdani, M. (1972) *The Myth of Population Control*. Monthly Review Press, New York

Mares, P., Henley, A. and Baxter, C. (1985) *Health Care in Multiracial Britain*, National Extension College, Cambridge

Menage, J. (1993) Post-traumatic stress disorder in women who have undergone obstetric and/or gynaecological procedures. *Journal of Reproductive and Infant Psychology*, **11**, 221–8

Melzack, R. (1973) *The Puzzle of Pain*, Penguin, Harmondsworth

Merskey, H. (ed.) (1986) Classification of chronic pain: descriptions of chronic pain syndromes and definitions of pain terms. *Pain*, Suppl. 3, S271

Morgan, J. and Sturdy, J. (1995) Breastfeeding in the 1990s. *Modern Midwife*, **5**(1), 19–22

Narang, I. and Murphy, S.(1994) Assessment of the antenatal care for Asian women. *British Journal of Midwifery*, **2**(4), 169–73

NAWCH (1993) *Achieving Health Care for Black and Ethnic Minority Children and their Families*, National Association for the Welfare of Children in Hospital, Argyle House, Euston Road, London NW1 2SD

NCT (1994) *HIV and AIDS Policy*, National Childbirth Trust, Alexandra House, Oldham Terrace, London W3 6NH

NHS Management Executive (1993) *Maternity Services for Asian Women*, Department of Health, London

Nicolaides, K. (1994) Interview broadcast in the *Everyman* series, BBC 1, 3 December 1994

Niven, C. (1992) *Psychological Care for Families Before, During and After Birth*, Butterworth-Heinemann, Oxford

Nolan, M. (1994) Effectiveness of antenatal education. *British Journal of Midwifery*, **2**(11), 534–8

Norton, D. (1994) Doula training. *MIDIRS Midwifery Digest*, **4**(4), 452

OPCS (1992) *Infant Feeding*, Office of Populations Censuses and Surveys, Social Survey Division, HMSO, London

Oxby, H. (1994) When do women decide? *Health Visitor*, **67**(5), 161

Paradice, R. (1993) How important are early mother/infant relationships? *Health Visitor*, **66**, 211–13

Parsons, L. and Day, S. (1992) Improving obstetric outcomes in ethnic minorities: an evaluation of health advocacy in Hackney. *Journal of Public Health Medicine*, **14**(2), 183–91

Phillips, D.P., Todd, E.R. and Wagner, L.M. (1993) Psychology and survival. *Lancet*, **342**, 1142–5

Prasad, S. (1994) Towards better health care provision for ethnic minorities in Britain: reproductive health and family planning in the Asian community. *British Journal of Family Planning*, **19**, 283–9

Price, S. (1989) Weaning practices of Asians in Britain. *Health Visitor*, **61**, 279–81

Priest, J. and Schott, J. (1991) *Leading Antenatal Classes: a Practical Guide*, Butterworth-Heinemann, Oxford

Raeburn, J. (1994) Screening for carriers of cystic fibrosis. *British Journal of Medicine*, **309**, 1428–9

Rajan, L. (1993) Perceptions of pain and pain relief in labour: The gulf between experience and observation. *Midwifery*, **9**, 136–45

Rajan, L. (1994) Social isolation and support in pregnancy loss. *Health Visitor*, **67**(3), 97–101

Ralph, K. and Alexander, J. (1994) Borne under stress. *Nursing Times*, **90**(12), 28–30

RCM (1991) *Successful Breastfeeding*, Royal College of Midwives, Churchill Livingstone, London

RCM (1994) *Men at Birth*, Press Office, Royal College of Midwives, London

RCN (undated) *Equality Matters*, Royal College of Nursing, London

Rogers, C. (1989) *Freedom to Learn for the 80s*, Charles Merrill, Ohio

Rogers, J. (1989) *Adults Learning*. Open University Press, Milton Keynes

Rothman, B.K. (1988) *The Tentative Pregnancy: Prenatal Diagnosis and the Future of Motherhood*, Pandora/Unwin Paperbacks

SANDS (1995) *The Management of Pregnancy Loss and the Death of a Baby: Guidelines for Professionals*, Stillbirth and Neonatal Death Society (SANDS), London (see Useful Addresses)

Salim, B.M. (1993) Pakistan Coin Pain Scale. *PAIN*, **52**(3), 373–4

Schott, J. and Henley, H. (1992) *Breaking the Barriers: a Training Package on Equal Access to Maternity Services*, Obstetric Hospital, University College London Hospitals NHS Trust, London

Seel, R. (1994) Men at the birth. *New Generation*, **13**(4), 16–17

Senior, P. A. and Bhopal, R. (1994) Ethnicity as a variable in epidemiological research. *British Medical Journal*, **309**, 327–30

SHARE (1992) Purchasing and contracts. Health and Race: Creating Social Change. *SHARE Newsletter*, Issue 4 (King's Fund Centre, London)

Smith, D. and Marteau, T. (1995) Detecting fetal abnormality: serum screening and fetal anomaly scans. *British Journal of Midwifery*, **3**(3), 183–6

Smith, D., Shaw, R. and Marteau, T. (1994) Informed consent to undergo serum screening for Down's syndrome: the gap between policy and practice. *British Medical Journal*, **309**, 776

Smith, D., Shaw, R., Slack J. and Marteau, T. (1995) Training obstetricians and midwives to present screening tests: an evaluation of two brief interventions. *Prenatal Diagnosis*, **15**(4), 317–24

Sosa, R., Kennell, M., Klaus, M. *et al.* (1980) The effects of a supportive companion on perinatal problems, length of labor, and mother-infant interaction. *New England Journal of Medicine*, **303**(11), 597–600

Steer, P. (1993) Rituals in antenatal care – do we need them? *British Medical Journal*, **307**, 697–8

Sutton, J. and Scott, P. (1994) Optimal fetal positioning: a midwifery approach to increasing the number of normal births. *MIDIRS Midwifery Digest*, **4**(3), 283–6

Thorley, K. and Rouse, T. (1993) Seeing mothers as partners in antenatal care. *British Journal of Midwifery*, **1**(5), 216–19

Thornton, J. and Lilford, R. (1994) Active management of labour: current knowledge and research issues. *British Medical Journal*, **309**, 366–9

Torkington, N. P. K. (1987) Racism and health. *Women's Health Information Centre (Newsletter)* Spring, p. 7

Trevelyan, J. (1994) Please tell mother. *Nursing Times*, **90**(9), 38–9

UK Amniotomy Group (1994) A multicentre randomised trial of amniotomy in spontaneous first labour at term. *British Journal of Obstetrics and Gynaecology*, **101**(4), 307–9

Urwin, J. (1994) Choice advice. *Nursing Times*, **90**(26), 56

Van den Akker, O. (1993) Prophylactic benefits of antenatal screening: helpful or harmful? *British Journal of Midwifery*, **1**(5), 220–3

Vyas, S. (1994) Screening for Down's syndrome: ignorance abounds. *Student British Medical Journal*, **2**, 400–1

Vincent Priya, J. (1992) *Birth Traditions and Modern Pregnancy Care*. Element Books Ltd, Shaftesbury

Walsh, M. and Ford, P. (1990) *Nursing Rituals, Research and Rational Actions*, Butterworth-Heinemann, Oxford

Walshe, J. and Warrier, S. (1993) *Dates and Meanings of Religious and Other Festivals*, Foulsham Educational, London

Weller, P. (1993) *Religions in the UK: a Multi-Faith Directory*, University of Derby/Inter-Faith Network for the UK, 5–7 Tavistock Place, London WC1 9SS

Whittle, J. (1993) Screening for Down's syndrome. *British Journal of Midwifery*, **1**(3), 109

Williams, R. (1992) The health of the Irish in Britain. In *The Politics of Race and Health* (ed. W.I. U. Ahmad), Race Relations Research Unit, Bradford University

Wilson, S. (1994) Obstetric anthropology. *Student British Medical Journal*, **2**, 477

Woollet, A. and Dosanjh-Matwala, N. (1990) Postnatal care: the attitudes and experiences of Asian women in East London. *Midwifery*, **6**, 178–84

Worden, J. W. (1991) *Grief Counselling and Grief Therapy: a Handbook for the Mental Health Practitioner*, 2nd edn, London

Part Four

Specific Health Issues

INTRODUCTION

In this section we examine some health issues that have specific relevance to certain religious and cultural minority groups. We have not included health issues that are common in the general population.

Differences in disease prevalence

The prevalence of certain diseases also common in the general population is significantly increased in some minority ethnic populations. It is important that health professionals should be aware of these so that they can provide appropriate care and give accurate information to clients.

Diabetes   The incidence of insulin dependent and non-insulin dependent diabetes is greater in populations of Asian and African-Caribbean origin (Kumar and Clark, 1994; Mather and Keen, 1985; Samanta *et al.,* 1987). Women of ethnic groups other than Northern European have been shown to have a higher incidence of gestational diabetes (Dornhorst, *et al.,* 1992), and Asian women have a significantly higher prevalence of abnormal glucose tolerance during pregnancy (Samanta *et al.,* 1989).

Hypertension   Hypertension is more common in people of African descent (Kumar and Clark, 1994). In the USA, hypertension is more common, more aggressive and less well managed in African-Americans than in white Americans (Kaplan, 1994). It has been suggested that an internalised response to race and gender discrimination may be a contributory factor to high blood pressure amongst black women (Krieger, 1990).

24 Female circumcision – female genital mutilation

Female circumcision is more correctly known as female genital mutilation (FGM) because:

- it involves removing healthy tissue
- it has no health benefits
- in its more radical forms it results in significant long-term morbidity.

It is estimated that over 100 million girls and women throughout the world have been genitally mutilated (RCN, 1994).

FGM in varying degrees is common in half the countries of Africa, particularly across central Africa from west to east. In some African countries it is traditionally carried out on all women, in others it has been performed on fewer than 5 per cent of women. FGM is also practised to some extent in a few areas of the Middle East and South East Asia (Hosken, 1994; Jordan, 1993). It is not practised in Saudi Arabia. In those countries where FGM is traditional, many members of the educated elite are abandoning it (Hedley and Dorkenoo, 1992).

There are three types of FGM:

- Removal of the clitoral hood. This is the only type that can correctly be called circumcision.
- Excision of the clitoris and part or all of the labia minora (clitoridectomy).
- Infibulation, the most extensive form of FGM in which the clitoris and the labia minora are removed and the labia majora are reduced and then stitched together, leaving a small opening so that urine and menstrual fluid can escape. Occasionally infibulation is performed over an intact clitoris.

FGM is carried out on babies or young girls before the onset of puberty, often by older women or traditional birth attendants. It is usually done without anaesthetic, using a range of implements which are often unsterilized. Surgery under such conditions carries considerable risk of infection, haemorrhage, damage to surrounding organs and even death. Even the less severe forms of mutilation can cause heavy scarring, especially if there have been additional infections (Ladjalin et al. 1993).

Infibulation, in particular, causes numerous long-term medical problems. A woman who has been infibulated may be left with an orifice no bigger than the diameter of a pencil. As a result, it can take some women up to 20 minutes to empty their bladders, leaving them prone to recurrent urinary tract infections and often with irregular, prolonged and painful periods. Intercourse is impossible. When they marry, some women may have to be cut open by their husbands to make intercourse possible. This may result in infection.

> 'Some women would rather be divorced than have to have sexual intercourse.' Somali woman

The law

Under the Prohibition of Circumcision Act, 1985, it is illegal to perform FGM in Britain (Jordan, 1994). Performing FGM is punishable by a fine or imprisonment. Nevertheless, the practice is known to continue. In some cases girls are taken abroad for FGM to be carried out. In 1993 the French courts convicted and imprisoned a woman who paid for her two daughters to be circumcised, and a man who ordered his wives to circumcise their daughters.

Understanding why

FGM is deeply embedded in certain African cultures. It is done to ensure virginity and chastity. It is considered to be more aesthetic and hygienic. Women who have not undergone FGM may be unable to find a husband in a society in which marriage may be their only option. They may be stigmatised and assumed to be promiscuous.

FGM continues because parents feel it is the right thing to do and because they want their daughters to be marriageable and acceptable within their own community. Many see FGM as a positive and normal part of their heritage and identity.

Some people cite religious requirements as a reason for performing FGM. However, there is increasing awareness, for example in the Somali community, that FGM is a local cultural tradition rather than an Islamic requirement. There is no reference to female circumcision in the Quran, the Muslim holy book, nor in the Bible. FGM is not practised in the Middle-Eastern Muslim states and is known to pre-date Islam (Dorkenoo and Elworthy, 1994).

FGM and maternity care

Not all women whose families originated in those countries where FGM is practised are affected. However, since the more severe forms of FGM present special problems during birth and make some aspects of routine care impossible, it is important to find out if a woman has been circumcised, and if so to what degree. This should be done with extreme tact and sensitivity, especially as many women are fearful of health professionals' reactions and feel vulnerable to criticism.

Gentle and sensitive physical examination may also be required. It is important, for example, to check whether the introitus of a woman who is pregnant is large enough to give birth. Some women with a very small introitus conceive without full sexual intercourse. Where there is heavy scarring, labour may be more likely to be prolonged. Once the situation is known, an appropriate plan for care can be worked out with the woman and, where appropriate, her husband or partner. This may involve reversal during pregnancy (see below) or an anterior episiotomy at birth. It should not automatically include a caesarean section; many women fear that this will be imposed upon them simply because they have been infibulated. It is also necessary to discuss the fact that the woman will not be completely re-stitched after the birth (see below).The degree of mutilation and the agreed plan for care should be recorded so that women are not subjected to repeated questioning or examination, and so that staff know in advance of women who have undergone FGM.

Physical examination

Women who have undergone any form of FGM are even more likely than most to be embarrassed about exposing their genitals, especially in a society that openly disapproves of what has been done to them. For religious reasons, many women who have undergone FGM may also be unwilling to be examined by male doctors. In addition they are likely to be extremely frightened about having to open their legs and being touched during vulval or vaginal examination since this can evoke terrifying flashbacks of the mutilation itself. It is therefore very important to build a calm, trusting relationship beforehand and to minimise the number of examinations. Careful explanation should always be given about what is and is not going to be done. It is essential to be gentle and understanding if a woman is reluctant, resists examination or finds it difficult to cooperate. If she does not speak English a professional female interpreter must be available.

Women in communities where FGM is practised are often concerned that medical students and student nurses and midwives might be called in during examinations 'to have a look'. Some have heard stories of women being photographed during examination for research purposes. Such fears add to women's reluctance and fear of examination. It is very important that properly informed consent is obtained before any non-essential staff are allowed to be present, and before any action (such as photography or involvement in research) is taken which does not directly benefit the woman.

Health professionals

Health professionals, especially those who have not previously seen a woman who has been infibulated, are often deeply shocked or disgusted on discovering that a woman has undergone FGM. Some convey this to women in their care.

> 'I am appalled by some of the things health professionals say to women who have had FGM. After all it is not her fault this was done to her. We don't express shock, horror or disgust when we see a grossly obese woman even if we do have strong views about her size and the implications for her health.' Obstetrician

It is unacceptable for women who have undergone FGM to be treated in any way differently or seen as oddities. Their feelings and self-respect should be considered at all times.

> 'We know that people here think that it is wrong and we are beginning to see that it is not a good idea. But all the publicity is terrible for us. Every time someone looks at us in the street we feel as though they are wondering what our genitals look like. It is very humiliating'. Refugee worker and mother of five

It is most important that health professionals give every woman sensitive and respectful care. Those who are understandably distressed by what they see need to postpone their reactions and to deal with their feelings in a confidential setting, well away from the women they care for (see also Chapter 15).

Reversal

Reversal operations are sometimes performed for women who request them. Although tissue that has been excised cannot be replaced, infibulation can be reversed in order to allow the free passage of urine and menstrual fluid and to make sexual intercourse possible. Some doctors advocate reversals during pregnancy, so that anterior episiotomies are avoided at the birth, and the labial edges are already healed. Reversal during pregnancy also makes it possible to take fetal blood samples and apply scalp monitors if problems occur during labour.

However, reversal should not be carried out without first ensuring that the woman has thought through the potential social implications and considered how her family and, if she is married, her husband might react. In conservative families and communities that practise FGM, a woman who is not infibulated can become a social outcast. If a married woman is considering a reversal, her husband should be involved in the discussions. These should include information about how reversal can benefit the woman's health and make sexual intercourse easier and better for both of them. Women who undergo reversals should be given information about contraception.

Stitching after the birth

Infibulation, that is stitching the labia together so that intercourse is difficult or impossible, is illegal in the UK (see above). Consequently, complete repair of the vulva after birth so that it is restored to its infibulated state is illegal (Jordan, 1993). If the labial edges are left un-stitched it is usually important to oversew them so that they do not fuse together as they heal. However, if a couple specifically requests resuturing and the doctor is not prepared to do it, the labial edges could be left unstitched.

The fact that the woman cannot be re-stitched after the birth must be discussed with her, and whenever possible, her husband, during pregnancy, so that both of them have time to adjust to the idea and to raise their views and concerns.

Women who have undergone FGM may be terrified by having their genitals touched or by having their legs and thighs held and may be unable to cooperate if stitching of any kind is needed after birth. Local anaesthetic is inadequate under these circumstances and a spinal block is needed so that the woman can feel neither touch nor pain.

Breaking the cycle

In the UK, 10,000 girls are estimated to be at risk of FGM (Dorkenoo and Elworthy, 1993). Because FGM threatens the health and well-being of young girls and of women and because it is illegal, health professionals and others have a duty to protect babies and young girls from undergoing FGM in any of its forms.

The debate on how to do this is just beginning. Many hesitate to encroach on cultural practices and fear being seen as interfering or racist. Some believe that the best approach is non-confrontational, and that by avoiding conflict health professionals are in a better position to inform women about the law, and to educate and help them to realise how their daughters will benefit both physically and psychologically if they remain intact. Others believe that encouragement and education are too difficult and too slow and that the practice has to be stopped now by prosecuting those responsible, even at the risk of antagonising the community and driving the practice further underground.

Despite the fact that it is illegal to perform FGM and illegal for a parent to ask someone else to do it, it will probably take time to stop a practice that is deeply rooted in culture and history. Outside pressure alone will not put a stop to FGM. Community leaders and more importantly, women themselves need to decide to see that it stops. This is already happening amongst some groups of African women.

However stopping FGM is easier said than done. In order to break the cycle, women need the strength and courage to believe that their daughters will not be outcasts if they are not circumcised. They also need to be able to withstand family and social pressures to conform with traditional ideas of hygiene, acceptability and normality.

In addition, if a mother is to understand the reasons for not allowing her daughter to undergo FGM, she is likely to have to face the enormity of what has been done to her. Psychologically, this is asking a great deal. FGM is done with the consent of the parents and is sometimes performed by an older female relative. Although the motives of the adults were very different, coming to terms with FGM can be compared to acknowledging and trying to come to terms with the experience of incestuous abuse and violence.

Women who are caught between tradition and a growing awareness of the long-term trauma FGM is likely to cause their daughters, need continuing help and support while they come to terms with what happened to them and develop the strength and courage to break an age-old custom.

USEFUL ADDRESSES

FORWARD
(Foundation for Women's Health and Development)
38 King Street
London   WC2 8JT

Minority Rights Group
379 Brixton Road
London   SW9 7DE

The haemoglobinopathies are a group of autosomal, recessive, inherited disorders of haemoglobin. The most common are sickle cell disorder (sometimes called sickle cell disease or sickle cell syndrome) and thalassaemia. There are milder and more severe forms of both disorders. In the UK, the haemoglobino-pathies mainly, but not exclusively, affect minority ethnic groups. But no specific haemoglobinopathy is confined to a single group (Department of Health, 1993).

Recessive inheritance

People who carry a recessive disease (also known as carrying the trait) have no symptoms, though people who carry beta thalassaemia trait may have mild anaemia. Someone who carries the trait may pass it on to their children through their genes. If both members of a couple carries the trait, **each** of their children has:

- a one in four chance of being completely unaffected
- a one in two chance of inheriting the trait (and therefore having no symptoms)
- a one in four chance of having the disease.

THALASSAEMIA

Thalassaemia indicates either partial or no production of alpha and beta globin chains which are vital to the structure of the haemoglobin in the red blood cells (Anionwu, 1993).

Alpha thalassaemia major Alpha globin chains are essential for the production of haemoglobin needed for the unborn baby. A child with two parents who are carriers of alpha thalassaemia (that is, who carry the trait) has a one in four chance of inheriting the disease. The more severe form of alpha thalassaemia major is incompatible with life. The affected fetus develops hydrops fetalis and dies, usually during the second trimester. The mother is also at risk from toxaemia.

The trait for alpha thalassaemia occurs in people of Chinese, Vietnamese, Greek, Middle Eastern and Cypriot heritages (Anionwu, 1993; Department of Health, 1993).

Beta thalassaemia major   A child with two parents who are carriers of beta thalassaemia (that is, who carry the trait) has a one in four chance of inheriting beta thalassaemia major. A person with beta thalassaemia major is unable to make enough of the beta haemoglobin chain which is essential for the production of haemoglobin after birth. This results in a life-threatening haemolytic anaemia which is treated with regular blood transfusions combined with treatment to prevent iron overload. People with beta thalassaemia major are likely to have delayed puberty, to be infertile and to develop heart failure and diabetes. At present, the complications associated with beta thalassaemia major and iron overload often lead to an early death. There are about 600 people with beta thalassaemia major in the UK, and several thousand carriers (Department of Health, 1993).

The trait for beta thalassaemia (Hb AB Thal) occurs in varying rates among people of Mediterranean, Southern European, South Asian, Chinese, Vietnamese and African-Caribbean heritages. The gene occurs very rarely in people of white British heritage (Department of Health, 1993).

In Britain, the two main groups affected by thalassaemia are the Cypriot and South Asian communities. Levels of awareness and the uptake of premarital and antenatal screening are generally high in the Cypriot community, which is relatively small and concentrated (Anionwu, 1993). However, sections of the South Asian community are also severely affected, and these are generally more scattered and less well-informed. Studies indicate that many people of South Asian descent know little or nothing about the disease or how it is inherited, nor about the possibility of antenatal screening (Anionwu, 1993).

SICKLE CELL DISORDER, DISEASE OR SYNDROME

Sickle cell disorder (or sickle cell disease) is among the most common genetic disorders in Britain. Some affected people prefer the words 'disorder' or 'syndrome' to 'disease'. They point out that many other inherited conditions such as haemophilia do not have the word disease, with all its connotations of sickness, attached to them.

There are approximately 6,000 people with sickle cell disorder (SCD) in the UK, as well as many thousand more who carry the trait (Anionwu, 1994; NHS Management Executive, 1994). The different kinds of sickle cell disorder include sickle cell anaemia (Hb SS), haemoglobin SC disease (Hb SC) and sickle beta thalassaemia, (Hb S Beta-thal), and vary a good deal in their severity and symptoms. Sickle cell anaemia and one form of sickle beta thalassaemia are usually the most severe.

Sickle cell trait (Hb AS) occurs in varying rates in people of African-Caribbean, West African, Cypriot, Mediterranean, South Asian and Middle Eastern heritages. C trait (Hb AC) occurs in varying rates in people of African-Caribbean and Ghanaian heritage. D trait (Hb AD) occurs in varying rates in people of Chinese and Cypriot heritage and, very occasionally, in people of white British heritage.

Sickle cell disorder is caused by an abnormality in the structure of the haemoglobin in the red blood cells. This results in a tendency for the red blood cells to change temporarily into a sickle shape when they are deprived of fluids or oxygen. The sickle-shaped cells block peripheral venous blood flow, resulting in venous occlusion and pain which is often excruciating. In addition to painful sickle crises, in the most severe forms of SCD, people may suffer from infections, anaemia, damage to their joints and eyes, strokes in childhood, and pulmonary infarcts. Their life expectancy is shortened. The highest death rate due to SCD occurs in children under the age of five because of their susceptibility to infections, especially pneumococcal infections. Prophylactic antibiotics are given to reduce the incidence of infections.

Sickling of the red blood cells can be precipitated by a range of factors, including pregnancy. Sudden changes in temperature, dehydration, fever, infection, alcohol, strenuous exercise, emotional stress, hypoxia and acidosis are also implicated. Affected individuals can try to minimise the likelihood of crises by avoiding precipitating factors, but sickling is often unpredictable. Some people go through long periods with few or no crises, and then periods with frequent, severe crises (Anionwu, 1994).

Care during pregnancy and birth

Sickle cell disorder increases both maternal and fetal mortality and morbidity. Mothers with SCD have an increased incidence of pre-eclampsia, impaired placental function, intra-uterine growth retardation, premature labour, fetal distress and stillbirth (Eboh and Van den Akker, 1994).

Pregnancy also increases the risk of sickle cell crises. Women experiencing a crisis must receive prompt and expert care. They urgently need rest, warmth, support and reassurance, as well as fluids and analgesics of appropriate strength.

A number of studies have shown that people with a sickle cell crisis are thought to exaggerate the severity of their pain and are often given lower levels of pain relief that they need. However, most people with sickle cell disorder manage painful crises at home and only go to hospital when they have tried everything else and are desperate (Anionwu, 1983). Some profesionals worry that people with SCD and other painful conditions will become addicted if opiates are given too freely. These worries are unfounded. People in pain and addicts show very different emotional and physiological responses when given opiates. For example, people in pain are much slower to develop a tolerance to opiates and have no difficulty in giving them up when they are no longer needed (Consumer Association, 1989; Vallerand, 1994).

Women with SCD should receive specialist care and monitoring during pregnancy. This should include regular haemoglobin checks and assessment of fetal growth, and urine cultures to check for infection.

During labour it is particularly important to avoid dehydration and hypoxia. Anaesthetics can precipitate sickling and women with SCD need skilled management during and after receiving anaesthesia.

After the birth, women remain at extra risk of sickling. They should be encouraged to drink plenty of fluids and should be protected from temperature changes and stresses. There are no contra-indications for breast feeding.

Contraception

There is evidence that injectable progestagens are safe for women with SCD and that they may reduce the incidence of sickle crises. The IUD and other barrier methods also appear to be safe. Although combined oral contraceptives may increase crises in women with SCD, they are not contra-indicated (Howard, 1994).

THE OFFICIAL RESPONSE AND ITS CONSEQUENCES

The health service in the UK has been slow to acknowledge and respond to the needs of people with SCD and thalassaemia. The haemoglobinopathies have been described as 'a pointer to' the impact of institutionalised racism within the NHS (Anionwu, 1993).

- Although the number of people with haemoglobinopathies is similar to the numbers with cystic fibrosis- or haemophilia, **services** for people with haemoglobinopathies are much more haphazard and less well funded (Davies, 1986).
- In most areas there is no routine **screening of neonates** for SCD and thalassaemia although the incidence of SCD is 500 per 100,000 people of African and African-Caribbean heritage (Anionwu, 1994), and one in every seven people of Cypriot heritage carries the gene for beta thalassaemia (Department of Health, 1993). And yet there is routine universal screening of neonates for phenylketonuria (10-12 per 100,000) and for hypothyroidism (20 per 100,000).
- In 1993, a Department of Health Working Party confirmed that people with haemoglobinopathies were not always given the best possible care, even in regions where these disorders are common. The Working Party made a series of recommendations for improving services (Department of Health, 1993). However no extra **funding** was provided.

This lack of resources, as well as a lack of awareness and information among health professionals, has serious consequences for people with haemoglobino-pathies and their families.

- Many people who are carriers have never heard of sickle cell disorder or thalassaemia. In one survey of ten women, none knew anything about SCD at the time when they were told that they had an affected child (Midence, *et al.* 1992). There is very little outreach work to increase understanding in the communities most affected.
- Screening programmes are inadequately publicised and people who may carry a trait are frequently not offered screening.
- Appropriate counselling, information and support are not always available to people who carry or have SCD or thalassaemia.
- People who are tested are sometimes given inaccurate or confusing information about the result and its implications.

  'People who have milder forms of SCD, for example sickle beta + thalassaemia are sometimes told they have sickle cell trait and are therefore horrified when they are screened in pregnancy and are told that in fact they have a mild form of the disease.' Nurse lecturer practitioner/Specialist in haemoglobinopathies.

- People who need medical help, for example with an acute sickling crisis or with a blood transfusion, are not always appropriately or sympathetically treated.

The physical, practical and emotional consequences of having a haemoglobin-opathy or loving someone who has one are enormous. Every member of the family has to adjust emotionally, and to learn practical ways of helping and supporting the person with the condition. When a child is affected, parents commonly feel shocked, guilty, angry, fearful, helpless and ashamed (Sickle Cell Society, undated). These practical and emotional difficulties are compounded when services are inadequate and when health professionals lack information, understanding and empathy. For some people they are also exacerbated by poverty, lack of social support and language barriers (Eboh and Van den Akker, 1994).

SCREENING

All screening and diagnostic tests must be combined with non-directive counselling. Ideally, screening should be offered to everyone at risk of carrying a haemoglobinopathy before pregnancy, so that they know well in advance of any potential risks to their children. However, in most cases screening only takes place in pregnancy, if at all.

Screening in pregnancy

It has been recommended that information about and screening for haemoglobi-nopathies should be routinely offered to all women in areas where black and minority ethnic groups form more than 15 per cent of the population (Department of Health, 1993). Despite this, screening is still haphazard almost everywhere. In most cases, individual health professionals have to decide to whom they will offer screening. This can be very difficult and encourages professionals to base their practice on assumptions and stereotypes. A policy of offering screening to all women would reduce the pressure on health professionals and improve services.

Although screening for haemoglobinopathies is generally desirable, a good deal of information is needed when deciding whether to offer screening to an individual woman. The woman needs to be able to identify the origins of her parents, grandparents and great-grandparents, a total of fourteen people. Many people do not have accurate, detailed information about their ancestry. There may have been adoptions, mixed marriages or mixed relationships in previous generations of which they may be unaware. Adoptees may have no idea of their genetic heritage.

Some people may fear that questions about their heritage and origins are discriminatory or racist. They may suspect that their right to be in the country and to use health services is being questioned. Since these are delicate issues, especially in a climate of racial discrimination and suspicion, it is important to begin by explaining why you are asking about people's origins. Particular care should be taken to maintain people's confidentiality as, for example, some may not have told their partners about their family history or that they were adopted.

The sequence of testing in pregnancy

- If a woman is tested and does not carry a haemoglobinopathy trait, no further steps are necessary.

- If she is found to be a carrier, she and her husband or partner should be invited for counselling with a view to screening the father. Tact and sensitivity may be required as some men may be reluctant to attend appointments or be screened. They may resent the implication that there could be something 'wrong' with them and see this as a threat to their self-esteem.
- If the father is tested and is negative, no further action is needed, though a woman who is a carrier may benefit from opportunities to discuss the potential implications.
- If the father is found to be a carrier, the couple may want to consider further investigations to assess the baby's Hb type. The possible methods will depend on the stage of the pregnancy, and further counselling should be offered so that parents can decide whether to accept diagnostic tests such as chorionic villus sampling, amniocentesis or fetal blood sampling. Parents will also need opportunities to think about what they will do if their baby is affected. The variability of sickle cell anaemia, for example, makes the decision on whether to terminate an affected pregnancy very difficult (Anionwu, 1993).

The length of this process can present problems if the woman is carrying an affected child and decides to terminate the pregnancy. It becomes even more critical if a woman has booked late, possibly because she views pregnancy as normal and only wants 'to book a bed for the birth'.

Infant screening

Infant screening should be combined with the Guthrie test in areas where more than 15 per cent of population are members of black and minority ethnic groups. Cord blood should not be used since there is a risk of contamination with maternal blood (Department of Health, 1993). In many areas, however, individual practitioners are again left to decide to whom to offer infant screening, and there is a danger that some babies with a haemoglobinopathy may be missed. Children with undiagnosed SCD and their parents may not get the care, information and support they badly need.

HIV and AIDS confront health professionals and society with a unique combination of most of the taboos that exist in varying degrees in every culture; sex, intravenous drug use, homosexuality, bi-sexuality, variations in sexual practices, disease, disability and death.

HIV AND AIDS AND MINORITY GROUPS

Because AIDS raises so many fearful issues it is often a vehicle for irrational and discriminatory attitudes and behaviour against groups which are already the targets of prejudice and discrimination. Much of the media attention has concentrated on where AIDS is supposed to have come from, seeking to find someone to blame. When AIDS was first recognised amongst gay men in the USA it was labelled the 'gay plague'. In the 1980s it was said to have originated among people of African descent on the Caribbean island of Haiti. Later, widespread publicity was given to claims that the disease originated in Africa (Patton, 1990). Haemophiliacs and other people who do not belong to stigmatised groups are described as 'innocent victims'. In fact there is no conclusive evidence about the origins of HIV (BHAN, 1991).

In such an atmosphere, many people are labelled 'high risk' (and, often more important, a risk to others) simply on the grounds of the group they are perceived to belong to, rather than because of their actual lifestyle or participation in risk behaviours. As a result of such assumptions cases have occurred of black people being assumed to be infected, being pressurised into accepting HIV tests, and being subjected to elaborate barrier precautions, purely on the grounds of their skin colour.

Both the media and society as a whole tend to vacillate between irrational prejudice and panic, and sweeping the whole issue of AIDS and HIV under the carpet. But where AIDS has come from is not nearly as important as where it is going and what needs to be done. The emphasis on membership, actual or assumed, of a 'group' rather than on individual behaviour as an indication of risk is racist, homophobic and offensive. It is also dangerous since it creates a false dichotomy between so-called 'high-risk groups' and the rest of the population who may be assumed to be free of infection and not at risk. Focusing on minority groups and on 'who is to blame' allows many people whose behaviour does in fact place them at risk to deny the relevance to themselves of HIV and AIDS. The staff who care for them may also become unjustifiably complacent and so may place themselves in danger.

WOMEN AND AIDS

Infection rates in heterosexuals are increasing throughout the world. AIDS has become the leading cause of death for women aged between 20 and 40 in some major cities throughout the Americas and Western Europe as well as in sub-Saharan Africa (Chin, 1990).

The position of each woman in relation to HIV and AIDS has to be considered in the context of her individual social and personal situation. Some women are well aware of how HIV is transmitted; some know very little or are beset with social and emotional problems against which the possibility of HIV and AIDS pales into insignificance (Positively Women, 1994). Some women are monogamous and are confident that their partner is too; some have their doubts but do not want to face reality, or may find the possible consequences too difficult to deal with. Some women feel able to say no to unprotected sex, carry condoms and insist that their partners use them; others may not have the power or the authority to protect themselves against possible infection. Many women in all cultures are financially dependent on their partners and often rely on them for their sense of identity and security. Some may be too vulnerable to be able to insist on using condoms or on knowing about their partner's behaviour in relation to sex or drugs. Some women risk violence if they question their partner's fidelity.

Despite moves towards equality between the sexes, Western society still holds very different standards for men and women, especially in relation to sexual behaviour. As a result, women with HIV and AIDS are likely to experience even more disapproval and less support than men in a similar situation. They may also be caring for family members with AIDS-related illnesses. Women with HIV or AIDS who are pregnant often attract extra censure and hostility from people who see them as having put their unborn child at risk. Concern for infected women is 'overshadowed by apprehension about the fate of their potential children' (Levine and Dubler, 1990).

Women of minority ethnic groups who are HIV positive or have AIDS face additional prejudice, in some cases from their own community as well as from society at large (Positively Women, 1994). They are likely to find it more difficult to get access to services, are often poorer, more isolated and less supported. They may be burdened with several extra layers of stigma and discrimination rather than receiving the care and support they need.

The prevalence of HIV and AIDS in pregnant women

The true spread of HIV infection among women in the UK is not known. A large-scale anonymous testing programme in London in 1991 showed that in certain antenatal clinics approximately 1 in 500 women were HIV positive. Only one quarter of these had informed the health professionals caring for them that they were infected (Banatvala and Chrystie, 1994). It is not known if the remaining three-quarters of the women knew that they were HIV positive. A study by Davison and others (1993) concluded that there is evidence of under-recognition of HIV in pregnancy, particularly in England and Wales.

HIV testing in pregnancy

In 1992 the Department of Health recommended that, providing informed consent was obtained first, HIV tests should be offered to all pregnant women in areas in which a higher prevalence of HIV infection was known about or suspected (Department of Health, 1992). By 1994, however, named HIV tests were routinely available in only four hospital-based antenatal clinics in the UK (Banatvala and Chrystie, 1994).

The potential consequences of accepting an HIV test are enormous, especially for pregnant women. Testing must always be a matter for personal choice. However, where the test is not routinely offered antenatally, each health professional has to decide whether to broach the subject and with whom. This raises particular issues when caring for women of minority ethnic groups. Some women are assumed to be at risk of HIV (and a risk to others) simply because of their skin colour or origins. Others are assumed not to be at risk, and HIV and AIDS may not be discussed with them, because they belong to a religious or cultural community that is considered to have a strict code of conduct with regard to sexual behaviour. But assumptions are dangerous and offensive; individuals in any community, however conservative, may behave in ways that put them, and therefore their partners, at risk. All women need to know about maintaining sexual health and how to protect themselves against AIDS and other sexually transmitted diseases.

> '*I am a Muslim woman who is a representative of a growing number of Muslim women throughout the world who is a recipient of HIV. I was never a drug user and was in a long term monogamous relationship for 18 years. I thought I would never get this virus, because not only do these things happen to other people, but I am a Muslim and I believed that Muslims didn't get HIV.*'   (From Rahman, 1994, by permission of the Naz Project)

> '*It is important to strike a balance between adding to prejudice, racism and stereotyping and ignoring the issue of HIV and AIDS which is a form of inverse racism. By colluding with taboos within a community we are jeopardising people's health. It is important to recognise and work with people's fears and to give clear information so that they can make informed choices.*'   South Asian AIDS worker

Testing for HIV in pregnancy raises complex issues (Shepherd, 1994). Anonymous antenatal testing for example may help epidemiologists gain a picture of the prevalence of HIV in sexually active women of childbearing age, but it is of no benefit to individuals. And testing purely to protect staff is irrational, since women whose test result is negative may sero-convert after the test. Such testing is also unreasonable if health professionals are not also tested. The only way to protect both staff and clients is to adopt universal infection control precautions.

For individual clients there may be physical, emotional and practical advantages in being tested. But there may also be disadvantages. Simply having the test and waiting for the results may cause anxiety and stress. Some people may have false positive results, others false negative; both of these have major long-term consequences. The mere fact that a person is known to have been tested may lay them open to prejudice and abuse (Department of Health, 1994; Mercey et al., 1993; Shepherd, 1994). Sensitive, non-directive pre-test counselling – which means giving balanced, objective information about risks and potential advantages and disadvantages – is therefore essential, so that each woman can evaluate her own situation and reach her own informed decision.

It is unacceptable to put pressure on anyone to accept a test. Consent is a matter of personal choice which must be respected. Women who refuse an HIV test should receive exactly the same level of care as everyone else and should not be assumed to be infected or to be at risk of being infected (Department of Health, 1994).

It is also important that women receive post-test counselling and support. Nobody should assume that a pregnant woman who is HIV positive will decide to terminate her pregnancy or should put pressure on her to do so (Positively Women, 1994). There are many reasons why women choose to have babies and for some, these may be more powerful than the fear of passing on the virus (Levine and Dubler, 1990).

BARRIERS TO COMMUNICATING ABOUT AIDS

Talking about HIV and AIDS is never easy. Few people, even those who know themselves to be at risk, find it easy to discuss the issues surrounding HIV and AIDS or to face the possibility that they might be infected. Most people see AIDS as a remote issue that has nothing to do with them. For many women of black and minority ethnic groups, issues such as poverty and racism are much more pressing.

> 'If a family has to ensure that someone stays up all night to watch in case someone puts a fire bomb through the letter box, the distant possibility of HIV pales into insignificance.'   South Asian AIDS worker

People who experience frequent discrimination may be reluctant to disclose information that will attract further prejudice against themselves or their families. Asylum seekers and refugees may be particularly wary of discussing HIV since they may fear that infection or the possibility of infection could be used as a pretext for deporting them (see also Chapter 27).

Women of African heritage are often very aware of the media picture of AIDS as an African issue and of policies which treat certain people as high risk on the basis of their skin colour or origins. They may have heard of hospitals pressurising black women to accept testing, or carrying out testing without consent. They may also have heard that African women have been routinely isolated in some UK maternity units and subjected to elaborate barrier precautions.

Many women, especially those from religious or cultural backgrounds with a strict moral code, may not consider AIDS or AIDS testing relevant. Some may feel offended and upset that their behaviour or that of their husband or partner is being questioned.

Some health professionals are equally reluctant to raise the subject of AIDS. In order to be able to handle the needs and feelings of each client appropriately, health professionals need a level of self-awareness and to have had opportunities to think through their own attitudes and feelings about HIV, AIDS, sexuality and substance mis-use. They need to be able to talk about these difficult issues in an open and balanced way. Their knowledge base must also be kept up to date so that they can meet the needs of all their clients, and they need to review and develop their communication and non-directive counselling skills.

Health professionals also need to work on and deal with their attitudes and feelings towards people of different cultural and religious groups so that they can see beyond stereotypes and relate to the individual for whom they are caring. 'If staff do not explore their own subjective value system and culturally based pre-conceptions and assumptions, they cannot give accurate, objective information and therefore cannot meet the client's potential needs' (Aston, 1993).

Non-directive pre-test counselling should precede all the tests women are offered during pregnancy. However, enough time is rarely allowed and not all health professionals feel equipped to carry out such counselling, particularly in relation to HIV and AIDS. It may, therefore, be appropriate in some cases to refer women to specialist HIV and AIDS services for pre- and post-test counselling until adequate resources and skills are made available in antenatal clinics.

Language

The advent of HIV and AIDS means that we have to learn to talk about things that were formerly taboo and secret. We have had to develop a new, socially acceptable language. Words and phrases such as penetrative sex, safer sex and condoms are now in common usage, and bi-sexuality and alternative sexual practices are talked about in ways that would have been unthinkable a decade ago. But even though these issues are now discussed more openly, many people, including many health professionals, find them embarrassing or distasteful and have difficulty in raising them or dealing with them in a calm and objective way.

Language can be even more of an obstacle in more conservative communities. In most South Asian languages, for example, there are no socially acceptable words for parts of the body between the waist and knees and no appropriate words other than offensive slang for different sexual identities and sexual activities. Where such words have not become at least partially accepted, it can be very difficult to discuss intimate personal and sexual matters. In communities where homosexuality is taboo, lack of vocabulary may not be the only problem. Men who have sexual relationships with men may simply not identify with terms such as gay, homosexual or bi-sexual. It is important to think in terms of behaviour rather than labels, and to talk, for example, about 'men who have sex with men'.

Interpreters

It is important to take great care over the choice of an interpreter for discussions about HIV and AIDS and related issues. It is inappropriate to use the woman's husband as it may be his behaviour that is in question, and it is clearly unacceptable ever to allow a child to interpret (see also Chapter 11). Women may also feel unable to talk freely through an interpreter who is older, or through a man. Confidentiality is vital and some women may be worried if the interpreter is a member of their own community. It is also very important that the interpreter has had opportunities to deal with her own attitudes and feelings about HIV and AIDS and the issues surrounding it, and that she is trained in the skills of non-directive counselling.

IMPLICATIONS FOR POLICY AND PRACTICE

Given the rapidly changing knowledge base and the complexity and sensitivity of the issues surrounding HIV and AIDS in relation to pregnancy and childbearing, it is not surprising that it is difficult to reach consensus or consistency in policy and practice. There are plenty of problems and, as yet, few sound solutions. However, this should not be an excuse for inaction. The problems will not go away. In order to avoid discrimination and to ensure that all women benefit equally from the service, managers and individual practitioners need to devise, implement and monitor rational policies and practices on screening and non-directive counselling. Universal infection control precautions must be in place at all times and invasive procedures kept to a minimum in order to reduce the risk of vertical transmission (Shepherd, 1994).

USEFUL ADDRESSES

AVERT (Aids Education and Research Trust)
11 Denne Place,
Horsham
West Sussex RH12 1JD.
Publishes *AIDS and Childbirth*, an information leaflet for parents.

BHAN (Black HIV and AIDS Network)
41 St Stephen House,
Uxbridge Road,
London W12 8LH
Supports people of Asian, African and African-Caribbean descent.

Blackliners
49 Effra Road,
London SW2 IBZ
Run by black people for black people.

Positively Women
5 Sebastian Street,
London EC1V OHE
A self-help group run by and for women living with HIV and AIDS.

The NAZ Project
Pallingswick House,
241 King St,
London W6 9LP
HIV/AIDS and sexual health service for the South Asian, Turkish and Arab communities.

The Jewish AIDS Trust
HIV/AIDS Education Unit,
Colindale Hospital,
Colindale Avenue,
London NW9 5HG
Education, counselling and support.

Refugees are likely to have been through many stressful experiences, both before emigration and since their arrival in the receiving country, and this will have implications for their health and health care needs. Under the 1951 United Nations Convention Relating to the Status of Refugees (the Geneva Convention), a refugee is defined as a person who has fled their home country, or cannot go back to it, because of a well-founded fear of persecution for reasons of race, religion, nationality, membership of a particular social group or political opinion.

The number of refugees and displaced people in the world has risen dramatically in recent years. In 1987 about 12 million people were recognised as refugees by the United Nations High Commissioner for Refugees (UNHCR) (Finlay and Reynolds, 1987). By 1993 this number had risen to approximately 18 million with another 20 million 'internally displaced' people who had fled their homes but had not crossed an international border. Only about 5 per cent of displaced people seek asylum in European countries. Britain has a smaller proportion of people seeking asylum in relation to its population size than any comparable European country (Refugee Council, 1992). A high proportion of adult refugees and asylum seekers are women of childbearing age.

Current British legislation

The Geneva Convention contains certain basic regulations for the protection of refugees. It prohibits, for example, the coercive return of people to a country where they fear persecution. Although the UK is a signatory, the details of the Convention have not been incorporated in British law and its interpretation therefore depends to some extent on the attitude of the government in power (Finlay and Reynolds, 1987). Nevertheless, the 1993 Asylum and Immigration (Appeals) Act states that 'no removal or application of the Immigration Rules may be contrary to the UK's obligations under the Convention'.

In the UK a **refugee** is legally defined as a person who has been granted refugee status by the Home Office. People who have applied for refugee status and are waiting for a Home Office decision, and people who have been refused refugee status but granted 'Exceptional Leave to Remain' (which must be re-applied for every year), are known as **asylum seekers**. The process of applying for refugee status can take many months and even years (Runnymede Trust, 1994). Until the Home Office confirms a person's status as a refugee, their future and that of their dependants is uncertain. The status and rights of any children of asylum seekers born in the UK depend on those of their parents.

A person who has been granted refugee status may apply to bring in their family immediately (though the process may then take a long time), and may apply for settlement after four years. A person who has been granted Exceptional Leave to Remain (ELR) may apply to bring in their family after four years, and may apply for settlement after seven years (Refugee Council, 1992). The family is defined in Western European cultural terms, that is, as spouse and dependent children. It does not include adult children, parents and other people whom many refugees regard as their close family.

Increasingly strict laws to control the numbers of asylum seekers coming have been passed in Britain since the beginning of the twentieth century. Current legislation in this area is extremely tight and probably cannot be tightened any further without contravening international law. Under the Asylum and Immigration (Appeals) Act 1993, people who have travelled through a 'safe' country since leaving their home can be refused asylum and immediately deported back there. There is no guarantee that they will not then be deported back to the country from which they first had to flee. Although this practice is not acceptable under the terms of the Geneva Convention, according to Refugee Council statistics in the last six months of 1993 Britain deported 745 asylum seekers under the terms of this act.

The 1993 Act also introduced restrictions on the rights of people applying for refugee status, and measures designed to reduce the numbers of asylum seekers. People from 'refugee-producing countries' coming to or passing through Britain must have valid entry documents. Airlines and other carriers are deterred from bringing people into the UK without such documents by a summary fine of £2,000 per person. This makes it impossible for most people fleeing persecution and torture to get to Britain to ask for asylum, since, by definition, most are unable to obtain such documents without risking their lives. Asylum seekers who miss two interviews with the Asylum Screening Unit may be refused refugee status and deported even if, for example, they simply have not received the appointment letters.

Such treatment by the authorities increases the fear and insecurity under which many asylum seekers and refugees live. Many are resentful and hostile as a result of their own experience and that of their families and friends.

Diversity of background and experience

People have come to Britain seeking asylum throughout history, and in the 1990s come from a wider range of countries than ever (Table 27.1). Despite their shared legal status they are clearly not one homogeneous group. They come from many different areas of the world, cultures and religious groups. Some come from urban areas, some from rural, some are intellectuals, some are political activists, some simply belong to a religious or ethnic group that is being persecuted and murdered. Many refugees have been in Britain for many years; others have just arrived. A few have lived here for years and then suddenly become refugees because they cannot return home (Finlay and Reynolds, 1987). Some people have been granted refugee status and know that they can stay; others are waiting for their status to be decided and live in constant uncertainty and worry. Most newly arrived refugees settle in London since this is where the majority of refugee advice and support services are situated and where they are most likely to find other people of their own community.

Table 27.1 Origin of refugees and asylum seekers entering Britain

Period of immigration	Main countries of origin	Approx. numbers
c. 1880–1914	Eastern Europe (esp. Russian Empire)[a]	2 500 per year
1930s–1940s	Germany[a]	–
Post-1945	Poland Other Eastern Europe[b]	200 000 50 000
1956	Hungary	15 000
1968	Czechoslovakia	5 000
1972	Uganda[c]	30 000
1973	Chile	3 000
1970s–1980s	Vietnam Iran Poland	19 000 20 000 1 500
1980s–present	Iran, Turkey (Kurds), Iraq, Ghana, Palestine, Ethiopia, Eritrea, Afghanistan, Sri Lanka, Zaire, Somalia, India, Pakistan, Sudan, Uganda, Rumania, Togo, Ivory Coast, Yugoslavia	–[d]

[a] Mostly Jewish people: many deported from Britain under anti-alien legislation (see Foot, 1965).
[b] Workers allowed into Britain to help with post-war reconstruction.
[c] Expelled Ugandan Asians, many with British passports.
[d] See Refugee Council, 1992.

A survey conducted by the Home Office Research and Planning Unit in 1994 found that most people seeking asylum in Britain were urban in origin with good educational backgrounds, often with a degree or a professional qualification. The survey also found that most refugees were unable to use their skills and experience in Britain. Over half had never been able to get paid employment in Britain and a third had had only a series of patchy temporary unskilled jobs. The report stated that 'overall there is a wealth of talent and skills among refugees in Britain that is failing to be employed to good effect ... this is to the detriment of the whole country, refugees and non-refugees alike' (Runnymede Trust, 1994).

REFUGEES AND MATERNITY CARE: PSYCHOLOGICAL AND PRACTICAL ISSUES

Before a refugee leaves their own country, there may be little time to think or to express their shock, terror and grief. These may only emerge once they are physically safe, or at a crucial event such as the birth of a new baby. Many refugees have experienced or witnessed intimidation, violence, torture and rape and have been emotionally if not physically scarred by the events that led to their flight. Many are bereaved by the loss of the lives they have known, their friends and close family and familiar surroundings. Many worry about those they have left behind. Arriving in the UK brings initial relief and safety. But this may be undermined by experiences of hostility and suspicion, racism and racial violence, poverty and isolation. Depression and anxiety are common among refugees and asylum seekers. Some also experience the symptoms of post traumatic stress disorder (Beiser, 1990). Support and help are essential if people are to overcome the enormous problems they face and be able to nurture and support a new family member.

> ' ... people coming here had the problem of a civil war at home; people had been traumatised and lost everything; moved from their home without warning; lost friends; lost environment; lost loved ones. Those who were lucky enough to come here, when they knew they were coming to the UK were full of hope. They thought they would forget all problems behind. But when they came here in fact the more problems started ... the promised land is not here, it is not there! ... They ended up in the inner city ... yesterday's refugee is tomorrow's ghetto dweller. This is all very sad because you don't see any way to run away from the situation ... they are on their way to this situation!'   Somali refugee (from Amidu, 1994, by permission)

Asylum seekers waiting for a decision on whether they can stay also face complete uncertainty about their future. They cannot plan ahead in any way or take any steps to improve their situation. They cannot begin to make commitments or put down roots. They are not allowed to work. Existing in a kind of pointless limbo is devastating to most people's self-confidence and self-esteem. Some are held in a detention centre or prison for several months while their cases are considered. This is acutely distressing for people who, having fled from oppression and danger to what they hoped would be safety, find themselves imprisoned by their 'host' country. Some attempt suicide.

Women who arrive pregnant or with children are often more isolated and more vulnerable than their male counterparts. Women who have been separated from their husbands and are unsupported face particular problems. Women with children are often so pre-occupied with their children's needs that they do not seek help in dealing with their own needs. Of all immigrants, refugees and asylum seekers generally have the least support. Many have no family or community to whom they can look for companionship or help (Goodburn, 1994). High stress levels are known to affect pregnancy outcomes (Niven, 1992).

Practical issues

Refugees and asylum seekers have to adjust to the practicalities of daily life in a completely different culture. Most also face a language barrier. Health professionals working with clients in this situation may need to take on a wider role which may include helping clients find out about and use the different services and facilities available, ensuring that they are getting all the benefits to which they are entitled, and helping them with the basics of running a home and family in a completely strange place.

Most refugees and all asylum seekers are unemployed, living on low incomes in the most deprived areas (BHAN, 1991; Goodburn, 1994). Housing is a serious problem for almost all of them (Runnymede Trust, 1994). Asylum seekers are usually housed in temporary accommodation with little space or privacy and the additional uncertainty of knowing that they can be moved to a completely different area with little warning. Kitchen facilities are usually poor and often open for only a few hours every day. Often it is impossible to leave food in the kitchen fridge in case it is stolen. It can be very hard for people to prepare nutritious and comforting food (Schott and Henley, 1992).

Both refugees and asylum seekers are entitled to statutory health services, including free medical treatment under the NHS and registration with a GP. Gaining access to services can however be difficult because of language problems and unfamiliarity with the British system (Goodburn, 1994). People living in bed and breakfast hotels may find it particularly difficult to register with a GP since some practices are reluctant to accept patients in temporary accommodation. They may also not know how to change GPs when they are moved on. Many people may not use services appropriately simply because they do not know how. For example, those who do not understand the role of the GP may go straight to an accident and emergency department for minor or chronic problems. Many asylum seekers are reluctant to complain about services or to demand even those benefits to which they are fully entitled in case they jeopardise their chances of being granted refugee status (BHAN, 1991).

Even when accessible care is offered, some women may be distrustful and defensive. Their experiences both before and since they left home may have made them reluctant to give people in authority personal information or to discuss physical or emotional problems. Some women may need special counselling and support to help them overcome memories of traumatic physical and emotional experiences, and also to come to terms with their new situation. Women who have been raped or tortured need extremely sensitive and thoughtful care during examinations and other procedures. Some physical symptoms are the result of torture and may not make sense to health professionals. Specialist advice should be sought (see Useful Addresses).

It is particularly important in such cases to build up a relationship of mutual trust and to try to ensure the greatest possible continuity of care. It is also necessary to be aware of possible cultural and religious issues that may be important for each woman and to find out from her what she needs and wants in relation to her pregnancy and new baby. Where there is a language barrier a professional interpreter will be required (see also Chapter 11). There may, however, be particular issues of confidentiality and security when selecting an interpreter for a refugee or asylum seeker.

USEFUL ADDRESSES

The Refugee Council
3 Bondway
London SW18 1SJ

Refugees Advisers' Support Unit offers advice and information, bulletins, translated leaflets on women's health and other issues.
Community Development Team provides information on locally-based refugee consortia, local refugee-geared health material and initiatives.

Medical Foundation for the Care of Victims of Torture
96–98 Grafton Road
London NW5

Range of professional services, including consultation, counselling for people who have been tortured, training for professionals, uses in-house trained interpreters.

Immigration Law Practitioners Association (ILPA)
115 Old Street
London EC1V 9JR

In every culture there are people who use substances which may affect their health and the well-being of their unborn children. The effects of substances that are commonly used within the general population, such as tobacco and alcohol, are well documented elsewhere. This chapter focuses on three substances used by some people of certain cultural or religious minority groups.

Attitudes to substance use

Most people consider it risky to take any unnecessary drugs during pregnancy. People who use illegal and other substances are often stigmatised and marginalised. Women who are pregnant and who misuse substances face additional social disapproval and are often terrified that their children might be removed. For many women of black and minority ethnic groups, this fear is compounded by experiences of discrimination, stereotyping and racism. These may deter them from discussing substance use or from accepting health care.

When substance use is an accepted part of a culture, people may be unaware of any risk and may see no reason to change their habits. Giving up something that is accepted and familiar from one's own culture is especially hard when living in another culture. There may be little motivation to do so if the pressure to change comes from outsiders who may be thought prejudiced or ill-informed. Whatever personal feelings and beliefs health professionals have about substance use, it is important to avoid alienating clients and to maintain good relationships. Sensitivity and a supportive approach are essential if there is well-founded concern for the health of a woman or her unborn child because of substance use.

KHAT/QUAT

Khat (also spelled quat) consists of the leaves of the shrub *Catha edulis,* which is found and used mainly in East Africa and in the Arab peninsula. The leaves contain an amphetamine-like substance and are chewed. In Somalia and most other places chewing khat is mainly an accepted recreation for men, like having a smoke or a drink together. The use of khat by women is often considered socially unacceptable and is less common. Chewing khat is one of the few familiar social activities which people who have been uprooted and traumatised by civil war can maintain. There is no legal prohibition against the importation or use of khat in the UK.

The recreational use of khat does not seem to be harmful. However, over-use seems to depress the appetite, leading to listlessness and malnourishment. Khat is also expensive. Long-term over-use of khat can result in gastric disturbances, male sub-fertility and impotence. In the UK, over-use is mainly a problem among young men seeking asylum who often feel isolated and demoralized because they have nothing to do.

Pregnant women who chew khat may have raised blood pressure and smaller babies (Abdul-Ghani *et al.*, 1987). There is no evidence of increased mortality or morbidity in babies exposed to khat antenatally (Eriksson *et al.*, 1991).

MARIJUANA

The use of ganja, a form of marijuana, is part of Rastafarian religious practice. Marijuana is also used by many non-Rastafarians. It is widely believed to be beneficial and certainly to do far less harm than alcohol (Cashmore, 1992). Because marijuana is illegal in many parts of the world, under-reporting of use is common and it has not been possible to do large-scale, controlled studies on the effects of marijuana during pregnancy.

Although some adverse effects have been reported, the results of those few small studies that have been carried out are conflicting (Brust, 1993; Priest, 1990). Unlike cigarette smoking and high alcohol consumption, there is no conclusive evidence that intra-uterine exposure to marijuana has any long-term effects on the baby (Fried *et al.*, 1992; Husain and Khan, 1985). One small study of poor women in rural Jamaica has suggested that the reduction of psychological stress and physiological symptoms which women associate with marijuana use may actually mitigate any potentially harmful effects (Dreher, 1989). Further research is needed to assess suggested links between maternal marijuana use and low birth weight, and to establish whether marijuana predisposes users to malignant disease. Women who believe that marijuana use is beneficial, for whom it has religious significance, or who gain pleasure or relief from it, are unlikely to give it up.

PAN

Pan is a green leaf, mixed with betel nuts and limestone to which other substances including nuts, grains and tobacco leaves may be added (HEA, 1994). This mixture turns bright red when chewed. Pan chewing is common among men and women in many parts of the Indian sub-continent and South East Asia. There are no legal restrictions on pan or its constituents.

There are various health risks associated with pan chewing. These include tobacco addiction, mouth ulcers and oral cancers. The betel nut contains addictive substances and can cause dizziness and sweating. Studies have shown lower birth weight and delayed skeletal maturity in mice who were exposed to betel antenatally (Sinha and Rao, 1985). A controlled study of the effects of betel on pregnancy outcome in humans showed that the babies of mothers who chewed betel had lower birth weights and a lower incidence of jaundice than the control group (De Costa and Griew, 1982).

Tay–Sachs is a recessive genetic disease causing progressive, degenerative brain disease from the age of six months, resulting in death by the age of three or four. One in twenty-five Ashkenazi Jews (see Chapter 39) carries the disease, compared with one in 250 of the non-Jewish population. Carriers are perfectly healthy and there may be no history of Tay–Sachs disease in their family. The child of two carriers has a one in four chance of developing Tay–Sachs disease.

Since the 1980s there has been an active campaign to raise awareness of Tay–Sachs disease within the Jewish community, and to encourage young people of Jewish descent to be screened before marriage and before pregnancy. This is especially important for Orthodox Jews because they are unlikely to accept a termination of pregnancy if the baby is found to have the disease (see Chapter 39). In communities where marriages are arranged, the families of young people who have been tested and found to be Tay–Sachs carriers can prevent introductions to potential partners who are also carriers.

Because of the distress and stigma that can be experienced by carriers, some communities have set up a screening programme in which young people are tested but not told the result. Instead, their test results are held in a central file identified by number only. Before a couple is introduced with a view to marriage, their numbers are checked. If they are both carriers the introduction is not made.

Screening in pregnancy

A pregnant woman who is Jewish or whose partner is Jewish should be asked if she and her partner have been screened for Tay–Sachs. If not, screening should be offered simultaneously to both partners. If both partners are carriers they should be offered specialist genetic counselling. The choices that a couple make will depend on their degree of religious observance and their individual views. Some may choose to take the risk of having an affected child. Others may opt for chorionic villus sampling or amniocentesis with a view to termination if the baby is affected.

References and further reading

INTRODUCTION

Dornhorst, A., Paterson, C., Nicholls, J. *et al.* (1992) High prevalence of gestational diabetes in women from ethnic minority groups. *Diabetic Medicine* **9**, 820–25

Kaplan, N. (1994) Ethnic aspects of hypertension. *Lancet,* **344**, 450–52

Krieger, N. (1990) Racial and gender discrimination: risk factors for high blood pressure. *Social Science Medicine* **30**(12), 1273–81

Kumar, P. and Clark, M. (1994) *Clinical Medicine,* Baillière Tindall, London

Mather, H. and Keen, H. (1985) The Southall Diabetes Survey: prevalence of known diabetes in Asians and Europeans. *British Medical Journal,* **291**, 1081–84

Samanta, A., Burden, A. and Fent, B. (1987) Comparative prevalence of non-insulin-dependent diabetes mellitus in Asian and White Caucasian adults. *Diabetes Research and Clinical Practice,* **4**, 1–6

Samanta, A., Burden, M., Burden, A. and Jones, G. (1989) Glucose tolerance during pregnancy in Asian women. *Diabetes Research and Clinical Practice,* **7**, 127–35

24 FEMALE CIRCUMCISION – FEMALE GENITAL MUTILATION

Adamson, F. (undated) *Female Genital Mutilation: Counselling Guide for Professionals,* FORWARD, London (see Useful Addresses)

Dorkenoo, E. and Elworthy, S. (1993) *First Study Conference of Genital Mutilation of Girls in Europe,* FORWARD, London

Dorkenoo, E. and Elworthy, S. (1994) *Female Genital Mutilation: Proposals for Change,* Minority Rights Group, London

Hedley, R. and Dorkenoo, E. (1992) *Child Protection and Female Genital Mutilation: Advice for Health, Education and Social Work Professionals,* FORWARD, London

Hosken, F. P. (1994) *Genital/Sexual Mutilation of Females,* 4th edn, Women's International Network, Lexington, Mass., USA

Jordan, J. (1994) Female genital mutilation (female circumcision). *British Journal of Obstetrics and Gynaecology,* **101**, 94–95

Ladjali, M., Rattray, T. and Walder, R. (1993) Female genital mutilation. *British Medical Journal,* **307**, 460

RCN (1994) *Female Genital Mutilation, the Unspoken Issue,* Royal College of Nursing, London (Order No. 000353)

25 HAEMOGLOBINOPATHIES

Anionwu, E. (1993) Sickle cell and thalassaemia: community experiences and official response. In *'Race' and Health in Contemporary Britain* (ed. W. I. U. Ahmad), Open University Press, Buckingham.

Anionwu, E. (1994) Women and sickle cell disorders. In *Healthy and Wise: the Essential Health Handbook for Black Women*, Virago, London

Consumers Association (1989) Sickle cell disease and the non-specialist. *Drugs and Therapeutics Bulletin*, **27**(3), 9–12

Davies, S. (1986) Comprehensive care for sickle cell disease. *THS Health Summary* **3**(12), 7

Department of Health (1993) *Report of a Working Party of the Standing Medical Advisory Committee on Sickle Cell, Thalassaemia and Other Haemoglobinopathies*, HMSO, London

Eboh, W. and Van den Akker, O. (1994) Antenatal care of women with sickle cell disease. *British Journal of Midwifery*, **21**, 6–11

Howard, R. (1994) Contraception and sickle cell disease. *IPPF Medical Bulletin*, **28**(4), 3–4

Midence, K., Davies, S. and Fuggle, P. (1992) Courage in the face of crisis. *Nursing Times*, **88**(22), 46–8

Modell, B. and Berdoukas, V. (1984) *The Clinical Approach to Thalassaemia*, Grune and Stratton, London

NHS Management Executive (1994) *Asian Women and Maternity Services*, Department of Health, London

Searjeant, G. R. (1992) *Sickle Cell Disease*, 2nd edn, Oxford University Press, Oxford

Sickle Cell Society (n.d.) *A Handbook on Sickle Cell Disease: a Guide for Families*, Sickle Cell Society, London

Vallerand, A. (1994) Street addicts and patients with pain: similarities and differences. *Clinical Nurse Specialist*, **8**(1), 11–15

26 HIV AND AIDS

Aston, J. (1993) *The Construction of Pregnant Women and HIV*. MA thesis (unpublished), London University

Banatvala, J. and Chrystie, I. (1994) HIV screening in pregnancy: UK lags. *Lancet*, **343**, 1113

BHAN (1991) *AIDS and the Black Communities: Policy Report 1*, Black HIV and AIDS Network, London (see Useful Addresses)

Chin, J. (1990) Current and future dimensions of the HIV/AIDS pandemic in women and children. *The Lancet*, **336**, 221–4

Davison, C. F., Holland, F. J., Newell, M. L., *et al.*, (1993) Screening for HIV infection in pregnancy. *AIDS Care*, **5**, No. 2

Department of Health (1992) *Department of Health Guidance PL/CO(92)5, Appendix 2*, Department of Health, London

Department of Health (1994) *Guidelines for Offering Voluntary Named HIV Anti-body Testing to Women Receiving Antenatal Care*, Department of Health, London

Khan, S. (1994) *Contexts: Race, Culture and Sexuality, as Assessment of Our Communities* NAZ Project, (see Useful Addresses)

Levine, C., and Dubler, N. (1990) HIV and childbearing I. Uncertain risks and bitter realities: the reproductive choices of HIV-infected women. *Millbank Quarterly*, **68**(3), 321–51 (Millbank Memorial Fund, London)

Mercey, D., Bewley, S. and Brocklehurst, P. (1993) *A Guide to HIV Infection and Childbearing*, AVERT (see Useful Addresses)

Patton, C. (1990) *Inventing AIDS*, Routledge, New York and London

Positively Women (1994) *Women Like Us: a Survey on the Needs and Experiences of HIV Positive Women*, Positively Women (see Useful Addresses)

Rahman, T. A. (1994) *AIDS and the Muslim Communities*, The Naz Project (see Useful Addresses)

Shepherd, C. (1994) *HIV Infection in Pregnancy*, Books for Midwives Press, Cheshire

27 REFUGEES AND ASYLUM SEEKERS

Amidu, E. (1994) *Somali refugees in London's East End: An investigation into livelihood*, MSc dissertation, University of London (Unpublished)

Beiser, M. (1990) Migration: opportunity or mental health risk? *Triangle, Sandoz Journal of Medical Science*, **29**(2/3), 83–90 (Sandoz Medical Publications, Basel, Switzerland) **29**(2/3), 83–90

BHAN (1991) *AIDS and the Black Communities*, Black HIV and AIDS Network (see Useful Addresses)

Finlay, R. and Reynolds, J. (1987) *Social Work and Refugees: a Handbook on Working with People in Exile in the UK*, National Extension College, Cambridge

Goodburn, A. (1994) A place of greater safety. *Nursing Times*, **90**(28), 46–8

Mares, P. (1982) *The Vietnamese in Britain: a Handbook for Health Workers*, National Extension College, Cambridge

Niven, C. (1992) *Psychological Care for Families Before, During and After Birth*, Butterworth-Heinemann, Oxford

Refugee Council (1992) *UK Asylum Statistics 1982–92*, Refugee Council, London

Runnymede Trust (1994) Refugees: Home Office research. *The Runnymede Bulletin*, July/August p. 8

Schott, J. and Henley, A. (1992) *Breaking the Barriers – a Training Package on Equal Access to Maternity Services*, Obstetric Hospital, University College London Hospitals NHS Trust, London

Spencer, S. (1994) *Strangers and Citizens: a Positive Approach to Migrants and Refugees*, Institute for Public Policy Research/Rivers Oram, London

28 SUBSTANCE USE

Abdul-Ghani, N., Eriksson, M., Kristiansson, B. and Qirbi, A. (1987) The influence of khat-chewing on birth-weight in full-term infants. *Social Science Medicine*, **24**(7), 625–7

Brust, C.(1993) *Neurological Aspects of Substance Abuse*, Butterworth-Heinemann, Oxford

Cashmore, E. (1992) *The Rastafarians*, Minority Rights Group, London

De Costa, C. and Griew, A. (1982) The effects of betel chewing on pregnancy outcome. *Australian and New Zealand Journal of Obstetrics and Gynaecology*, **1**, 22–4

Dreher, M.C. (1989) Poor and pregnant: perinatal ganga use in rural Jamaica. *Advances in Alcohol and Substance Abuse*, **8**, 45–64

Eriksson, M., Abdul-Ghani, N. and Kristiansson, B. (1991) Khat chewing during pregnancy, effect on the off-spring and some characteristics of the chewers. *East African Medical Journal*, **68**(2), 106–11

Fried, P.A., O'Connell, C.M. and Watkinson, B. (1992) 60 and 72-month follow-up of children prenatally exposed to marijuana, cigarettes and alcohol: Cognitive and language assessments. *Journal of Developmental and Behavioural Pediatrics*, **6**, 383–91

HEA (1994) *Black and Minority Ethnic Groups in England: Health and Lifestyles*, Health Education Authority, London

Husain, S. and Khan, I. (1985) An update on cannabis research. *Bulletin of Narcotics*, **37**, 3–13

Priest, J. (1990) *Drugs in Pregnancy and Childbirth*, Pandora Press, Unwin Hyman Books, London

Sinha, A. and Rao, A. (1985) Embryotoxicity of betel nuts in mice. *Toxicology*, **37**(3–4), 315–26

29 TAY–SACHS DISEASE

Ellis, I. (1991) Carrier screening for Tay–Sachs. *Nursing*, **4**(41), 16–18

Feldman Paritzky, J. (1985) Tay–Sachs: the dreaded inheritance. *American Journal of Nursing*, **85**, 26–4

Part Five

Specific Cultures and Religions

INTRODUCTION

This section looks at five cultures and seven religions in relation to daily living and childbearing issues. The information it contains may be relevant, in varying degrees, to clients and their families who identify themselves as belonging to one of these.

We are only too aware that there is a fine balance between what may be considered 'useful information' and damaging generalisations. Writing anything about the beliefs, practices and needs of different groups is like walking a tightrope. We are conscious of the ever-present danger of reinforcing myths, prejudices and stereotypes. On the other hand, we have found that our own thinking and our understanding of the way that culture and religion work in people's lives, as well as our understanding of practical ways of improving care, have been enhanced by learning more about specific cultures and religions and about how people see them from the inside. But this process must start with ourselves. Reflecting on our own personal beliefs, values and practices enables us to respond respectfully and flexibly to those of other people. This section is only valuable or valid if it is read in this light and with this understanding. **So, if you have turned to this section without first reading the rest of the book and, in particular, Parts One and Three, it is very important that you turn back to the beginning and read the earlier sections first.** You will also find that Parts One and Three deal in more detail with many of the themes that are, to avoid duplication, outlined only briefly below.

Most of the content of the following chapters is based on what we have learnt or confirmed during our meetings with women, and some men, of different cultural and religious groups. We have included Christianity among the religions because it is as inappropriate to assume that all health professionals know about Christianity as it is to assume that they all know about Islam or Judaism. We have chosen five traditional cultures on the basis of the numbers of people who may be influenced by them in the UK, or because they cover specific issues relevant to health and maternity care. We have discussed traditional South Asian culture in some detail, both because people of South Asian heritage make up the largest minority ethnic group in the UK, and also because in many ways traditional South Asian culture illustrates very clearly some of the greatest contrasts with current Western European culture, values and lifestyles.

In some cases ethnic identity and religious identity overlap. For example, most, though not all, people of Pakistani heritage are Muslims. However, most major world religions, by definition, include people of many different cultural heritages. It is no more possible or useful to generalise about Somalis, Hindus or African-Caribbeans than to generalise about English people or Europeans. Cultures that outsiders may assume to be unified and similar are often extremely diverse. Particular beliefs, practices, values and traditions may be more important to some people than to others. People in rural isolated areas may have very different values, ways of life and traditions than those in urban areas. When people migrate they maintain certain aspects of their culture but may adapt or lose others. The children and grandchildren of immigrants may feel very strongly about certain aspects of their heritage and may reject others, or may find them irrelevant. Within each community each person will have specific individual needs. It is extremely important not to categorise people, to make assumptions or to generalise. Culture is a framework, not a straitjacket (see Chapter 1).

We have written in this section about Judaism, not Jews, about traditional Chinese culture, not Chinese people. Not everyone will identify with what we have written about Judaism or Chinese culture, but we offer a framework for understanding some of the factors that may be important to some people. We make no apology for including frequent reminders that the only way to provide high quality care is to find out from each person about her own needs and wishes.

'Behind any label is an individual human being who can think and speak for herself. Listen to her, give her time and space, don't assume you know what she needs or wants.' Director of midwifery education

30 **Traditional African-Caribbean culture**

INTRODUCTION

The term African-Caribbean is used here to mean people whose families are of mainly African descent and came to Britain from the West Indies in the Caribbean. Some people use the historical term West Indian. Others may refer to themselves as Black, Black British or Afro-Caribbean. This chapter discusses those aspects of traditional African-Caribbean culture which **may** be important to some people in Britain whose families originated in the Caribbean. For specifically religious traditions and practices see the relevant chapters.

The West Indies

The West Indies is made up of more than twenty-two countries, mainly islands or groups of islands, which stretch over a 2,000 mile curve from near the southern tip of Florida to Guyana on the mainland of South America. Each country has a different history and its own distinct culture.

The Caribbean is a multiracial society, the majority of people being the descendants of Africans who were removed by force from their homes in West Africa in the seventeenth and eighteenth centuries and transported to work as slaves on sugar plantations in the Caribbean. At that time sugar was extremely valuable and a source of great wealth for the plantation owners. During the eighteenth and nineteenth centuries people from southern China and from southern India were also brought to the West Indies as indentured labourers to perform various functions under the British and other colonial governments. The cultures of the Caribbean are therefore extremely diverse and many Caribbean people are also of South Asian, Chinese, European or mixed heritages.

Although most of the West Indian countries that had been part of the British Empire obtained their independence in the 1960s and 70s, their economic dependence on and links with Britain remained strong, since their economies had been based entirely on British needs. Their systems of government, schools, police and judiciary were also based on British systems. Many people in the West Indies were brought up to think of Britain as the mother country, caring, responsible and welcoming towards her subjects of all races. The political and cultural climate has changed considerably in the Caribbean over the past thirty years and most countries now have stronger local links, in particular with the USA (Coombe, 1986).

Traditional African-Caribbean culture is very much influenced by the history of its people and by the strengths needed to survive appalling cruelty, injustice and hardship. It is also influenced by the many different cultures from which its people originated and by the experience of being part of the British Empire and of a British-run colonial system for almost 300 years.

Emigration to the UK

The main period of African-Caribbean immigration occurred in the 1950s and early 1960s. People from the West Indies arrived in Britain to work in the burgeoning post-war reconstruction industries and in the public services. Some had fought with the Allies in the Second World War and stayed on in Britain to provide desperately needed labour. Others were recruited through special government and private recruitment programmes. London Transport, the British Hotels and Restaurants Association and other employers sent recruiters out to the West Indies to fill vacancies in the UK (Peach, 1968). In the early 1960s the National Health Service recruited African-Caribbean nurses and midwives with the active support of Enoch Powell, then Conservative Minister of Health (Larbie et al., 1987).

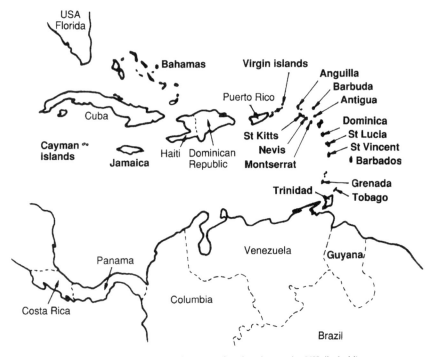

Figure 30.1 The Caribbean, showing main areas of emigration to the UK (in bold)

People came to Britain from various parts of the Caribbean, including in particular Jamaica (the largest number), Guyana on the South American mainland, Trinidad and Tobago, and Barbados (see Figure 30.1). Because of the very strong historical and cultural differences between the different Caribbean countries, people tended to settle and socialise separately during the early days. Unlike most other immigrant groups, a large number of African-Caribbean women came on their own to find work, sometimes leaving children in the care of other relatives until they were able to send for them.

British-born

Well over half the African-Caribbeans in the UK were born and brought up here and are the children and grandchildren of the immigrant generation. A key issue for British African-Caribbeans is the experience of persistent racial discrimination (see Chapter 4).

Despite the fact that most people of African-Caribbean heritage are British-born, there are certain practical aspects of traditional African-Caribbean culture which **may** still be important to some people. **Since it is not possible to predict to whom they will and will not be important, the only way to find out is by listening sensitively to each individual and asking when appropriate.**

LANGUAGE

In the West Indies most older people speak a patois; a complete language that combines features of the vocabulary, grammar and intonation of West African languages and, depending on the island, of English, French or Spanish. There is a good deal of variation in the patois of different islands. Until relatively recently, patois was often frowned upon as being the language of the 'less educated' and many parents discouraged their children from speaking it. Some older British African-Caribbeans still feel uncomfortable about the use of patois. The official written language of most West Indian countries is English, though this may be influenced to some extent by the local patois.

Many British African-Caribbeans are bilingual, speaking a form of patois at home and with friends, and standard English at work or with non-African-Caribbean friends. Since patois is not normally written it is very flexible and open to new influences. Patois as spoken by younger British African-Caribbeans often has special features that mark it out from a traditional West Indian patois. It is sometimes referred to as Black English (Sutcliffe, 1982). (See also Chapters 8 and 40.)

TRADITIONAL FAMILY STRUCTURES AND RELATIONSHIPS

There is a wide diversity of family patterns in the Caribbean, depending to some extent on factors such as class, family heritage and religion. There is historically a relatively high proportion of lone-parent families and families where the parents are not married. This has as its basis the systematic and calculated destruction of the African family system in the West Indies over a period of 200 years by white slave-owners. Slaves were not allowed to marry. Husbands were forcibly separated from their wives, parents from their children, and siblings from each other. African slaves were also used as breeding stock and for the sexual satisfaction of their white masters (Hiro, 1973). When slavery was abolished in the early nineteenth century most ex-slaves were turned out of their 'homes' and were without work. Once the 'free' labour on which the sugar plantations had depended was no longer available, the economy of the islands collapsed and has remained in most cases poor. Many men had to emigrate to other islands or to the American mainland to find work. Women were not able to rely on men for security or financial support for themselves and their children.

Traditional West Indian society is therefore strongly matriarchal, with mothers, grandmothers and other female relatives often forming the core of the family and providing advice and strong practical and emotional support, especially around pregnancy, childbirth and the care of children. Female family support remains important for many African-Caribbean women in Britain. Older female relatives may expect to have a major say in, for example, the care of a new-born baby. Many girls are brought up to be independent and self-sufficient and not to rely on men for practical and emotional support and protection. Nevertheless, both in Britain and in the West Indies there is now increasing involvement of men with their families.

Marriage   Marriage is traditionally a serious and responsible step and the confirmation of a long association. In the West Indies, once a couple are married, the husband is generally considered responsible for the support of his wife and children. Some couples therefore only marry when they have lived together for many years and have children. A wedding may be a large and expensive celebration and therefore a major expense for which a couple may save for several years (Mares *et al.*, 1985).

Views on marriage and children within the British African-Caribbean community are likely to vary a good deal, particularly in view of changing attitudes and expectations in the majority community. In some cases a single woman who becomes pregnant, especially if she is very young, may be seen as bringing shame on her family and community and letting down her parents who have worked hard to provide her with chances that they did not have. Although most parents accept and support a young woman in such a situation, some may reject her (Larbie, 1985). As in traditional English society, class and religion influence people's views about marriage. Middle-class African-Caribbean people may be more likely to feel that it is important that a couple should be married before they have children. Many Christians and Muslims also hold traditional views about cohabitation and marriage.

RELIGION

Many African-Caribbeans are Christians belonging to many different denominations: Pentecostalists, Seventh Day Adventists, Anglicans, Baptists, Methodists and Roman Catholics. In Britain, African-Caribbean people may join black-led Pentecostalist churches, often because they feel unwelcome in 'white' churches and find them too conservative. Some people are also very aware of the role of the older-established churches in the history of European colonialism.

A large number of Jehovah's Witnesses in the UK are of African-Caribbean descent. A small but increasing number of young African-Caribbeans are Rastafarians, or are influenced by Rastafarism. Some are Muslims. (See the chapters on these religions below.)

CARIBBEAN FOODS AND DIETS

Food is very important in traditional African-Caribbean culture. A great deal of emphasis is placed on eating a healthy nutritious diet, and putting good food on the table may be a family's first priority. Sharing food brings families together and is a vital part of family life.

Caribbean cooking methods and ingredients have been influenced by the diets of many areas, including West Africa, Western Europe, China and India. There is a good deal of variation in flavours and cooking methods between the different islands. The main staple starches are yams, sweet potatoes, rice, breadfruit and plantain. Fish is traditionally a major source of animal protein and the seas surrounding the West Indian islands are full of many kinds of tropical fish. Fish and red meat or chicken are often marinated with herbs and spices before cooking. Tropical fruits and vegetables form an important part of the traditional diet but some of these are expensive in Britain. The main pulses used are kidney beans, black-eyed peas, gunga peas and split peas. Many traditional dishes are baked or stewed. (Hill, 1990; Mares *et al.*, 1985). Food is generally spicy and even many British-born African-Caribbeans find British hospital food bland and unhealthy (Larbie, 1985).

In the West Indies there is a strong emphasis on a balanced diet, and on traditional herbal and dietary remedies for common conditions. Although much of this is now dying out, certain traditions are still strong and may influence some African-Caribbean women in Britain. For example, some women may eat green bananas as a source of iron during pregnancy and may drink nutritious drinks such as milk mixed with stout. Some African-Caribbean women may also follow specific religious food restrictions.

PHYSICAL CARE

As with most people whose families originated in hot climates, physical cleanliness and frequent washing are very important. Most people are accustomed to showering or bathing and changing their clothes frequently. Many women prefer to wash and change before attending a clinic. Black or dark skin is often prone to dryness and can easily become uncomfortable especially in areas with hard water. Most people rub oil or moisturiser into their skin after washing to keep it supple and smooth. Many parents oil their babies' skin after a bath.

In hospital some African-Caribbean women may find the washing facilities inadequate and feel that they are not keeping themselves as clean as they would wish. It is particularly important to be able to wash frequently after giving birth. Women who are unwell may need help with applying moisturiser. It is traditional in the West Indies to add an antiseptic to the bath water.

PREGNANCY ISSUES

Antenatal care and education   Pregnancy is traditionally regarded as a normal process during which women are expected to maintain their everyday routines. Female family members and friends are often an important source of information and support. Although most young British-born women of African-Caribbean heritage are perfectly familiar with the idea of antenatal classes they may be reluctant to attend; they may fear feeling conspicuous as the only black woman there, or may feel excluded by the cultural assumptions and norms that are likely to underlie the classes.

Some people may try to avoid focusing on anything negative during pregnancy. It may be important to be sensitive to this during antenatal classes and clinics (see Chapter 19).

Antenatal screening   The increased incidence of hypertension and diabetes in people of African-Caribbean descent means that it is important to check for these carefully antenatally (see also the Introduction to this section). Haemoglobinopathies are also relatively common among people of African-Caribbean descent (see Chapter 25).

LABOUR AND BIRTH

Traditionally labour and birth are considered natural processes which women usually accept with stoicism and little pain relief. Support is provided by older women in the family and, until recently, most people in the West Indies had their babies at home. Younger African-Caribbean women in Britain are, however, likely to have very much the same attitudes and expectations as their white contemporaries. Husbands and partners are increasingly likely to wish to be present during labour and birth. Some women may want their mother or a female friend as well.

In traditional African-Caribbean culture it is generally far more acceptable for people to express and show how they are feeling than in, for example, traditional English culture. Some women may be expressive and noisy during labour. It is important neither to assume that this indicates an urgent need for pain relief, nor that it is merely an expression of feelings and does not (see also Chapter 20).

Some women of African descent have a pronounced tilt to their pelvis and it may therefore be particularly important to remain upright and mobile as far as possible during labour (see Chapter 20). There is a high rate of spontaneous multiple births among women of African descent.

POSTNATAL CARE

Rest and recovery   Traditionally women are expected to rest for two weeks after the birth and to avoid anything that might cause a chill. Few women in Britain follow this tradition, though older relatives may encourage them to. A few women may not wash their hair for some days after the birth.

In traditional African-Caribbean culture, some women do not handle or cook certain foods while bleeding after giving birth or while menstruating. Although it is difficult to follow such traditions in Britain, some women may still wish to. Most couples avoid sexual intercourse until the woman has stopped bleeding.

Feeding the baby   Breast feeding is traditionally regarded as best for the baby. Bottle-fed babies may occasionally be given diluted evaporated or condensed milk, a custom that arose in the Caribbean when refrigeration was scarce.

Eye infections in the baby are traditionally treated by squirting a little breast milk into the eye.

Contraception   Historically in the Caribbean families were large, though family size is now falling. Women are traditionally responsible for contraception and methods are generally a matter of personal choice and religion. A few women may believe that breast feeding provides protection against conception (see also Chapter 21).

CHILDBEARING LOSSES

Infertility   In African-Caribbean culture fertility is traditionally important for both women and men. Infertility is stigmatized. For some people it may be important to prove their fertility by having a baby before they enter into marriage or a permanent relationship. Some women may fear that their partners will leave them if they are infertile. Men may fear that they will not be able to develop a permanent relationship or be seen as a real man. They may become anxious and may sometimes refuse to consider the possibility that they are 'at fault'. Both men and women are likely to need very sensitive support and understanding if infertility is suspected. Strict confidentiality is essential.

Miscarriage, stillbirth and neonatal death   Requirements when a baby dies during pregnancy or around the time of birth will vary a good deal depending on religion, family and community traditions, and personal preferences. As always, bereaved parents will need full information about their choices, and support and time to decide what is best for them.

DEATH OF AN ADULT

Some of this may also apply in the case of a miscarriage, stillbirth and neonatal death, but there are usually significant differences. It is always important to check everything with the parents.

In the West Indies people are normally buried, though customs are changing in Britain. Mourning and funeral rituals vary between families, communities and religious groups. However, in many communities (except perhaps among Rastafarians, see Chapter 40), funerals are traditionally big events with as many members of the family and friends as possible attending. The body may be brought home before the funeral service so that people can come and pay their last respects. If the family wishes the coffin may also be kept open in the church during the early part of the funeral ceremony. Family members may wish to fill in the grave themselves. In some families relatives gather for nine nights after a death to say prayers for the person who has died (Green, 1992). Some families may wish to fly the body to their country of origin for burial. (See also the chapters on specific religions.)

31 Traditional Akan (Ghanaian) culture

The continent of Africa covers an area of nearly 12 million square miles and has a population of about 500 million people. It contains many different countries, regions, religions, climates, histories, heritages, languages and ways of life. It is clearly impossible to write anything useful about the culture, values and needs of Africans as a group, just

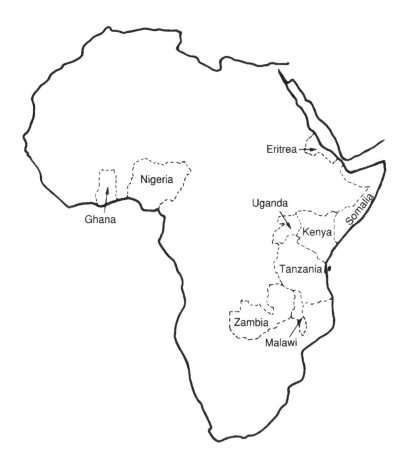

Figure 31.1 Africa, showing the main countries of emigration to the UK

as it is impossible to write anything useful about the culture, values and needs of Europeans, who inhabit a land mass of only about 4.5 million square miles. We have chosen to focus on two African cultures: the traditional Akan culture and, in Chapter 33, traditional Somali culture. The Akan people form the largest group within Ghana, from where the largest number of African people in the UK originated.

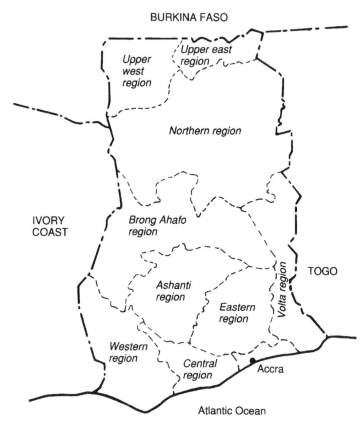

Figure 31.2 The regions of Ghana

Table 31.1   The languages of Ghana

Region	Language
Upper West region	Fafra
Upper East region	Moshie
Northern region	Hausa and Dabgani
Brong Ahafo region	Brong (like broken Twi)
Western region	Ahanta, Nzema
Ashanti region	Twi
Eastern region	Twi, Kwawv, Akim and Akwapim
Volta region	Ewe, Krobo and Ada
Central region	Fanti and Efutu
Accra	Ga

Ghana

Ghana lies on the west coast of Africa on the Gulf of Guinea. It was formerly known as the Gold Coast, became a British colony in the late 1800s and gained independence in 1957. Ghana is divided into ten regions. Each of the tribes living within the different regions has their own values, beliefs, culture, customs and way of life.

Because of the diversity of religions, languages, cultures and traditions in Ghana, it is not possible to describe 'Ghanaian culture' with any degree of accuracy. This chapter focuses mainly on traditional Akan culture, the tribe to which the majority of Ghanaians belong. Most Akans live in parts of the Eastern and Central regions and in the Ashanti region. **The extent to which an individual woman of Akan heritage and her family in Britain follow these traditions will vary. Since it is not possible to predict to whom they will and will not be important, the only way to find out is by listening sensitively to each individual and asking when appropriate.**

Emigration to the UK

People from Ghana came to the UK mainly between the late 1950s and the early 1980s. Most came as students to study medicine, dentistry, law, engineering or accountancy, or to train as nurses, midwives, caterers and pharmacists. Many Ghanaians have lived in the UK for much of their lives, and a growing number of people of Ghanaian heritage were born here. More recently a few Ghanaians have come to Britain seeking asylum (see also Chapter 27).

LANGUAGES

Ghana is a multilingual country with eight different languages. There are also a large number of different dialects.

English is the official national language and is used for administration and bureaucracy. People from different regions who do not share a common language speak English with each other. English is taught in all schools and most people who come to the UK speak English.

THE NAMING SYSTEM

The name order is similar to the British system, with the surname last. When a woman marries she keeps her own family name. It is therefore important to ask and record her husband's name so that he can be properly addressed (see Chapter 14).

The baby is given the father's family name. Traditionally it is the father's prerogative to choose the baby's personal name which is given at the naming ceremony (see below).

TRADITIONAL FAMILY STRUCTURE AND RELATIONSHIPS

The role of women   Most Ghanaian women, like other women in West Africa, have a great deal of autonomy and control over their own lives. They run businesses, own land and conduct financial transactions such as buying property without needing to defer to their husbands. Ghanaian women may feel restricted and insulted by attitudes to women in the UK in relation to independence, money, business and obtaining a mortgage.

'The thing I found hardest was adapting to the marriage culture of the British where the husband controls the finances of the family and the wife is an extension of the man. And also the problems working mothers have with child-care facilities.'   Akan mother of two

Puberty   A woman's fertility and potential for motherhood is considered very important and is a source of pride. In Akan culture, a girl's first menstrual period is usually marked with ritual and celebration as it heralds the onset of womanhood. This contrasts strongly with the secrecy and embarrassment common in the UK.

Traditionally, an Akan girl is the first to wash on the morning after her first period starts. The senior women in the family bathe her and teach her about personal hygiene. Ritual food is prepared by boiling and mashing yam, some of which is dyed yellow with palm oil. The yellow and the white yam are mixed to symbolise an egg, and are shaped into a ball into which a hard-boiled egg is inserted. This food symbolises fertility and fruitfulness.

When she has washed, the girl sits down facing the senior woman of the family. The next girl due to reach puberty sits behind her. The senior woman throws the yam containing the egg over the shoulder of the newly initiated girl to the young girl behind her. The latter eats the yam as a preparation for her own approaching womanhood and fertility.

In the evening it is traditional for the family to eat a celebration meal. They may also hold a ceremony in which the young woman is dressed in her best and presented in public.

Once a girl has reached puberty she is respected as an adult and is given more responsibility in preparation for her future role as a mother. She may also be given a sum of money so that she can start trading or learning a skill in order to support herself.

Marriage   The ability to have children is part of people's self-esteem in traditional West African culture, and proving fertility may be very important for both men and women. Marriage may take place after a child is born. Married couples do not always live together. Traditionally they take joint responsibility for the children, the father being the provider and the mother the carer. In traditional Akan culture, an aspiring husband asks the bride's parents for her hand and pays them a dowry. The groom's parents visit the bride's parents three times to request the marriage. Some marriages are arranged, but only if both young people are willing.

Most families have very strong ties. Older people are generally respected, listened to and cared for by their families in their old age. Since it is generally the women who care for elderly relatives, it is important that a bride gets on with her in-laws.

Polygamy is common in Ghana, including among some Christians. Polygamy is not usually practised in the UK, however some married men will also have girlfriends (see Chapter 17).

Visiting people at home   It is considered polite in many Ghanaian households to take off one's shoes at the front door.

RELIGION

Ghana is a mainly Christian country. The main Christian denominations in Ghana are Anglicans, Catholics, Methodists, Pentecostalists and Baptists. Some Ghanaians are Muslim. Some follow traditional African spiritual practices. They worship ancient gods and ancestors and consult their own 'fetish' priests and priestesses.

Festivals   In addition to the different religious festivals, each region has its own festivals, in particular to celebrate the harvest and to mark the changing seasons. These emphasise renewal and encourage people to start each new season with confidence and hope. There are also different traditional rituals to mark important life events such as naming a child, the onset of puberty (see above), marriage, multiple births, the birth of a tenth child and death.

AKAN FOODS AND DIETS

Traditional staple foods in the Akan diet include yams, plantains, cocoyam, maize, corn and rice. Most of the ingredients used in traditional cooking are available in cities in the UK. Fish is eaten, especially by people who originated from coastal areas. Chicken and lamb are also eaten. Some people eat beef and a few eat pork. Food is often spiced with chilli and black pepper.

During pregnancy some Akan women avoid fatty foods in order to reduce nausea. It is traditionally believed that it is important for women to eat the foods they crave during pregnancy. In northern Ghana some women may avoid eggs during pregnancy as they are traditionally believed to cause a difficult labour. This is based on the similarity between egg white and a heavy show.

Fasting   Some women may observe religious fasts. It is also traditional to fast during the forty days of mourning following a death in the family. This may involve restricting food intake rather than abstaining from food and drink altogether.

PHYSICAL CARE

Cleanliness   Most people have a complete wash at least once or twice a day. Many prefer not to sit in a bath of water but to shower or pour water over themselves. After bathing people may oil their skin to keep it supple. They may also oil their scalp and their hair. Some women wrap their heads in a scarf before going to bed in order to avoid getting oil on the bed linen.

Clothing   Many Akan women in the UK wear Western-style clothes. Some prefer to wear traditional dress during labour and in hospital, especially in hot weather. This consists of a blouse and a wrap-around skirt, usually of brightly coloured, patterned cotton. After initiation at puberty (see above) women traditionally wear an additional wrap over the skirt and around the waist. This is similar to the cloth traditionally used to make a carrying sling for a baby, and symbolises a woman's potential for motherhood.

Jewellery   Some Akan women wear weddings rings. Some people may wear charms with religious or protective significance. If there are medical reasons for removing jewellery, permission should always be sought. Items that the woman does not want to remove should be taped.

PREGNANCY ISSUES

Pregnancy is traditionally viewed as normal and healthy. Many women continue working until labour starts.

Antenatal care   Traditionally, women are cared for by their local midwife who is likely to be well known in the community. Often she has delivered several members of the family, sometimes over two generations. In contrast, UK patterns of care may seem unfamiliar and impersonal. Most women are, however, happy to accept the care they are offered.

It is traditional for women not to announce their pregnancy in case something goes wrong, especially if there have been previous childbearing losses. For this reason, some Akan women may not come for care until their pregnancy is well established. Women whose legal status in the UK is uncertain may also be reluctant to seek antenatal care in case their right to be here is questioned.

It is traditional in Akan culture for pregnant women to avoid sitting where someone could walk behind them since this could bring bad luck. A woman may prefer to sit with her back to a wall, and may be unwilling to sit in an open row in a waiting area, or with her back to a door in a consulting or examination room.

Many Akan women prefer to be examined by women. Individual preferences should be respected (see also Chapter 19).

Antenatal screening   Many women are likely to feel very positive towards Western medical practice and to accept whatever is offered without question. However, some may not understand the potential implications of some screening tests. It is important that all women receive clear information about the benefits and drawbacks of screening so that they can make informed decisions about their care (see also Chapter 19).

There is a higher than average incidence of hypertension and diabetes in women of African descent. Haemoglobinopathies, especially as sickle cell anaemia, are common and all women should be counselled and offered appropriate screening (see Chapter 25).

Antenatal education   Most Akan women in the UK do not attend antenatal classes. This may sometimes be because the idea of formal classes is unfamiliar and they expect to learn everything they need to know from their female relatives. Women who are working long hours may also not be able to attend. Some women may also fear that they will be conspicuous as the only black woman present, or that the content and approach of the class will be irrelevant.

LABOUR AND BIRTH

Traditionally, Akan women move around freely during labour, and may prefer to make a noise rather than to keep quiet. Women's attitudes to pain relief vary and the decision is a matter of personal choice.

In Akan culture a difficult labour is traditionally seen as a punishment for a former misdeed. A woman who does not give birth spontaneously may be judged, by herself and by others, to be not 'a proper woman'. Attitudes are changing as women's knowledge about childbearing increases. However it is important to bear in mind that for some women it may be especially important to have a normal delivery, and that interventions such as the acceleration of labour, a forceps delivery and a caesarean section can have profound long-term emotional and social consequences for some women. Particular care should be taken to assess the necessity for such procedures and, when there are clear clinical causes for concern, to make sure that the woman fully understands the reasons for recommending intervention.

Some African women have a pronounced tilt to their pelvis and it may therefore be particularly important to remain upright and mobile as far as possible during labour (see Chapter 20).

Support during labour   Traditionally, Akan women have several female supporters during labour and birth. Some women may therefore want more than one labour companion. Although this is not part of traditional practice, Akan men are increasingly attending births, especially if their wife or partner has no female relatives or friends to call on. However, some men who accompany their wives may not feel prepared or equipped for this role. They may need considerate and tactful support to put them at their ease (see also Chapter 20).

Muslim families may wish to whisper the call to prayer immediately after the birth (see Chapter 37).

The placenta   The placenta is usually disposed of. Some traditional families may want to keep the cord stump. This may be buried or kept in a special place so that the child will know where he or she belongs.

The sex of the baby   Traditionally the birth of a son, particularly if it is the first baby, is particularly welcomed. He will carry on the family traditions, and will provide for the family. However attitudes are changing with changes in the roles of men and women.

Twins   Twins are considered a special blessing from God. At the following harvest a special twin celebration is held. The babies may be given special bracelets made of coloured beads. There is a high rate of spontaneous multiple births.

POSTNATAL CARE

Rest and cherishing   In the first week after the birth it is traditional for older Akan women to look after the new mother and baby. The baby's head, body and limbs may be massaged at least once a day using specially prepared oils. This is done to increase the baby's suppleness and flexibility, and to encourage healthy development.

By giving birth a woman proves her womanhood. After the birth, she is the centre of attention. In order to ease her aches and pains, to help her relax and to cherish her, she too is oiled and massaged regularly in the first week or two after the birth. Hot compresses and binders may be applied to her tummy which is also massaged. As the weeks pass this care gradually tails off and the woman resumes her normal activities.

Akan women in the UK who do not have female relatives to care for them in this way can feel very isolated and uncared for.

'I can't really describe it. I was lonely and the joy and pride were lost because there was nobody there to care for me. Who could I turn to?'   Akan mother of two

Postnatal depression   In traditional Akan culture people with mental problems are more likely to seek help from spiritualists than from the medical profession. Mental illness of any kind may be considered shameful and stigmatising. As a result, women may be less likely to seek medical help for emotional problems.

Feeding the baby   Most women breast feed their babies. There is no prohibition against colostrum. Sterile sugar water may be given on a teaspoon until the milk supply is established

Naming the baby   A naming ceremony is traditionally held on the eighth day after the birth. Various other traditional ceremonies may be performed, including placing the baby by the door and symbolically sweeping away any negative influences. The baby may also be given, in turn, tiny amounts of salt, pepper, sugar and gin mixed with water and enjoined to identify each: 'If it is salt, say it is salt'. This is to encourage the baby to begin to learn about differences and always to tell the truth. The baby may also be thrown up and then caught in order to provoke a startle reflex. This is believed to 'shock' a new-born baby into realizing where he or she is and to focus the baby's attention on his or her new surroundings.

Depending on the family religion, other ceremonies may also be performed.

Circumcision   Circumcision is traditionally performed on all male infants, regardless of their religion, on the eighth day following the birth (see above).

Female circumcision (female genital mutilation) is not traditionally practised by Akans, but is practised by some Ghanaian Muslims (see Chapter 24).

Contraception   Traditionally, Akan women go home to their parents and live separately from their husbands for three months after the birth. In polygamous families women are not usually expected to resume sexual intercourse for some time. Traditionally the issue of postnatal contraception is therefore not so pressing in Ghana.

For some women the decision on contraceptive methods is influenced by religious factors (see Chapter 21).

CHILDBEARING LOSSES

Infertility   Infertility carries a major stigma. For some people it may be important to prove their fertility before they marry. Confidentiality may be a major concern for many people. Religious considerations may influence some people's decisions on the kinds of investigations and treatment that are acceptable.

Miscarriage, stillbirth and neonatal death   A woman who cannot bear children is traditionally considered not to be 'a proper woman'. This may add to the devastation women feel when they lose a baby at any time during pregnancy or afterwards. Women who have had a miscarriage may not talk about it and may sometimes not mention it when a history is taken.

In contrast to the traditional mourning rituals for adults (see below), those for a baby are minimal, especially for a first child. Mourning the loss of the first child is traditionally forbidden as it is considered to be a bad omen for future births. Gentle explanation should be given to parents of the choices available when their baby has died. Some may not wish to see, hold or name the baby and may not wish to attend a funeral. There is no prohibition against taking photographs. Some parents who chose not to see their baby may want to see photos at a later date.

DEATH OF AN ADULT

Some of this may also apply in the case of a miscarriage, stillbirth and neonatal death, but there are usually significant differences. It is always important to check everything with the parents.

When an Akan adult dies, the funeral is traditionally very elaborate. The mourning period lasts for forty days, during which the bereaved are expected to mourn and are offered support. Family and friends gather to view the body and it is customary for people to express their feelings vocally and openly. Burial is generally preferred to cremation. The precise nature of any ceremonies will depend on the family's religion.

The Chinese community in Britain

Chinese people have a strong and long-standing tradition of emigration to work at sea and on land. Although there have been Chinese people in some areas of Britain, particularly the ports, since the early nineteenth century, the main period of Chinese immigration occurred in the 1950s and 1960s. At this time there was an economic boom in Britain, a collapse in traditional agriculture and fishing in the New Territories, and political uncertainty in China (Au and Au, 1992; Li, 1992).

Most of the first group of immigrants set up and worked in laundries, restaurants or lodging houses in the major ports, initially serving mainly Chinese seamen. As domestic washing machines became more common in Britain, and eating out and 'foreign food' more popular, many Chinese people moved into the restaurant trade and the number of Chinese restaurants and take-aways increased rapidly. The restrictions imposed by British immigration law (which meant that immigration vouchers were granted chiefly to employers wishing to bring in named individuals for work) and the Chinese tradition of family support, mean that many employed Chinese people of the immigrant generation still work in the restaurant or retail trades. In many of these families, the men came first to find work and save, sending for their wives and children after a few years. Most families were reunited in the 1960s and 1970s (Au and Au, 1992).

A small number of people from Malaysia and Singapore came to Britain originally to study, or to work in the health service (Li, 1992).

During the late 1970s and 1980s about 20,000 Vietnamese people came to Britain as refugees. Roughly 80 per cent of these are ethnic Chinese. As part of deliberate government policy Vietnamese refugees were initially dispersed around Britain, especially into rural areas. Some have since moved to urban areas with existing Chinese communities for essential support, and to gain access to familiar food and other commodities (Mares, 1982).

Although there are now sizeable Chinese communities in a few British cities, most Chinese families are fairly isolated, running perhaps the only Chinese restaurant or take-away in a small town. As a result their existence and needs may not be noticed or taken seriously by service providers (Au and Au, 1992).

Diversity

The origins, educational and occupational backgrounds of Chinese people in Britain vary widely. According to the 1991 census, almost a third of the Chinese people in Britain were born here (OPCS, 1993). Among the immigrant generation most people came from conservative farming areas in the New Territories, though some came from urban and often Westernised backgrounds in Hong Kong and elsewhere. There are also families from other areas of the Far East including Malaysia, Singapore, the People's Republic of China,

Vietnam, Taiwan and Indonesia (see Figure 32.1). There are also a small number of Chinese families from Mauritius, the South Pacific islands and the Caribbean.

All these Chinese families originally emigrated from other areas of China, often many generations ago. China is a huge and diverse country containing twenty-three provinces and fifty-six nationalities (Neile, 1995) and embracing many different cultures and traditions. These have influenced the traditions and preferences of the different Chinese families and communities in Britain. In addition, those Chinese families who have come to Britain from other areas of the world have been influenced by other local traditions and experiences.

Many Chinese people arrived in Britain with little or no formal education and have had little opportunity to learn English since; some arrived with a high level of education and excellent English. Some are professionals, for example, nurses, doctors, accountants and

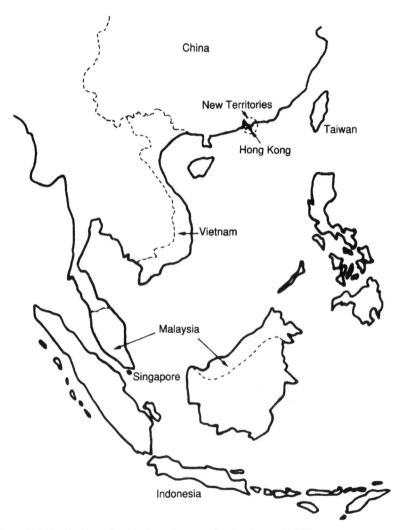

Figure 32.1 The Far East, showing the main areas of emigration to the UK

engineers, businessmen and women. Others do unskilled or semi-skilled work, particularly in the restaurant and allied trades, often working long, unsocial hours.

Despite the diversity of the Chinese community in Britain, there are aspects of Chinese culture relevant to childbearing which transcend differences of background and experience and which **may** still be important for some people, particularly for those who have come to Britain as adults. Some of them may also matter to a greater or lesser extent to British-born Chinese people. **Since it is never possible to predict to whom they will and will not be important, the only way to find out is by listening sensitively to each individual and asking when appropriate.**

LANGUAGE

There are many different Chinese dialects, most of which are not mutually comprehensible.

- Most people from Hong Kong and the New Territories speak Cantonese, Hakka, Toi-Shan or Chiu Chao.
- Most Chinese people from Malaysia and Singapore speak Hokkien, Cantonese or Chiu Chao.
- Most Chinese people from Vietnam speak Cantonese and Vietnamese, though some speak another Chinese dialect.
- Most people from Taiwan speak Mandarin.
- The official language of the Chinese People's Republic is a version of Mandarin called Pu Tong Wa.

There is only one written Chinese language. Everybody who can read and write the Chinese script can understand it whichever Chinese dialect they speak.

Although most younger Chinese people in the UK speak English, a survey in 1985 found that 75 per cent of Chinese adults spoke little or no English (Home Affairs Committee, 1985). This situation is maintained by the hours that many Chinese people work (see Chapter 9). In a survey among Chinese adults in Central London at about the same time, most said that language problems were the main barrier to their finding out about and getting health care (Bloomsbury Health Authority, 1984).

THE CHINESE NAMING SYSTEM (See Chapter 14)

TRADITIONAL FAMILY STRUCTURE AND RELATIONSHIPS

The traditional Chinese family is an extended family with a large number of people of several generations all living under one roof or in close contact. When a couple marries, the wife traditionally moves in with the husband's family, at least for a few years. Marriage is considered the point at which a person takes on adult status. Within the family, older people and their views and opinions are respected and obeyed. As a sign of respect, for example, younger people usually address their elders by titles such as mother, auntie or grandfather, rather than by their name.

The reputation and honour of the family are traditionally very important. They are the responsibility of and affect all the family members. People are generally expected to seek help within their own family and may be reluctant to mention problems to non-family members both within and outside the Chinese community in case this should affect their family's reputation. Some people may also be ashamed to claim benefits due to them for the same reason. Confidentiality is therefore most important. Good manners, filial piety and family and social harmony are highly valued in traditional Chinese culture. For example, Chinese children may be encouraged from an early age to hide personal feelings for the sake of politeness, and to avoid disputes that could disrupt social harmony (Shang, 1986).

Within the extended family, the paternal grandmother is likely to be most influential and to play a large part in caring for a new baby and in bringing up children. Although most Chinese families in Britain no longer live within such a family, the wishes and views of older relatives are still likely to be important, especially if they are in this country. Nowadays a grandmother, if she is available, may care for the children while the mother returns to work.

Traditional Chinese attitudes to sexual morality are strict. Premarital sex may be strongly frowned upon.

RELIGION AND PHILOSOPHY*

Traditional Chinese society does not contain an organised or formal religion in the way that most people accustomed to Western religious traditions find easy to understand. Instead, the Chinese philosophy and way of life are based on three main philosophical strands – Confucianism, Buddhism and Taoism – which also contain certain mystical aspects which may be important to some people. The main emphasis of traditional Chinese philosophy and beliefs is on people's behaviour in their daily life.

Although many Chinese people are not religious in a formal sense, these three philosophies are very important in forming the basic values and principles of Chinese society. For most people it is neither necessary nor possible to distinguish the three philosophies; they base their lives on a combination of the three according to family traditions and personal choice.

Some Chinese people are Christian, mainly Roman Catholics or Baptists. Some are Muslims. (See the sections on these religions below.)

Confucius was an ethical philosopher who lived about two and a half thousand years ago. He taught social harmony through a code of personal and social conduct which emphasises virtues such as sincerity, loyalty, honesty, respect for older people and traditions, obligations to parents and other family members, self-control and self-reliance.

Taoism is an ancient Chinese mystical philosophy which sees humankind has having a fixed place in the natural order of the universe and contains the idea of a unifying force or impersonal God which underlies all reality. Tao (pronounced 'dow') means 'the way'. Taoism stresses the perfection and beauty of nature and the importance of achieving purity and union with the natural world through meditation. In their daily lives people should attempt to achieve a state of harmony and balance within themselves, with nature and within their society. Harmony may be obtained by avoiding conflict and confrontation. If the immediate course of action is blocked, other alternatives may be tried. Taoism also contains a number of deities and saints, to whom people may pray for different causes. In Taiwan, Taoism is the leading religion.

Buddhism became established in China about 1,700 years ago. Buddhist philosophy is concerned with achieving an understanding of the human situation and the means whereby suffering and death can be transcended so that a new state of being is achieved. Most Buddhists believe in reincarnation (the cycle of death and rebirth) and in the ultimate aim of being released from this cycle and ceasing any kind of life comparable with earthly existence. Buddhism emphasises moderation and good conduct, and the performing of good deeds for others through which people build up spiritual merit. Many Chinese people pray to Buddhist deities and saints for different causes.

In traditional Chinese culture respect for older people also extends to deceased ancestors. Prayers may be said to ancestors at special festivals. Graves may be visited and

---

* Adapted from Mares, 1982, by permission of the author and the National Extension College.

cleaned during these festivals, food and other symbolic offerings made, and ancestors' achievements and good deeds celebrated.

Good and bad luck The concepts of luck and bad luck are important in traditional Chinese culture and may influence some people's behaviour and decisions. Certain times, dates and numbers are auspicious. For example, some people consider the number three lucky because in some Chinese dialects it sounds similar to the word 'life'. Four on the other hand sounds like 'death' and may be considered unlucky. Eight sounds similar to the word for 'prosperity'. For some families it may be important to carry out elective interventions on an auspicious day.

Festivals Chinese New Year is the most important Chinese festival. The date is calculated according to the lunar calendar and falls in January or February. Celebrations usually last two or three weeks, the first week being the most important. New Year is a time when people can start afresh, and signifies family reunion and harmony. It is a time of celebration when relatives gather and friends visit each other and when the dragon and lion dances may be performed to bring luck to the community. Couples traditionally visit the husband's parents on the eve of New Year. There are strong traditions about what should be done or avoided during this time to ensure good fortune in the coming year. For example, some families regard the third day as only for family visiting since, by tradition, friends who visit on that day will argue for the rest of the year.

New Year can be a tiring time for women. Before the festival most women clean and decorate their homes and prepare special dishes. Parents may prepare 'lucky money' in little red envelopes to give to children and grandchildren and sometimes to unmarried people. Women in hospital during New Year may have extra visitors to wish them good luck and to bring lucky red packets and gifts for the new baby. It is polite to wish Chinese people a happy new year in the first week of their New Year. Visitors to Chinese homes at this time may be offered special cakes and sweets.

The lantern festival is held on the first full moon of the New Year. It marks the end of New Year celebrations and welcomes the coming of spring. People may decorate their homes.

Chung Yeung is a family autumn festival, celebrated at the full moon in August. Traditionally fruit and moon cakes are eaten, children carry lanterns and the lion dance may be performed.

Qingming (pronounced Chingming) occurs in spring and is a solemn day when the whole family visits the graves of their ancestors. Buddhists traditionally burn simulated money in front of the graves and bring food and other symbolic offerings. Some women may take their babies to the graves of their ancestors. (For more on the dates of Chinese festivals see Walshe and Warrier, 1993.)

PRINCIPLES OF CHINESE MEDICINE*

Chinese medicine is a well-organised and highly respected system of medical knowledge based on recorded observations, experiments and trials and on a rigorous body of theory. It is based on maintaining a natural balance or harmony within the human body. According to Chinese medical theory, illness is an impairment of balance or harmony in the body due to internal, external, physical or mental causes.

Chinese medicine has certain key concepts including chi, yin and yang, and five elements of matter. Chi is vital energy and gives life to all living matter. It is believed to circulate along fourteen channels or meridians, twelve of which influence or are influenced by major internal organs. The strength, flow and distribution of chi in the body

---

* Adapted from Mares, 1982, by permission of the author and the National Extension College.

depends on a proper balance of the elements of yin and yang. Acupuncture may be used to stimulate the flow of chi along the meridians of the body.

In Taoist tradition, harmony only exists in the natural world and in the human body when there is a balance between two vital opposing forces or energies known as yin and yang. Yang is seen as hot, fiery male energy while yin is seen as cold, dark, watery female energy. The interaction of yin and yang produces change, birth, growth and death. Disease occurs when there is a deficiency of yin or yang in the body. There are also five elements of matter which are believed to influence health and illness and the functioning of the major organs.

The aim of the traditional Chinese medical practitioner is to correct the imbalance of all these vital forces in the body. Once equilibrium has been restored, the person will be able to overcome their illness. Diagnosis is traditionally made through visual observation, discussion, palpation and percussion, and the taking of pulses. Medical practitioners are traditionally given great respect in Chinese culture.

Treatments may include exercise, observance of dietary rules, herbal treatment, acupuncture and moxibustion, a form of acupuncture which involves burning dried herbs often in a cradle on top of an acupuncture needle. In contrast to Western medicine, there are few if any major invasive procedures in Chinese medicine. Cutting the body open as in Western surgical procedures is not part of traditional Chinese medicine.

For minor illness and at times such as pregnancy, people may also use traditional home remedies and tonics based on herbs and other substances available from Chinese shops, as well as self-prescribed dietary remedies.

Traditional Chinese medicine and the principles on which it is based are likely to be important for many Chinese people in Britain. Older people may rely entirely on Chinese medicine. Many younger people who are familiar with the basic biomedical concepts of Western medicine may nevertheless accept the principles of Chinese medicine and may use it in parallel with Western treatments or when Western medicine appears ineffective or invasive. Although some Chinese medical treatments are very effective, others may not be, or may lead people to delay seeking other medical treatment, occasionally with serious consequences. A few medicines are thought to be harmful during pregnancy or to interact with Western medication. It may be helpful to ask Chinese women antenatally whether they are taking traditional medicines, while indicating respect for their choices and willingness to work as far as possible with their preferences (Fong and Watt, 1994).

CHINESE FOODS AND DIETS

Since China is a huge country with tremendous variations in climate and agriculture there is no one traditional Chinese diet. People in different communities are likely to eat different diets depending on their family's area of origin within China.

Rice is the staple food of most Chinese families in Britain, and is traditionally eaten at every main meal, sometimes in the form of rice noodles or rice gruel. It is generally regarded as an essential source of energy and nutrients and many people feel that a meal is incomplete without it. However, people whose families originated in Beijing and northern China may eat mainly wheat-based dishes such as noodles and dumplings. Some people eat all kinds of meat, including offal; some avoid pork or beef. Dishes may be steamed, stewed or stir fried depending on the family's area of origin. Onions, ginger and garlic are often used to add flavour, as well as soy sauce and chilli sauce rather than salt. Vegetables are usually cooked. (Salads with dressing or mayonnaise are not part of traditional Chinese cooking.) Plain boiled vegetables (including potatoes) may not appeal to people used to a more flavoured diet.

Soup is eaten with many meals, often as one of the main dishes, and is usually based on the water in which the vegetables or meat have been cooked. Noodles, vegetables and other ingredients may be added. Food is traditionally eaten with chopsticks or a spoon (for soup) and so is usually served in bite-sized pieces. Chinese tea is usually drunk without milk.

Milk and dairy products are not traditionally part of most Chinese diets and some people may dislike the taste. Some Chinese people are also unable to digest lactose because they lack the enzyme lactase. For people with lactose intolerance, large quantities of dairy products may cause cramps, a bloated feeling, belching and diarrhoea. Small quantities of dairy products, if liked, can be digested even by people with lactose intolerance and may be a valuable source of calcium. Lactose intolerance usually develops, if at all, between the ages of one and four (Mares, 1982).

Food and health Food is very important in Chinese culture. Traditional Chinese medicine also places great emphasis on diet in health care and in restoring physical and emotional harmony.

In order to maintain harmony within the body and to avoid damaging extremes it is traditional to balance foods that are yin (hot) with foods that are yang (cold). Yin and yang foods are defined by type not temperature, thus, most fruit and vegetables are cold while red meat and spices are hot. Different cooking methods also affect the attributes of food, for example, boiled and steamed foods may be considered cold, and fried foods hot. Rice is a balanced or neutral food. Different illnesses and conditions are considered hot or cold and an appropriate diet of heating or cooling foods may be chosen to restore the balance (Mares, 1982). Although some people think consciously in terms of yin and yang foods and other dietary categories, most people take them into account automatically in selecting a balanced and nutritious diet. Some younger Chinese people may disregard some or all of these beliefs, but others may still be influenced by them.

In hospital, a range of food and drinks should be available so that most women can select items that will meet their dietary needs. Cold meat and salad, or sandwiches may not be seen as adequately nourishing. Some women will require rice with both main meals. This must be long grain, not pudding rice, ordered specially if necessary. Younger women are more likely to be familiar with English food. If families are bringing food in for women in hospital they are likely to bring chopsticks but may need a spoon, bowls and a plate.

Diet in pregnancy and after childbirth According to Chinese tradition, diet is very important in ensuring a healthy pregnancy and recovery after birth. Both before and after the birth some women may choose or avoid certain foods. Pregnancy, particularly from the beginning of the second trimester, is traditionally regarded as a yang (hot) condition. Women who follow traditional practices may cut down on yang foods such as red meat and fried dishes and eat more cold foods to maintain their own health and that of the baby. This may be particularly important if they feel unwell or if there are problems with the pregnancy. After the birth the mother is traditionally regarded as being in a yin (cold) condition and requires yang (hot) foods for at least a month to build up her health. Hot foods are often high in protein. Foods to be avoided during this period may include boiled and steamed foods, green vegetables, salads, ice cream and all cold drinks. Some women may prefer to have a vacuum flask of hot water by their bed rather than a jug of cold water.

Chinese people whose families originated from different regions of China may also follow other traditional beliefs and avoid particular foods. For example, during pregnancy Chinese women from Vietnam may avoid certain starchy foods in case the baby grows too large risking a problematic birth, cabbage because it causes flatulence, and eggs and prawns (Mares, 1982). Beliefs about what constitutes a healthy diet vary a good deal so it is important to check when discussing dietary changes that each women feels able to eat any foods that are recommended.

After the birth some women may be given a special thick broth to promote well-being and milk production. This is made with sweet black vinegar, ginger and stewed pigs' trotters and served with a freshly boiled egg for extra protein. It is an important part of

Chinese tradition surrounding childbirth and may be fed to her symbolically on a spoon. In some homes female visitors may also be offered this broth.

Religious restrictions   A few people may follow the Buddhist tradition of abstaining from meat on the days of the new and full moon.

PREGNANCY ISSUES

Antenatal care   Historically, pregnancy and birth are considered to be women's business, though attitudes are changing among the younger generation. It is traditionally believed that women should try to avoid stress, strain and anything unpleasant during pregnancy, and should think positively. Some pregnant women may, for example, decide not to attend sad events such as funerals during pregnancy. Some may also try to avoid moving house or renovating their home in order to cut out unnecessary work and stress. A few women may be reluctant to go out in late pregnancy.

In traditional families, issues such as pregnancy, childbirth and contraception are not discussed between the sexes. Many women prefer to say little about their pregnancy in the first few months both out of modesty and for fear of attracting bad luck.

Some conservative women from rural areas may also worry about certain symbolic articles or actions that are traditionally believed to cause harm to the baby. For example, in Chinese tradition scissors on the bed may cause a cleft lip or cleft palate, and cutting the wings and legs off a chicken when preparing food might harm the baby.

The system of provision of antenatal care in Britain is usually acceptable though some people find it unfamiliar and bewildering. Men who wish to accompany their wives or partners may find the timing of antenatal appointments difficult if they work long or unsocial hours.

Some Chinese women may not wish to be examined by a male doctor. A female doctor should always be available in such cases (see also Chapter 19).

Antenatal screening   People are likely to vary in their attitudes to antenatal screening. Blood samples are not normally taken in Chinese medicine and some Chinese women may be frightened and reluctant to give blood. Careful reassurance and explanation may be needed. Since the discussion of problems and negative events is traditionally believed in Chinese culture to bring bad luck, it may be important to talk about possible problems with particular care and sensitivity.

Women of Chinese descent should be offered screening for haemoglobinopathies and especially for thalassaemia (see Chapter 25).

LABOUR AND BIRTH

Labour   Traditionally men are not present during labour and birth. Instead a woman is normally supported by her mother or other married female relatives. Among Chinese men in Britain, views are likely to vary. In some families the husband's mother may put pressure on her son not to attend on grounds of modesty. Some men may prefer to leave the room while the woman is examined.

In traditional Chinese medicine women's health is extremely vulnerable during labour and birth and it is important to keep warm and avoid draughts. Some women may prefer to have windows closed even in warm weather.

If labour must be induced or an elective caesarean carried out, some parents may ask that it is done on an auspicious day (see above).

Pain in labour   Traditionally, Chinese women are expected to be stoical and not to show pain during labour. Some women may feel inhibited about asking for pain relief until it is too late, particularly if they do not fully understand what is available. It is important to find out what each women feels and needs.

The birth   Astrology is an important part of Chinese traditional belief. Some families may want to know the precise time of birth so that the child's horoscope can be drawn up. In Chinese tradition, a child is a human being from the moment of conception and his or her age is calculated to include the pregnancy. Thus, based on the lunar calendar, a Chinese baby may be considered be one year old at birth.

Some families may want to take the placenta home to bury it.

The sex of the baby   All through history Chinese families have relied on sons for the family's income and survival and to take care of them in their old age. This was particularly important for farming families who needed as many sons as possible to work on the farm. Sons also carry on the family name. Historically, therefore, the birth of a son was particularly highly valued and in some cases daughters were regarded as inferior and rejected. Although attitudes have changed, for some parents the birth of a son may still be a matter for particular celebration.

Couples from the People's Republic of China in the UK for a temporary period, for example to study, may be restricted by Chinese law to having one child only. They may wish particularly strongly for a son to support them in their old age and to carry on the family name.

Multiple births   It may be considered very lucky to have twins, especially a boy and a girl. They are known as 'the dragon and the phoenix'.

POSTNATAL CARE

Rest and warmth   Traditionally a woman should rest for one month after giving birth while other women care for her and her baby. Serenity and harmony are considered very important and care should be taken to avoid any stress. In Britain few new mothers are able to rest for a month. Women who have been taught from childhood that this period of rest and protection is essential for their long-term health and well-being may sometimes be distressed and worried about the possible consequences.

It is also considered vital to keep warm and wrap up well. Some women may cover their heads and wear cardigans even in warm weather. Some women believe that it is most important to avoid bathing or showering during the first month as this could cause serious health problems later. They wash by sponging themselves down in hot water. Ginger may be added to the water since it is believed to have healing properties and to help clear wind from the body. Some women also avoid washing their hair after giving birth.

Traditionally both mother and baby should avoid draughts or fresh air which may be believed to carry infection and cause problems such as arthritis later. The baby should also be kept well wrapped up. Some women do not go outside or take their baby outside during this month.

Some women may take Chinese medicines to increase uterine bleeding after the birth and ensure that the uterus is properly cleansed.

Care for the baby   Traditionally the baby's umbilical area is bound to prevent bleeding. Some women may be reluctant to bathe the baby until the cord stump has separated for fear of introducing infection. Some women may also fear that the baby will become chilled.

Some Chinese babies may be born with or may develop patches of bluish skin known as Mongolian spots. In the past some health professionals have mistakenly assumed that these were bruises.

Feeding the baby   Although there is a strong tradition of breast feeding in China, some Chinese women in Britain may, for a variety of reasons, prefer to bottle feed their babies. Some may worry that breast feeding will over-tire them and restrict their activities. Some, perhaps influenced by baby milk advertising and images of happy white babies, may feel that Western scientifically-produced bottle milks are best for their baby. Bottle feeding may also be seen as indicating good financial status in contrast to breast feeding which is the only option for poorer families. In traditional families the grandmother may have most influence on how the new baby is fed and cared for. If so, it is important to include her in discussions on infant feeding and care. Some women do not breast feed in the presence of men.

Some women may feel that a healthy baby should be fat and 'bouncing' since extra weight may help a baby withstand gastro-intestinal and other infections.

Increasing awareness of the benefits to the baby has resulted in increased breast feeding among Chinese women in Britain. Some women may be reluctant to give the baby colostrum. They may express and discard it, giving the baby sugared water until the milk comes in (see Chapter 21).

Naming the baby   In Chinese tradition the husband's father normally chooses the baby's personal name though nowadays many parents choose their baby's name themselves (see Chapter 14). Children are not normally named after relatives or ancestors since this would be considered presumptuous. Some families ensure that the name they choose is compatible with the child's horoscope. In Hokkein tradition, for example, it is considered lucky to name a baby boy after an animal associated with strength, courage and luck, such as Loong (dragon) or Foo (tiger). There is no specific naming ceremony.

Welcoming the baby   When the baby is around one month old, there may be a family celebration, the scale of which varies from family to family. Some families give thanks for the baby's safe arrival, some pray to their ancestors. Buddhists may burn incense. Relatives and friends may be given boiled eggs dyed red to symbolise happiness, good luck and fertility. Sometimes the baby's head is shaved to encourage strong hair growth.

CHILDBEARING LOSSES

Miscarriage, stillbirth and neonatal death   People who see the death of their baby as the will of God may in some cases feel that they should not grieve openly. They may feel that they should not express or talk about their feelings even though they are deeply distressed and as one Chinese woman put it 'crying inside'. For some people, however, the sense of a divine purpose may help them to accept their loss.

Most Chinese parents are unlikely to have any objection to hospital staff washing and wrapping the baby's body. It is always important, however, to check first to see if the parents have any particular wishes. Because of the apparent complexity of traditional Chinese religious beliefs to outsiders it may sometimes be particularly hard for Chinese parents to explain their wishes. (See also Chapter 22.)

In Chinese tradition, association with death and misfortune may be considered unlucky. In some cases the parents of a baby who has died may avoid celebrations such as weddings in order not to bring bad luck.

DEATH OF AN ADULT

Some of this may also apply in the case of a miscarriage, stillbirth and neonatal death, but there are usually significant differences. It is always important to check everything with the parents.

Members of the immediate family usually come and sit beside the dying person. Unless the person is Christian or Buddhist there are normally no special rites or ceremonies.

Last offices   Traditionally, the body is brought home and laid out in a coffin dressed in formal clothes or traditional dress. In hospital last offices should be carried out as normal, provided the family has no special wishes. Some families may bring a special shroud to wrap the body in. In some families it is traditional to put a coin or a nutmeg in the dead person's mouth.

Burial is traditional but rising costs have made cremation more common. Providing a lavish funeral for someone who has died is a sign of respect. Some families may wish for a traditional Chinese priest to conduct the burial but this can be difficult to organise in Britain. Christian families are likely to want a Christian funeral service and burial, usually conducted by their own minister. White is the traditional Chinese colour of mourning.

A wake may be held for several days, though this is becoming less common. Some people may consider it important to grieve loudly, believing that the louder the crying the sooner the gods will hear. Some families may employ professional mourners for this purpose. Some people from conservative, rural areas may believe that contact with death brings bad luck and may sometimes avoid a family in which a death has occurred recently.

Post mortems   There is no specific prohibition against post mortems but some people find them distressing. It may be important to reassure families that the body will be complete and repaired before burial or cremation.

Traditional Somali culture

The Somali Democratic Republic lies above the Equator on the east coast of Africa, with a long coastline forming what is known as the Horn of Africa (see Figure 33.1 and also Figure 31.1). To the east, Somalia faces the Indian Ocean; to the north it faces the Gulf of Aden on the other side of which is the Arabian peninsula. For centuries there has been commercial, cultural and religious contact between the people of Somalia and the people of the Arabian peninsula.

Somalia became independent in 1960. Before then it was divided into two colonial territories, British Somaliland and Italian Somaliland. In recent years Somalia has been severely affected both by drought and by civil war. Between the outbreak of the civil war in 1988 and 1991, approximately 600,000 Somali people fled to Ethiopia to escape the conflict. It has been estimated that by 1993 three-quarters of the roughly eight million Somalis had been displaced by the war (Lem, 1994).

The Somali community in Britain

There have been small Somali communities in the UK, mainly in East London, Cardiff, Hull and Sheffield since the end of the nineteenth century. Initially they consisted largely of merchant seamen (Karmi, undated). However, most people of Somali origin in Britain arrived as refugees and asylum seekers after the outbreak of the civil war in Somalia.

Somali refugees are at present concentrated mainly in Tower Hamlets, East London, Brent, Sheffield, Ealing and Brighton (Refugee Council, 1994). Although some Somalis in Britain are highly educated, many have had little education, particularly since their country has been severely disrupted for some time. English is not taught in Somali schools, so few Somalis speak English when they arrive. Many Somalis arriving in the UK are disorientated and traumatised. Many have seen family members killed and suffered violence themselves. The experience of coming to the UK has also been traumatic for many people (see also Chapter 27).

An enquiry into the daily lives of Somali refugees in Tower Hamlets found a high level of poverty and disillusionment. Few people were receiving the benefits to which they were entitled. There were extreme difficulties in getting health care and very few interpreters to help. Of a random sample of 360 people, 88 per cent lived three to a bedroom in flats that were often damp and infested with vermin. Somalis were also frequently victims of racist attacks. Unemployment was the norm and despite strong attempts at community organisation by self-help groups, 'there is an atmosphere of despair and a pervasive sense of communal depression' (Refugee Council, 1994).

This chapter outlines aspects of traditional Somali culture relevant to childbearing which **may** be important to some people of Somali origin in Britain, particularly those who came to Britain as adults. **Since it is never possible to predict to whom they will and will not be important, the only way to find out is by listening sensitively to each individual and asking when appropriate.**

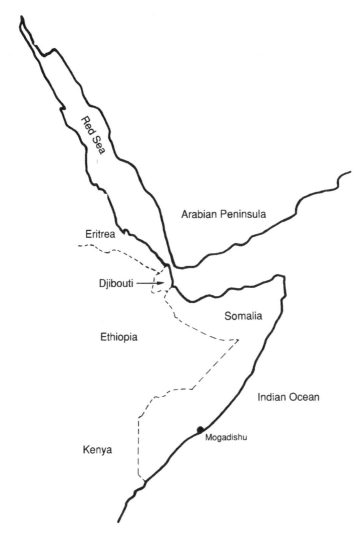

Figure 33.1 Somalia

LANGUAGE

The official language is Somali. People who have had secondary education in Somalia are also likely to speak Arabic. A few speak Italian, English or French.

THE SOMALI NAMING SYSTEM

The Somali naming system is different from the English naming system and there can be major confusion over records as well as how to address people correctly (see Chapter 14).

TRADITIONAL FAMILY STRUCTURE AND RELATIONSHIPS

The traditional family unit in Somalia is extended, with several couples and three generations living together or very close to each other. For most Somalis, relationships with other members of the extended family are very important. In rural areas of Somalia it is traditional for a bride to live with her husband in her in-laws' house. In the cities, couples who can afford it are more likely to live on their own but near to both sets of parents. For most Somali people in the UK who have been separated from their families it is very important to live near and spend time with other Somalis.

Most Somali men traditionally see their main role as provider for and head of the family, and main decision-maker. The primary traditional responsibility of most Somali women is to care for the home and the children. Differences in the roles of men and women are generally more marked in families from rural areas and among people who have had little formal education.

There are no formal restrictions on women other than those laid down in the Quran (see Chapter 37). However in many families, husbands or other male members of the family are likely to feel that it is their responsibility to know where a woman is going when she leaves the home.

Family loyalty is traditionally very important. People are expected to give unquestioning support to their family, especially in times of crisis.

The reputation of the family affects every member and is extremely important. Immoral or unacceptable behaviour by one member brings shame on the whole family and can affect the life chances of every other member. For example, an unmarried woman who becomes pregnant threatens not only her own future but that of all her unmarried female relatives. In such a drastic situation her family may reject her or punish her severely. Since the reputation of girls and women is particularly important, many families set close limits on their freedom, especially if they are unmarried. In the face of the very different pressures on young women in modern British society this may cause serious tension within families.

Marriage   Marriages are traditionally arranged by the family though the young people themselves make the final decision. Mothers may play a prominent role in finding suitable partners for their children. Marriage between cousins is common and is often seen as having many benefits both for the families and for the couple themselves (see also Chapter 37).

Visiting families at home   It is considered polite to remove shoes before entering a Somali home.

RELIGION

Somalia is an Islamic state. Almost all Somalis in Britain are strict Muslims and are likely to adhere carefully to the beliefs and practices of Islam (see Chapter 37).

FOODS AND DIETS

The main traditional sources of starch are sabayad, a form of unleavened bread made of wheat flour and fried, pasta and rice. In Britain many Somalis also eat UK-style bread and pitta bread. The main meats are lamb, beef and chicken (all halal). Somalis also traditionally eat some fish, especially tuna, eggs and baked beans. Cheese is not generally popular though many people drink warm milk and yoghurt mixed with water. Onions and tomatoes are used in many dishes and salads are popular (Northwick Park and St Marks NHS Trust, 1994).

The main meal of the day is traditionally eaten at midday and usually consists of meat or chicken cooked with vegetables, sabayad, rice or pasta, and salad. This is traditionally followed by the cooking liquid from the main dish (eaten as a soup), and then by fruit. Many women like their food hotly spiced with chillies, though they avoid chillies when pregnant or breast feeding. Women may eat porridge for breakfast, especially during pregnancy and after birth (Northwick Park and St Marks NHS Trust, 1994).

Religious restrictions   Most Somalis follow Muslim food restrictions strictly and also fast during the month of Ramadan (see Chapter 37).

PHYSICAL CARE

Clothing and cleanliness   Somali women traditionally wear a jelabi (pronounced jelahbi), also called a msar (pronounced masar). This is a long-sleeved, high-necked, full-length dress. The hair is normally covered with a hijab, a head scarf. Girls are likely to start wearing a jalebi from the age of 12.

Like most people from hot countries, most Somali women prefer a shower to a bath and to wash frequently.

Jewellery   Somali women are unlikely to wear jewellery with special religious or other significance. Some women wear earrings but are usually prepared to remove them if necessary.

Make-up   Many Somali women wear henna (a brownish-yellow dye) on their finger and toe nails. They may also decorate their hands and feet with henna. Once applied, henna cannot be removed but fades and grows out with time. In people with dark skins the colour of the skin under the finger and toe nails is particularly important in detecting cyanosis. Coloured nails may therefore cause problems if a woman needs a general anaesthetic or becomes seriously ill during pregnancy or labour. It may be advisable to explain to a women in early pregnancy that it would be easier for the midwife to keep a check on her during the birth, if she starts letting the henna grow out of her finger and toe nails.

PREGNANCY ISSUES

Antenatal care and customs

> *'Most Somali women feel extremely lonely, so bear with us if three or four of us come with a woman to support or interpret for her.'*   Somali woman

Many Somali women, especially those from rural areas, may find the British system of antenatal care unfamiliar and worrying. It is important to ensure that women understand what services are offered and why (see Chapter 19).

Some women may not prepare or buy clothes, equipment or nappies before the birth for fear of tempting fate.

Modesty and physical examinations   Modesty is extremely important. Most Somali women will want to keep their bodies covered as much as possible during examinations and treatment (see also Chapter 19). Unnecessary exposure of any part of her body including her legs is likely to cause a woman extreme anxiety and distress. If a woman normally wears a jelabi (see above), it may be helpful to suggest that she wears a top and long skirt for antenatal check-ups.

Most women will prefer to wear a jelabi during labour and to cover their heads with a scarf. Health professionals should help make sure that a woman's legs remain covered as much as possible.

Female circumcision – female genital mutilation Many Somali women have undergone some degree of genital mutilation. This has important implications for antenatal care and also for the management of labour and birth (see Chapter 24).

Antenatal screening See Chapter 19

Antenatal education Many Somali women, especially those from rural areas, find the idea of formal antenatal education strange. In Somalia, other women in the family give a new mother all the information she needs about pregnancy, birth and the care of a small baby, and support and advise her as her pregnancy continues (see also Chapter 19).

LABOUR AND BIRTH

Labour Labour and birth are traditionally seen as women's business. However, attitudes are changing both in Somalia and in Britain, and more men are staying with and supporting their wives during labour.

Traditionally Somali women are expected to accept pain stoically and quietly. Younger women may be more likely to want pain relief of some kind. It is important to check that each woman knows about the different types of pain relief she can choose and feels free and able to ask for help when she needs it (see Chapter 20).

Birth Parents may wish to whisper the Muslim call to prayer into the baby's ear (see Chapter 37).

The sex of the baby As in most societies, boys are often particularly welcomed. Fathers regard boys as adding strength and honour to the father's line. However it is important not to assume that daughters are not welcomed.

POSTNATAL CARE

Rest and recovery In Somalia, it is traditional for a woman to rest and to be cared for by her extended family for the first 40 days after the birth. Household chores are done for her and her other children looked after. In the UK this kind of support is seldom available and many women are anxious to go home to look after their families.

At the end of the forty days, the woman takes a ritual cleansing shower and then returns to normal life. Sexual intercourse is forbidden until this time.

Visitors Friends and relatives are under a strong obligation to visit a new mother and to bring her food and presents. Anyone who does not visit is considered very bad mannered. Somali women may therefore have a lot of visitors after the birth. If this distresses the mother or other women in the ward, restrictions should be imposed with tact and with an understanding of people's obligation to visit.

Feeding the baby Most Somali women breast feed their babies, putting them to the breast soon after birth. Those without extended family support may need to know where they can get help with any breast feeding problems.

Naming the baby The baby is traditionally named on the seventh day after the birth, and the name is usually chosen by the parents, sometimes with advice from other family members (see Chapter 14). In some families the naming ceremony is an occasion for celebration and feasting, though others wait for this till the fortieth day (see below).

Welcoming the baby   The fortieth day after the birth is traditionally an important time for celebration and feasting. Parents give thanks for the child by entertaining family and friends and by giving to charity. The mother and baby are the centre of attention. Although friends and family often help with preparations, these occasions involve hard work for the new mother.

Circumcision   Boys are circumcised according to Islamic law, usually during infancy. Somali girls are traditionally 'circumcised' before puberty (see Chapter 24).

Contraception   Contraception is largely a matter of personal choice though it is likely to be influenced by religious beliefs. Some younger women may be happy to discuss contraception openly. More conservative women are likely to be more reticent and may require more time and sensitive support to explore choices and reach their decisions.

CHILDBEARING LOSSES

Termination of pregnancy   Termination of pregnancy is prohibited in Islam (see Chapter 37). Somali women are likely to be influenced by this when considering the possibility of a termination, and may only decide on a termination when their situation is desperate. As always, the strictest confidentiality is essential.

Miscarriage, stillbirth and neonatal death   Requirements when a baby dies during pregnancy or around the time of birth will vary a good deal depending on religion, family and community traditions, and personal preferences. As always, bereaved parents will need full information about their choices, and support and time to decide what is best for them. See Chapter 37 for details of Muslim religious practices.

34 Traditional South Asian culture

Terminology

The term 'South Asian' is used here to refer to people whose families originated in the Indian subcontinent, that is, India, Pakistan, Bangladesh and Sri Lanka. It does not include people whose families originated in other Asian countries such as China, Hong Kong, Vietnam, the Philippines and Singapore.

The terms 'South Asian' and, more commonly, 'Asian' are widely used in the health service and elsewhere as labels for people whose families originated in the Indian subcontinent. However, these terms mask tremendous diversity in terms of national, regional, cultural and religious traditions. Few South Asian people in Britain identify with them in a meaningful way, any more than most English people reply European when asked what group they belong to (Bowler, 1993). It must be noted, however, that in the face of continued discrimination and racism, Asian has become a unifying political label for many people.

Most people are more likely to define themselves in terms of the region or country from which they or their family emigrated, as, for example, Indian, Pakistani, Gujarati, Sylheti, Mirpuri, and/or the religious community to which they belong. Nevertheless, because certain cultural traditions are important in most areas of the Indian subcontinent, the term South Asian has its uses. This chapter discusses those aspects of traditional South Asian culture which may be important to some people in Britain. It does not cover specifically religious traditions and practices. For these see the chapters on religions below.

A diverse community

The South Asian community in Britain includes people of all occupational and educational levels and lifestyles. It includes people whose families originated from several very different areas of the Indian subcontinent – a vast area as diverse as Europe – as well as from East Africa, and from towns and cities as well as from more conservative farming areas. It includes Hindus, Jains, Sikhs, Muslims, Christians, Zoroastrians and Buddhists as well as people with no religious affiliation. Although many people are fluent in English, there are also people whose first language is Punjabi, Urdu, Hindi, Tamil, Gujarati, Sylheti, Bengali, Pashto or one of the other over 800 languages and dialects of the Indian subcontinent.

The South Asian community in Britain includes people who came here as adults or as children thirty or forty years ago, a few people who have arrived more recently, and the children and grandchildren of the immigrant generation. Almost half the South Asians in Britain were born and brought up here (OPCS, 1993). For them in particular only certain aspects of traditional South Asian culture are likely to be important. **Since it is never possible to predict what will be important and to whom, the only way to find out is by listening sensitively to each client and asking when appropriate.**

Emigration to the UK

The Indian subcontinent   Most emigration to Britain from the Indian subcontinent took place in the mid-1950s and 1960s when Britain was suffering chronic labour shortages, and government and industry were recruiting workers in those areas that had strong traditional links with Britain. Most people came from a few specific areas of north-western India, Pakistan and Bangladesh (see Figure 34.1). These were areas from which men had historically migrated to join the British Indian Army or the Merchant Navy, or to work in other countries of the British Empire (Anwar, 1979; Rose, 1969). There were also a number of professionals, mainly doctors and nurses, who came to Britain from all over the Indian subcontinent (Vadgama, 1982).

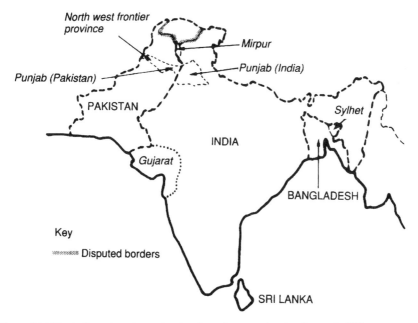

Figure 34.1 The Indian subcontinent showing the main areas of emigration to the UK

In most families, the men came to Britain first to find jobs and make provision for their wives and children to join them. Many families however had to wait many years to be able to come, often due to long delays by British authorities in processing their applications (Gordon and Klug, 1985). Some men also delayed sending for their wives and children because they planned eventually to return home.

Until 1962, all citizens of the British Empire or the Commonwealth had the right to come to Britain to work and to settle, and to travel in and out at will. After 1962, limited numbers of entry vouchers were granted by the Home Office to British Commonwealth citizens as and when their labour was needed to fill periodic shortages in Britain (Rose, 1969). In 1971 a further law was introduced to end immigration from the New Commonwealth. Since then almost all emigration to Britain from the Indian subcontinent has been of the wives and children of men working and settled in Britain, and, in some cases, of new spouses. In the Bangladeshi community, the reunions of wives and children with their husbands and fathers have continued into the 1990s.

East Africa   In the late 1960s and 1970s, the African countries of the old British Empire became independent. During the previous decades a large number of people of South Asian origin (mainly from Gujarat and Punjab – see Figure 34.1) had settled in British East Africa (Kenya, Tanzania, Malawi, Zambia and Uganda, see Figure 31.1) under the auspices of the British. They formed part of a commercial and professional middle-layer between the white colonisers and the African majority. They were generally identified with the unpopular colonial authorities and found themselves increasingly vulnerable as independence approached.

Recognising their vulnerability, the British government gave all the Asians in British East Africa the right to retain their British citizenship after independence. If they chose to remain British, the government guaranteed them the right to come to Britain at any time. However, in 1968, in response to media and public pressure, the government unilaterally withdrew this right. From now on, British East African Asians, like New Commonwealth citizens, would have to apply for entry vouchers to Britain. This led to an international outcry since it is illegal for any state to refuse entry to its own citizens. Following this, the British government set up a quota system under which 1,500 East African Asian families with British passports could enter the country every year. At that time there were still many thousands of Asian families stuck in East Africa, many of them forbidden to work, with no source of income and with nowhere to go except the UK (Tandon and Raphael, 1978).

In 1972, all the remaining Asians in Uganda were suddenly expelled and most were allowed to come to the UK. In the other East African countries, many Asians with British citizenship also had to leave. Although initially the British government refused to accept them except under the quota system, it was eventually realised that forcing people to wait years, penniless and unemployed, was pointless. Most East African Asians with British passports were allowed entry to the UK by 1980.

Other refugees   Since the mid-1980s a number of Tamil people from Sri Lanka have come to the UK as refugees (see Chapter 27).

LANGUAGES

There are fifteen official languages in India and more than 1,650 other languages and dialects (*Independent*, 5.11.94). In most areas of the Indian subcontinent people use several languages. They may speak a local language or dialect at home, the national and/or

Table 34.1   Main South Asian languages spoken in the UK

India
  People from Punjab speak **Punjabi**
  People from Gujarat speak **Gujarati**
  People from the northern part of Gujarat State speak a dialect of Gujarati called **Kutchi**
  The language of higher education in Northern India is **Hindi**

Pakistan
  People from Punjab Province speak **Punjabi**
  People from Mirpur speak **Mirpuri,** a dialect of Punjabi
  People from the North West Frontier Province speak **Pashto**
  The language of education in Pakistan is **Urdu**

Bangladesh
  People from Sylhet speak **Sylheti**, a dialect of Bengali
  The language of education in Bangladesh is **Bengali**

Sri Lanka
  Tamil people from Sri Lanka speak **Tamil**

	HINDI	URDU	PUNJABI	GUJARATI	BENGALI	SYLHETI	KUTCHI	PASHTO	TAMIL
HINDI	/								
URDU	almost all	/							
PUNJABI	quite a lot	quite a lot	/						
GUJARATI	a little	a little	a little	/					
BENGALI	nothing	nothing	nothing	nothing	/				
SYLHETI	nothing	nothing	nothing	nothing	quite a lot	/			
KUTCHI	a little	a little	nothing	quite a lot	nothing	nothing	/		
PASHTO	nothing	nothing	nothing	nothing	nothing	nothing	nothing	/	
TAMIL	nothing	nothing	nothing	nothing	nothing	nothing	nothing	nothing	/

Figure 34.2 How much speakers of one South Asian language are likely to understand of another

regional language at school or for contact with officials, and write in a third or even fourth language. In general, people with more education and more outside responsibilities speak more languages. In some communities this often means men.

Table 34.1 shows the main languages spoken by South Asians in the UK. South Asians from East Africa are also likely to speak Swahili (an African language) and, in many cases, English. Everyone born in the UK, and most people who came here as teenagers or young adults, also speaks English. (See Chapter 13 for more about written communication and the languages people read.)

Because they do not expect most outsiders to be well-informed about dialects, many Sylheti speakers say they speak Bengali, Mirpuri speakers say they speak Punjabi, and Kutchi speakers say they speak Gujarati. It may be particularly important to check when, for example, you are choosing an interpreter (see also Chapter 11). Figure 34.2 shows how much people who speak one language are likely to understand of the other languages.

NAMING SYSTEMS

Some of the naming systems in the Indian subcontinent are different from the British naming system. This can cause dangerous confusion with records. It is also important to address people acceptably (see Chapter 14).

TRADITIONAL FAMILY STRUCTURES AND RELATIONSHIPS

In the farming communities from which the families of most (but not all) South Asian people originally emigrated, the male head of the family and his wife, their sons and wives, and their grandsons, their wives and children, all traditionally live in one household and run the family farm. Daughters, when they marry, leave the family farm and go to live for the rest of their lives with their husband's family. Although this pattern is changing, the extended family, its values and responsibilities and the way that roles and responsibilities are still the norm for many people and are generally highly regarded.

Practical and economic factors in Britain mean that few extended families are able to live together under one roof. As early as 1984 a study found that only 18 per cent of South Asian households contained an extended family (Brown, 1984). Nevertheless, for most people the bonds remain strong and there is frequent, even daily, communication between different parts of the family. Many people also regard their community as an extension of their family and many communities are very close-knit.

Authority   The extended family system has several important features which contrast with those of the modern Western European nuclear family. For example, there is a more formal hierarchy; the male head of the household traditionally has overall authority. Beneath him, older family members normally have authority over younger family members, and men over women, at least in public matters. Within each generation, an older brother has authority over his younger brothers, and an older sister-in-law over her younger sisters-in-law. A young wife or mother may be very much under the authority of her mother-in-law. Older people have authority and influence, and are respected and deferred to by adults as well as by children.

Men and women   In the traditional South Asian extended family the roles of men and women are differentiated, though the degree of differentiation and the way it is expressed varies a lot between different communities. In some communities men are traditionally responsible for all matters outside the home, for all contact with non-family members, with people in authority and with institutions, for the protection and financial support of the family, and for major and public family decisions. Women are traditionally responsible for all aspects of running the home and for day-to-day matters within it, and for the practical, emotional and spiritual care of the children.

In some more conservative families and communities women spend almost all their time in the home and rarely go out into the outside world. In the farming communities from which most families originated, homes are larger and are surrounded by a large private area in which all the women and children of the extended family normally spend their days. Men may do any shopping that is necessary and women may only need to leave their homes on a few occasions each year. Some people in the UK still feel that a good husband should protect his wife from the risks of the outside world and from the public gaze and that women should remain in the safety of their home.

In many communities there is a strict code of behaviour between the sexes, both in public and within the extended family. In an extended family household, where several adult couples and any unmarried adults all live together, the women and children usually spend their days apart from the men. The code of behaviour also covers matters considered suitable for discussion in the presence of the opposite sex. Matters such as sexual intercourse, menstruation and the physical aspects of pregnancy and childbirth are not normally discussed between men and women, and in conservative communities may not be discussed between husbands and wives.

Family duties and responsibilities   Each member of a South Asian extended family is traditionally seen and sees themselves primarily as a family member rather than as an independent individual. Individualism and independence may be seen as selfish, unloving and disrespectful. Mutual dependence (generally a negative idea in the individualistic culture of modern Western society) is valued. For example, people may not be expected to live alone, family members in financial need are normally supported by the rest of the family, and children are looked after by other family members. Emotional closeness and dependence are highly regarded. Traditionally, nobody ever is, or should be, entirely independent of their family at any age.

The needs and interests of the family are also generally assumed to be the needs and interests of the individual. Family duties and the need to ensure the family's well-being should take precedence over individual wishes and ambitions, but at the same time every family member is normally assured of lifelong social, emotional, physical and financial support. No one need ever be lonely. Each family member has formal duties and responsibilities, depending on their position within the family, age, sex and marital status. Although these are not rigid, and individual personalities always play a part, most people accept them. Family members have a duty to become involved in the lives and relationships of other family members, particularly when it comes to important decisions like marriage, childrearing, or marital problems. Children belong to the whole family, not just to their parents, and their upbringing, care and discipline are a matter for everyone.

Since, in the Indian subcontinent, the extended family is normally the only source of financial, physical and emotional support for elderly, frail or ill members, its maintenance and traditions are seen as essential, particularly by older people. Many South Asian parents who have emigrated to Britain may feel that their family is their only real source of companionship and support, especially as they get older. In addition, most South Asian families maintain strong links with their families 'back home' and the views of the head of the family and of older family members in the Indian subcontinent may still be important to them. People may write and ask for their decisions on important family matters.

The reputation of any individual is traditionally seen as affecting the whole extended family. Unacceptable or shameful behaviour by one family member may have a drastic effect on the futures of all other members, and on the marriage prospects of any unmarried members. In some cases, therefore, families react extremely severely to transgressions, either punishing the individual harshly or rejecting them. Such a response may be seen as the only way to rescue the reputation of other family members and so the survival of the family.

Marriage   Marriages in many communities are traditionally arranged by parents and other older family members, since it is believed that they have the wisdom and experience to make this crucial choice, and that they understand the young people involved and their long-term needs as well as the needs of the whole family far better than the young people themselves. In addition, a marriage within a South Asian extended family involves not just two independent individuals who will form a new independent unit, but all the members of two extended families. Marriage builds links between families. The young woman traditionally moves into the home of her husband's extended family and lives with his whole family for the rest of her life. It is important that she should be happy and well cared for there. It is also important that she should fit in well with the other members, especially the women, with whom she is likely to spend most of her time. Her relationships with them are in many ways almost as important as that with her husband.

The whole basis of marriage in this system is very different. The marital relationship is traditionally less exclusive and in many ways less pressurised. It is assumed that the two young people will gradually learn to love each other once they are married. This is generally seen as a far more reliable basis for the long-term survival of a marriage and a family than Western 'romantic love'. In addition, those members of the family responsible for the choice normally take an active part in guiding and supporting the young couple after marriage and in advising them if there are any difficulties.

Many older people still regard the involvement of the wider family in the choice of marriage partner as important and beneficial. They feel that it is important to help choose a partner who will support and maintain their values and traditions, and who will bring up their grandchildren to respect their family's culture. In some cases this may mean deciding to choose a spouse from the Indian subcontinent. Since the woman is generally regarded as responsible for ensuring the success of a marriage, there may be particular pressure on her to fit in and make it work (Aitchison, 1994; D'Alessio, 1993).

In most communities in the Indian subcontinent and in Britain young people are now given an increasing amount of say in the choice of a marriage partner, though this depends to some extent on issues such as class and education. Most parents now guide rather than arrange their children's marriages. Most young people accept their family's concern and advice and make successful marriages.

However, for some South Asian young people brought up in Britain, marriage is a time when they can no longer move between different cultures. What is crucially a family decision in traditional South Asian culture, in English culture is an independent decision taken by the young people alone. In addition, the demands and pressures on the new marital relationship are likely to be far more like those affecting other Western nuclear families.

Some young people may feel unable to accept their families' choice of partner and may refuse. The long-term consequence of this can be disastrous since they may lose the support and love of their family and community and have to survive alone in a racist society that will never completely accept them. Young people who make a 'love match' may also be less likely to receive support from their families should there be problems.

Throughout the Indian subcontinent it is generally regarded as extremely important that people should marry within their own religious and social community. For Hindus and some Sikhs caste and community considerations are also likely to be important in choosing a suitable marriage partner. Marriage between cousins is common in Pakistani Muslim communities and occurs to some extent in other Muslim communities (see Chapter 37).

Sexual morality   There is traditionally a very strict code of sexual morality to protect families and communities. Pre-marital and extra-marital sex are forbidden. As in many communities, higher moral standards are often expected of girls. It is traditionally very important that a girl should not go out with or be alone with a man before she marries and that her reputation should be spotless. Immoral or questionable behaviour by one young woman also affects the reputations of the other women in the family, and may ruin the chances of those who are not yet married. There may be particular restrictions on some girls and young women in Britain, where many parents feel that their daughters are in great danger from the pressure and 'looser morals' of majority English culture.

Some South Asian woman who become pregnant outside marriage may feel that a secret termination is their only option. Total confidentiality is clearly essential since their own and their family's reputation and future may be at risk.

Families and childbirth   Traditionally the bearing and raising of children are regarded as a woman's greatest fulfilment and highest duty. In many communities the birth of the first child is traditionally seen as cementing the marriage and marks a bride's final acceptance in her new family. In the Indian subcontinent, as in many other places, pregnancy, childbirth and the care of babies and young children are usually women's area of responsibility. The older women of the family are an important source of support and guidance and are likely to expect their advice to be followed (see also Chapters 17, 19 and 20).

TRADITIONAL SOUTH ASIAN MEDICINE

The Indian subcontinent contains three main traditional and influential systems of medicine, all of them over 2,000 years old. These are the Ayurvedic system, based originally on ancient Hindu texts and influenced over the years by medical knowledge from different cultures; the Unani system, which originated in Greece and is largely used in Muslim areas; and the Siddha system, used mainly by Tamils in Southern India and Sri Lanka. All three work on the basis of different elements and humours which make up the body and are believed to affect people's physical, spiritual, emotional and mental well-being. Imbalances within the body cause illness and distress and must be restored through treatment using changes in the diet as well as medication containing herbs, minerals and other substances. Traditional practitioners diagnose conditions mainly through observation, detailed discussion with the patient, and the taking of pulses.

These three medical systems are widely respected and influence the way many people in the Indian subcontinent think about their bodies and about health and illness and the way it should be treated. All three are recognised by governments in the Indian subcontinent where there are training colleges and systems of registration for practitioners. In rural areas in particular, trained practitioners of traditional medicine are far more accessible and less expensive than practitioners of Western medicine. There are also large numbers of untrained or semi-trained practitioners who are generally even cheaper. In addition preparations based on traditional South Asian medicine are sold across the counter in pharmacies and general stores.

Home remedies and ideas about the maintenance of health and the treatment of illness are often maintained when people migrate (see also Chapter 2). Many South Asian people in the UK think of health and illness in terms of the principles of South Asian medicine and use traditional medicines particularly for intractable conditions, for conditions that they feel are not treated or recognised in Western medicine, or where they do not know of a Western over-the-counter equivalent. People may also prefer to consult a traditional practitioner if they speak little or no English or over matters that are embarrassing or difficult to explain.

Although most traditional medicines are probably harmless, some may contain toxic substances. Others may interact with Western medication and may cause unexpected and often unrecognised problems (Atherton, 1994; Healy and Aslam, 1989). It may be useful to ask whether a woman is taking traditional medicines and what these contain, particularly if she is also on Western medication. Any enquiries should be carried out with great sensitivity. Some people may be reluctant to discuss their views openly since they are aware that some Western health professionals regard all other medical systems as worthless and bizarre.

SOUTH ASIAN FOODS AND DIETS

The staple foods and diets of people in the Indian subcontinent vary from area to area depending on local climate and agriculture. For example, Sylhet (see Figure 34.1) is one of the wettest places in the world. The climate is excellent for rice, and fish (often reared in the flooded rice fields) is plentiful. People in the fertile Punjab area (divided between India and Pakistan) eat chapatis made of wheat or maize. People in Gujarat eat both rice and chapatis as their staple starch.

Most of the fruits and vegetables that grow in the different climatic regions of the Indian subcontinent are different from those traditionally grown in Britain. Cooked food is usually fried briefly and then stewed, with none of the cooking water thrown away. Vegetables are never boiled. Pulses such as lentils and chickpeas are an important source of protein throughout the Indian subcontinent, especially for vegetarians. A wide variety of spices are used, and many people used to South Asian food find English food heavy and tasteless.

The rice or chapatis and the different dishes are normally laid out in the centre of the table and people help themselves to food as they wish during the meal. Salads (often of chopped up vegetables such as cucumber, onion and tomato with lemon juice squeezed over them) are served as a side dish and are not normally a meal in their own right.

South Asian food is normally eaten with the fingers, usually of the right hand which is reserved for handling clean things, or with a spoon. Women who cannot get out of bed in hospital need a bowl of water to wash their hands before and after eating.

Religious restrictions   In the Indian subcontinent, food traditionally has a spiritual significance that it has almost completely lost in the West. Certain foods are prohibited on religious grounds and few conservative or devout people would consider eating them (see the chapters on religions below). Among South Asian people in Britain, not everyone follows religious prohibitions on food and for each individual this may be a question of personal conscience. Women and older people are generally more conservative, and some communities are more conservative than others (see also Chapter 18).

Food and health   Like all cultures, traditional South Asian culture contains beliefs about what people should eat and avoid to keep healthy. Food affects not only people's physical health but also their emotional and spiritual well-being. Part of the South Asian tradition classifies certain foods as hot or cold in terms of their effects (the precise foods and their classification differ between communities). This has nothing to do with the physical temperature of the food. 'Hot' foods are generally salty, sour or high in animal protein. They are believed to raise the body temperature. They excite, and, in excess, may over-excite the emotions in a similar way to alcohol. 'Cold' foods are generally sweet, bitter or astringent, and are believed to cool the body temperature, calm the emotions, and make a person cheerful and strong.

An excess of either hot or cold foods can unbalance the body and the emotions and cause ill-health. Certain conditions are also thought to 'cool' or 'heat' the body and to require more or less of certain foods. For example, cold drinks, fruit juices, salads and yoghurt may all be avoided if a person has a cold or a sore throat which are both 'cold' conditions.

Although the tradition of hot and cold foods is followed in Britain mainly by older South Asian women, it may still influence family diets and the advice given when people are pregnant, breast feeding or ill. Some people automatically follow the principles outlined above in order to maintain a healthy diet although they do not necessarily think in terms of 'hot' and 'cold' foods.

Diet in pregnancy and after childbirth   Some women may avoid 'hot' foods in early pregnancy (a hot condition) in case they overheat the body and cause a miscarriage. At the end of the pregnancy 'cold' foods may be thought, for example, to increase the risk of premature delivery, or to cause joint pains and arthritis. Some women may also avoid foods that are believed to cause flatulence during pregnancy and while breast feeding. Traditions differ, but these may include, for example, potatoes, lentils, citrus fruits and certain vegetables.

It is considered extremely important for both mother and baby that the mother should eat a balanced and nutritious diet once the baby is born. Some women may avoid 'cold' foods (including cold drinks) and choose more hot foods to stimulate the milk supply and boost their energy levels. Some may also drink herbal teas, such as fennel, cloves or dill, which are widely considered to prevent wind in both mother and baby. Families may bring in high calorie sweetmeats such as panjiri, made of crushed almond and cashew nuts mixed with sugar, ghee (clarified butter) and flour. This is traditionally given to new mothers to promote lactation. Coconut and coconut milk also traditionally promote lactation. Some women may like porridge made of chapati flour for breakfast.

The digestive system is traditionally believed to be vulnerable in the days and weeks after childbirth. Some people may avoid all spicy or unfamiliar foods and eat a bland diet for the first forty days after the birth or for as long as they are breast feeding. Some women may prefer to eat only food brought from home, provided their family is able to do this. For some families, bringing nutritious meals from home for a newly delivered mother is a very important part of caring for her (see Chapter 21).

PHYSICAL CARE

Cleanliness   In traditional South Asian culture cleanliness is linked to a wider concept of pollution. Certain things are traditionally considered both physically and spiritually polluting, and people should either avoid them or, if they have come into contact with them, should wash thoroughly. All body fluids, saliva, sweat, urine, amniotic fluid, faeces, blood and semen are traditionally considered impure and polluting. Menstrual blood, lochia and the placenta may be regarded as particularly polluting. Running water is regarded as a very effective cleansing and purifying agent. The degree to which South Asian people in Britain follow these beliefs varies a good deal. For a few people they are extremely important, for others they are unknown or irrelevant. Cleanliness is, however, generally very highly valued. It is also important for many people to wash before praying. In Islam this is compulsory (see Chapter 37).

People in hospital who feel dirty and possibly polluted may become very distressed, particularly if they are bed-bound and cannot wash themselves, or if adequate washing and showering facilities are not available. It is important to identify and discuss any particular needs and wishes and to try to reach an acceptable solution.

The head is traditionally regarded as sacred and the hair should normally be washed frequently. Some women, however, do not wash their hair towards the end of pregnancy and for some time after the birth to avoid the risk of a chill. The feet are traditionally regarded as dirty. Shoes may be considered particularly polluting and should not be put with other possessions, for example, in a bag with other clothes or on a locker. At home, most people take their shoes off when they come into the house or when entering a room where prayers are said.

In South Asian tradition the right hand may be used wherever possible for touching food and other clean things. It is therefore important to position lockers and food trays within reach of the right hand.

Washing and showering   Many South Asian people, like other people whose families originated in hot countries, prefer to shower or wash thoroughly at least twice a day, though in some communities women may not shower daily at vulnerable times such as during illness or after giving birth. After having a baby, or at the end of their menstrual period, some women have a cleansing shower to purify themselves.

For reasons of modesty, some conservative South Asian women prefer to shower in their clothes. They put on fresh dry clothes when they have finished. If they are wearing jewellery with special religious significance, this may be kept on while showering but is normally kept dry.

Many people wash their hands and cleanse their mouth on waking and before and after eating and drinking. Some people clean out their nasal passages with water and spit out any phlegm, particularly first thing in the morning. Most people also wash before praying. Women who cannot get out of bed may need a glass of water, a tooth bowl, a bowl of water and a towel.

After using the lavatory, a few women may wish to wash their genital area with water. They may only use the left hand, since in Asia the right hand is traditionally used for touching clean things and for handling food. At home they may keep a jug with a long spout in the lavatory for washing. However, to minimise the risk of cross infection in hospital (if there are no bidets) each woman who wants to use a jug should be given her own or invited to bring one into hospital with her which she could keep in her locker.

Clothing   Although many South Asian women wear Western clothes, many wear traditional styles that reflect their background, culture and often, religion. Some South Asian women who wear Western dress may prefer to keep their legs covered with trousers or a long skirt.

Shalwar kameez   The kameez (shirt) is a long tunic with long or half sleeves. The shalwar (or salwar) are trousers. Shalwar kameez are the traditional everyday wear of most Punjabi women (in both India and Pakistan) and of most Muslim women in Gujarat. There is also a long scarf called a chuni or dupattah, which lies over the shoulders and across the breasts. Some women pull one end of the dupattah over the head as a sign of modesty and respect in front of strangers, older people or men. In less conservative communities the width of the salwar legs may vary according to fashion, particularly among younger women.

Sari   Most Hindu women and most Bangladeshi women traditionally wear a sari over a blouse and underskirt. A sari is about five or six metres long. Hindu women may sometimes leave the midriff bare. Tamil Hindu women may be more likely to wear Western clothing.

Jewellery and make-up   Various items of jewellery may be worn in different communities in the Indian subcontinent to indicate that a woman is married. The most common is glass or gold bangles. Others include a ring with a precious stone, rings on the toes, or a small jewel in the nose. Some Hindu women may wear a necklace of gold or black beads with a gold brooch. Most women never remove their wedding jewellery as long as their husband lives. Wedding jewellery should never be removed unless absolutely necessary, and then only with the woman's consent. (See also Chapters 18 and 36.)

Surma   is a fine black powder which is placed just inside the upper and lower eyelids with an applicator rod. It is traditionally used by both adults and children in many areas of the Indian subcontinent and is generally believed to be extremely good for the eyes, preventing infections and improving the eyesight. Many women traditionally put surma on their children's eyes every day. Unfortunately most brands of surma contain lead sulphide and this can be absorbed through drainage down the tear duct or from rubbing the eyes and then licking the fingers. Research findings on whether and how much lead from surma gets into the blood appear contradictory (Attenburrow *et al.*, 1980; Healy and Aslam, 1989).

Since 1968 there has a been a ban on the importation of surma and other related products into the UK as well as publicity campaigns aimed at the South Asian communities explaining the risks of traditional surma and recommending alternative products known to be safe. The use of surma or similar products has become far less common. Most families now use an alternative traditional cosmetic called kajil that does not contain lead, or a commercial British cosmetic product. Some surma still comes into the UK brought as a special gift by relatives or friends and may be used by people who do not realise that certain brands are dangerous. A few Muslim families may receive gifts of surma from Makka or other places of pilgrimage and these may also be believed to bestow special spiritual blessing. Some women in Britain make their own surma but if the ingredients are bought from a hakim (a Unani practitioner, see the discussion of traditional medicine above) they may also contain lead sulphide (Healy and Aslam, 1989).

It may be important to check sensitively if it is thought that a family may be using surma on a child's eyes.

PREGNANCY ISSUES

Antenatal care and traditions   Like all women who are unfamiliar with the British system of antenatal care, some women brought up in the Indian subcontinent are likely to find certain aspects of it strange and difficult to understand. Even women who have been through several pregnancies in Britain may have had little explanation of what goes on or its purpose (Narang and Murphy, 1994). It is an essential part of client-centred care that each women understands the services offered (see also Chapter 19).

Modesty is extremely important in many South Asian communities. Some women keep themselves covered at all times, especially in the presence of men. Physical examinations can be a major source of anxiety and distress (see Chapter 19).

Antenatal screening (see also Chapter 19)   People of South Asian descent may be affected by hereditary conditions such as sickle cell disease or thalassaemia depending on their family's area of origin (see Chapter 25).

LABOUR AND BIRTH

Labour   In many communities in the Indian subcontinent it is traditional for a young woman expecting her first child to go home to her parents' house towards the end of the pregnancy and to have her baby there. The village midwife, her mother and other married female relatives support and encourage her during labour and birth. Her husband stays at his home. The new mother then often stays with her family for several weeks, resting, while the other women in the family look after her and the baby. If it is possible, she may return home in this way for every birth. Some women who are unable to be with their parents at this important time may feel lonely and unsupported.

In the Indian subcontinent labour and birth are traditionally attended only by women, though some fathers are now becoming involved, especially in urban areas. Resources and practices vary, but in many places there is little or no analgesia available, women can usually move around freely, adopting whatever position is most comfortable, and vaginal examinations are rarely carried out unless there are problems (Sen, 1989). In Britain an increasing number of South Asian fathers wish to stay with their wives during labour and the birth of their baby. However, many men, particularly in the more conservative communities, are still reluctant, and many women prefer to have one or more female companions with them if possible. Husbands who are embarrassed or worried by the idea of being with their wives during labour and birth should not be required to stay (see also Chapter 20).

Immediately after the birth   The practice of placing the baby on the mother's tummy straight after delivery may distress some women. They may want the baby washed first to remove any impurity from the birth canal. Some Muslim parents may want to whisper the call to prayer into their baby's ear (see Chapter 37). It is important to find out antenatally whether parents will want the baby washed immediately, and whether they will want to carry out religious or other ceremonies after the birth.

The sex of the baby   In the Indian subcontinent, as in many societies, there is traditionally a strong preference for male children. Family wealth and traditions are handed down through sons. Sons are also potential breadwinners for the whole family, and are responsible for the financial and practical support of elderly parents and other family members for their whole lives. The eldest son has a particular duty to support his parents. Where there are no pensions or other means of support for the sick and elderly, having a son may literally be a matter of survival.

Daughters, on the other hand, however much they are loved, traditionally leave home when they marry and live with their in-laws for the rest of their lives. They take on responsibility for their husband's parents and his other relatives. They do not contribute to the family income, and, in some communities, require an expensive dowry if they are to make a good marriage.

Attitudes towards boys and girls are changing in the Indian subcontinent, especially with the increased education of girls and now that, at least in urban areas, many women go out to work and can help support the family. Nevertheless, views on their status and value are slow to change in conservative communities. In Britain, attitudes have changed or are changing in most communities. Girls have more or less equal opportunities, equal access to education, and can go out to work. In most South Asian families in Britain, girls and boys are welcomed equally. Nevertheless, some people may feel let down if their new baby is another girl, and it may take time to get over the disappointment.

The placenta   In some South Asian communities families traditionally bury the placenta and umbilical cord after the birth. In other communities the placenta is regarded as polluted. It is helpful to discuss antenatally whether parents have any special wishes.

POSTNATAL CARE

Rest and recovery   In the Indian subcontinent it is traditionally extremely important that a woman should rest at home for at least six weeks after the birth. She is considered physically and emotionally vulnerable and needs sleep, warmth and good food. The other women of the family normally care for both her and her baby and for any other children, and encourage her to stay in bed and to ask for help whenever she needs it. The baby is brought to her for feeds if it is not in her bed. All this is considered vital to a woman's long-term physical and emotional well-being. Failure to rest is believed to slow down recovery and to risk serious long-term damage to her health. Lack of exclusive, close physical contact between mother and baby in the first few days does not appear to cause any problems (Woollett and Dosanjh-Matwala, 1990) (see also Chapter 21).

Discussing the baby   In some communities it is traditional not to praise the baby's appearance, in case this attracts jealousy or misfortune. Some people may put black spots or marks on a baby's face or body to make the baby less attractive and reduce the risk of the 'evil eye' (see also Chapter 21). Some people may find comparisons between the baby and other members of the family offensive.

Lochia   Some women consider lochia to be bad blood which the body needs to get rid of and may worry if the flow seems light. Some may also feel embarrassed to show soiled sanitary pads to a midwife. Midwives should be sensitive to this and could, for example, only ask to see pads when the woman's description of her blood loss gives cause for concern. Some women may also be distressed and humiliated by perineal examinations. All unnecessary examinations should be avoided.

Feeding the baby   In the Indian subcontinent babies are traditionally breast fed, often for a year or more, and breast feeding is generally highly valued (Ahmet, 1990; Bahl, 1986). Nevertheless, where artificial milk has been heavily promoted and advertised, many women may feel that it would be better to give their baby bottled milk if they could.

In some communities colostrum is not traditionally given to babies. Babies are given a mixture of sugar and water or artificial milk until the milk comes in (see also Chapter 21).

Naming the baby   Traditions vary in different communities. In some families, for example, the name is normally chosen by older relatives, or by the father's sister. If the people responsible for the choice are in the Indian subcontinent the name may take some time to arrive. Meanwhile the family will use a nickname (see also Chapters 14 and 21).

Contraception   Historically, high perinatal mortality and morbidity rates in the Indian subcontinent mean that South Asian families have traditionally needed to be large to ensure the survival and well-being of the family (Ahmed, 1990; Mamdani, 1972). One study quoted by Mamdani found that seven pregnancies were essential to ensure the survival of one son.

In Britain, shortage of space, the cost of children, lower mortality rates, lack of extended family support, changed priorities and other factors mean that many families decide to have fewer children. For some people, however, it is a duty to accept as a blessing every child that God sends and contraception is not acceptable.

Some women may be reluctant to attend family planning clinics or to discuss contraception because they do not want to discuss intimate matters with a male doctor. It is important that women know beforehand that there are always female staff available to provide information and advice. In some couples men make the decision on contraception and take full responsibility for it (see also Chapter 21).

CHILDBEARING LOSSES

Infertility   See Chapter 22

Termination of pregnancy   Termination may be rejected by many people on cultural or religious grounds (see also Chapter 22). Some women will only consider a termination if their situation is desperate. For religious rulings on termination see the chapters on different religions below.

Miscarriage, stillbirth and neonatal death   Grave stigma is traditionally attached to childbearing loss in some conservative South Asian communities, especially if it is caused by an abnormality and/or if it occurs more than once. Some women may wish to keep their miscarriage secret. For parents whose baby dies at a later gestation or after birth it may be important to keep the cause of the baby's death secret and possibly not to mourn too openly. It is clearly important to maintain strict confidentiality, and also to ensure that the parents are well-informed about the cause of the death, where this is known, and equipped to inform others accurately should they wish to do so.

Following a miscarriage, stillbirth or a neonatal death, some mothers may wish to observe the traditional period of postnatal rest and seclusion (see above).

In the Indian subcontinent, as in many hot parts of the world, it is traditionally important that burial or cremation should take place as soon after death as possible. For some communities this has a religious imperative. Some families may need help in getting death certificates and other essential paperwork completed as soon as possible.

In some communities it is considered better that the mother should not attend the funeral in case she becomes too distressed. In such cases it may be important to help mothers or couples find acceptable ways to create other memories around their baby (see also Chapter 22 and the chapters on religions). In most South Asian communities white is the traditional colour of mourning.

Post mortems   See Chapter 22

Religions

35 **Christianity**

The information below will only apply to certain Christian clients. Never assume. Always check everything with the person concerned.

CHRISTIANITY – A BRIEF DESCRIPTION

Christians believe in a loving God who is known in three ways – as Father, Son and Holy Spirit. They believe that everything is created and given life by God the Father. He entrusted the world to humanity but people's deceitful and cruel behaviour led them away from Him. This story is told in the books of the Jewish scriptures known by Christians as the Old Testament. The Old Testament is also seen as predicting the coming of Jesus Christ, the Saviour of humankind.

Jesus Christ

Christians believe that God the Father eventually sent His son Jesus as a human being to save humankind and to show people the way back to God. Jesus was a Jew who lived in Israel at the time of the Roman Occupation about 2,000 years ago. The stories of Jesus' life and mission are recorded in the four gospels of the New Testament, the most important holy book for most Christians. Jesus, known as the Christ (the Anointed One), summed up the whole of God's law as to love God and to love one's neighbour as oneself.

Many of Jesus' contemporaries became his followers and believed in him as their Saviour; others saw him as a wise teacher and kindly prophet. However, to many of the religious leaders in his society he was a threat because he claimed to be the divine Son of God and the Saviour (Messiah) whom the prophets had predicted would deliver the Jewish people. He was accused by the religious leaders of blasphemy and high treason and was killed by crucifixion by order of the Roman governor of Jerusalem.

Most Christians believe that Jesus Christ rose from the dead three days later and remained on earth appearing and preaching for forty days. He then ascended into heaven. For most Christians the resurrection of Christ is central to their faith since it shows that Christ overcame death, redeemed humankind and brought the hope of eternal life after death. Many Christians believe in the Second Coming of Christ at the end of the world when Christ will come to judge all mankind. They believe in Heaven as the ultimate reward for those who follow God's commandments and live a good life.

The founding of the church

Before Christ died he held a meal with his closest followers, the twelve apostles. At this meal, known as the Last Supper, Christ entrusted his message to the apostles and in particular, to the apostle Peter. He named Peter as head of his church. He also blessed bread and wine and gave it to the apostles. He asked them to do the same in memory of him. This is the basis of the Christian communion (see below).

The apostles and the other men and women who had followed Jesus took up his message and travelled around, despite severe persecution, preaching salvation through belief in Jesus Christ and through good works. They formed the early Christian church. In the year AD 313 the Roman Emperor Constantine was converted to Christianity and Christianity became the official religion of the Roman Empire, including Roman-occupied areas of Britain.

In the 2,000 years since Christ's death the Christian church has divided into a large number of different churches with different practices and views, each generally believing it is the true inheritor of Christ's message. Christianity is a missionary religion and in its various forms has spread throughout the world, in particular to Europe, much of the old Russian Empire, North and South America, the Far East, Central and Southern Africa and Australasia. Roughly one third of the world's population professes a variety of Christianity (Green, 1992).

The Christian churches in Britain

It has been estimated that there are about seven million practising Christians in the UK, but that probably about 38 million people would categorise themselves as Christians (Weller, 1993). The main Christian churches represented in Britain are:

- The Anglican church (the Church of England and its sister churches), which separated from the Roman Catholic Church during the Reformation in the sixteenth century (see below).
- The Roman Catholic Church (see below).
- The free or non-conformist churches, whose forebears wished to take the Anglican Reformation further. These include, for example, the Baptist Church, the Methodist Church, the Seventh-Day Adventist Church (see below), the United Reformed Church, Pentecostalist Churches (including the Elim Church and the Assemblies of God) (see below), the Society of Friends (Quakers) and the Salvation Army.
- The Eastern Orthodox churches, including the Greek, Russian and Serb Orthodox Churches, which split off from the Roman Catholic church in the eleventh century.

Although all these churches share belief in God and the divinity of Christ, there are often major differences between them in terms of beliefs, practices and attitudes. They also attach different importance to the sacraments, sacred ceremonies such as baptism and communion ordained by Jesus Christ, which confer special blessings on those who receive them.

In the past thirty years there have been important attempts to try to increase unity and communication between the different churches though these have not always been successful. Nevertheless, inter-church relations are now generally positive and in many cases ministers cooperate, for example, in visiting and caring for people in hospital. Despite this, many Christians are very much attached to their own particular branch of Christianity and its practices.

Christian values

All Christians regard the books of the Old Testament and the New Testament as having a special significance. Some churches regard every word as the absolutely literal and sacred truth. They set detailed standards of belief, practice and behaviour for their members based on a literal reading of biblical texts. Other churches regard the Bible as a source of information about God's purpose for humankind which must be interpreted (especially the Old Testament) in the light of modern thinking and circumstances.

Christianity stresses the importance of living a good life according to God's law, and of virtues such as honesty, justice, peace, compassion and love. Most Christians regard this life as a preparation for life after death; those who have led a good life according to Christian principles and who have loved God will be rewarded by eternal life in heaven. For many devout Christians, therefore, the suffering and pain of this life are only part of the picture, and decisions are made within the wider framework of God's law. Most Christian churches regard marriage and the family as central to a good Christian life, but attitudes differ on issues such as divorce, premarital sex, contraception, homosexuality and so on. Some churches, including the Roman Catholic Church and the Greek Orthodox Church, forbid the termination of pregnancy. (For more about specific practices and beliefs see the sections on Anglicanism, Roman Catholicism, Seventh-Day Adventism and Pentecostalism in this chapter.)

Few of the Christian churches prescribe precise details of daily life such as daily prayer, diet and dress. These are generally, though not always, regarded as personal issues. In many churches, Christians are expected to make their own decisions based on their personal beliefs and values. Although these beliefs and values are individual they are not flexible. It is important to find out what each woman requires and to respect her decisions.

For most Christian churches (though not all, see Seventh-Day Adventists below) Sunday is a day of rest and church attendance (usually optional). Services on Sunday may include communion, in which bread (and sometimes wine) are blessed and shared among the congregation.

In Britain church attendance has generally declined in the past forty years. However, many people who no longer practise their religion still regard themselves as Christian and may be grateful for the offer of a visit by a minister at times of distress and worry (see also Chapter 16).

Prayer

Prayer, both formal and informal, is important to many Christians, and may become particularly so around important life events such as birth and death and at times of anxiety and sorrow. Some people may say the Lord's Prayer or other prayers in hospital, or read the Bible. Some may wish for a chaplain or another Christian to pray with them. Some may wish to pray out loud and may need privacy for this. Some people may bring religious items such as prayer books, statues, pictures or a rosary into hospital with them. These should always be treated with respect.

Holy Communion

Some people in hospital may wish to attend a formal service or to receive Holy Communion on the ward. This is consecrated bread, and sometimes wine, taken in memory of the Last Supper (see above). It is normally brought by a priest or minister. The significance attached to Holy Communion varies in the different Christian churches (see also Roman Catholicism).

Festivals

There are certain important Christian festivals related to the life and death of Jesus Christ which most Christians celebrate. The most important festivals for most people are Christmas and Easter. The dates of these and other festivals usually fall later in the Orthodox churches than in the Western churches.

Christmas celebrates the birth of Christ and is a time of rejoicing and thanksgiving. It is also a time of family reunions and visits and present-giving. Many Christians go to church and some attend a service on the evening of Christmas Eve. In most UK churches Christmas Day falls on 25 December.

Ash Wednesday marks the beginning of Lent, the forty days before Easter (see below). Traditionally this was a period of severe fasting and penance in preparation for Easter.

Nowadays, it is generally less strictly observed but many Christians give up something special or take on an extra task during Lent. This is intended to teach self-discipline and self-denial and to enable the person in a small way to imitate Christ's suffering in the saving of humankind. Very devout Greek Orthodox Christians may, for example, eat no meat during Lent, and eat a very restricted diet in the last week. Some Catholics may attend extra masses during Lent.

Easter begins on **Good Friday**, a sombre day on which Christians remember the suffering and death of Christ on the cross. Some devout Christians may go to church, especially in the afternoon around the time when Christ is known to have died.

Easter Sunday celebrates Christ's resurrection from the dead after his crucifixion and is extremely important and joyful for most devout Christians. Many Christians go to church. For Orthodox Christians Easter is generally a more important festival than Christmas. Easter Sunday in the Western churches usually falls in March or April depending on the lunar calendar.

There are other festivals which may be important to some Christians, for example, the Ascension, which commemorates Christ's ascension into heaven, Pentecost, which commemorates the descent of the Holy Spirit (one of the three aspects of God) to Jesus' apostles after his death, and the Assumption, or Dormition (on 15 August), which commemorates the ascension into heaven of Mary, the mother of Jesus. The latter is mainly celebrated by Catholics and members of the Orthodox churches. These and other festivals may be celebrated in different ways by members of different churches.

Jewellery

Some Christians wear religious jewellery, for example, a cross, a medal of Christ or a saint or a picture on a chain or thread around the neck. Some religious jewellery has been blessed and may sometimes be believed to protect the wearer especially at times of special vulnerability. Religious jewellery should be taped if at all possible. If this is not possible, find an acceptable alternative.

Priests and ministers

In most Christian churches there is a priest, minister or pastor (who may also have another title) who leads services, administers sacraments and carries out pastoral care and counselling for the community. In some churches, including the Anglican Church, the priest may be a woman. Many hospitals have an Anglican, a Free Church and a Catholic chaplain, all either part-time or full-time.

Baptism

The sacrament of Baptism or Christening is practised by nearly all Christians. It commemorates the baptism of Christ by his cousin John and is seen as the beginning of an individual's relationship with God through the Church. In some churches baptism takes place when an individual is old enough to understand the commitment they are making. In such cases baptism may involve total immersion in a special pool of water. Some churches baptise infants on the basis of the faith and commitment of the parents. Godparents or sponsors may promise to help with the spiritual education of the child, and in some cases to give practical and financial support.

Emergency baptism   Some parents may want a very premature or seriously ill baby to be baptised, in which case the appropriate hospital chaplain should be called. In an emergency, for example if a baby collapses and there is not time to call a chaplain, baptism may be performed by anyone, but preferably by someone who themselves has been baptised. However, **even in an emergency it is always essential to consult the parents first**. Their consent is important on theological as well as psychological grounds, because they are taking on the commitment to God on their child's behalf. Parents must also be asked what name they want to give their child since the child's name must be used during the baptism.

> *'Some years ago I met a women whose experience shows how emergency baptism can be appallingly mishandled. The woman had had a traumatic birth and was resting. A midwife came in and said, 'I baptised your baby because he is poorly. We decided to call him Roger.' The baby subsequently died and the mother was not only deeply shocked and distressed but carried the anger inside her for years. She had not been told his condition was so serious. She had not wanted him to be baptised, a sacrament which to her was about life not death. And the final agony was that no one had consulted her about the choice of name, which is always immensely important to the parents.'*   Childbirth educator

To baptise a baby the following words should be spoken: ' . . . . (the child's name), I baptise you in the name of the Father, the Son and the Holy Spirit, Amen.' At the same time a little water should be sprinkled on the child's head. If the baby is in an incubator, sterile water may be preferable. It may also be easier to administer on a teaspoon.

If a baby dies unbaptised or is stillborn, a chaplain may offer a naming and blessing ceremony soon after the death.

DEATH AND FUNERALS

Anointing of the sick   When a person is very sick or known to be dying, Christians of some denominations may wish a priest to say prayers. He or she may also anoint the body of the sick person with blessed oil while saying certain prayers to give the person courage for whatever lies ahead of them, for forgiveness, and for restoration to health or acceptance into heaven according to God's plan. Anointing of the sick is not usually carried out for babies.

Last offices   Most Christians are not particular about who touches the body after death. Provided the family wishes, the normal procedures should be carried out.

Funeral services   Funeral services usually begin with a service in church led by a priest. After this the family and close relatives and friends generally accompany the body to the cemetery or crematorium. Most Christian denominations permit both burial and cremation. It is traditional in some Christian communities for people to go to the home of the family after the service to express their sympathy and have something to eat and drink.

Post mortems   Most Christians have no religious objection to post mortems.

The Anglican Church

The Anglican Church, which includes the Church of England and its sister churches, the Church of Wales, the Episcopalian Church and the Church of Ireland, has been the established or official church in Britain since it separated from the Roman Catholic Church in the sixteenth century. There are also Anglicans in most other parts of the world, including the Indian subcontinent, Hong Kong, East, West and Southern Africa, and North and South America. Altogether, there are about 70 million Anglicans in the world.

The Anglican church contains a very broad range of beliefs, practices and attitudes and few regulations which bind members' daily lives. Each individual makes their own decisions on matters of personal morality. Anglicans whose families originated in other parts of the world may also be influenced in their religious practice by different local cultures. As always it is important to ask each person what they would like and to avoid any assumptions.

Because the Anglican church is the established church of Great Britain and Northern Ireland, most hospital religious provision has evolved on the basis of traditional Anglican practices. There is also an Anglican chaplain in most hospitals who offers pastoral care and comfort and administers the sacraments. He or she also offers care to members of other religious denominations or to people with no formal religious attachment if asked, and can liaise with representatives of other religious groups as necessary.

The information below will only apply to certain Anglican clients. Never assume. Always check everything with the person concerned.

CHILDBEARING ISSUES

Anglican clients are unlikely to have specifically religious requirements at the birth of a baby provided all is well. It is important, however, to ask each client beforehand.

The Anglican prayer book provides a service of 'Thanksgiving for the Birth of a Child' which is normally used with the whole family in church rather than at home or in the hospital. This has replaced the old tradition (now generally disapproved of) of the Churching of women after a birth, which was originally intended to remove the pollution of the birth process.

Almost all practising Anglicans will wish to have their baby baptised by a minister within the first few months of birth, usually in their parish church.

Infertility Most Anglicans do not have religious views on different methods of investigation and treatment. Some may, however, feel strongly about the destruction of 'unused' fertilised embryos and the 'selective reduction' of implanted embryos (see below).

Termination of pregnancy Practising Anglicans may disapprove strongly of abortion, though the teaching of the Anglican Church on this subject is not as explicit or publicised as that of the Roman Catholic Church (see below). Termination may be more acceptable if the baby has a serious or life-threatening abnormality, or in the case of rape.

Miscarriage There is no specific religious service for a baby that has miscarried. Some ministers will conduct a simple funeral service after a late miscarriage. Not all parents will be aware of this possibility and it may be helpful to suggest it.

Stillbirth and neonatal death A funeral service is normally held for babies who are stillborn or die shortly after birth. It is not necessary for the baby to have been baptised, though for some parents the fact that their baby was not baptised may heighten their grief. The prayers said at the funeral may differ slightly depending on whether the baby was baptised.

Contraception   Most Anglicans do not object to artificial methods of contraception. Some may object to the use of the coil and other abortifacients.

Roman Catholicism

The information below will only apply to certain Catholic clients. Never assume. Always check everything with the person concerned.

Roman Catholicism is a branch of Christianity and is in itself a major world religion. It is estimated that roughly one-fifth of the world's population is Roman Catholic (Green, 1993).

Roman Catholics in Britain

In the UK, Catholics make up about 13 per cent of the total population (Green, 1993) and have a very mixed heritage. There is a small number of old English Catholic families in Britain whose forebears survived the Protestant Reformation in the sixteenth century and its aftermath. In Northern Ireland Catholics currently make up 38 per cent of the population (personal communication, Northern Ireland Office, 1994). The families of most other Catholics originated elsewhere in Europe, including the Irish Republic (the largest number), Italy, Spain, Portugal and Poland. There are also smaller Catholic communities whose families originated in the West Indies, the Philippines, South America, southern India and Sri Lanka, Hong Kong, the Middle East, and central and southern Africa. A survey in the 1970s found that one-quarter of the Catholics in Britain were immigrants and another fifth were the children of immigrants (Hornsby-Smith, 1991).

Within the overall unifying framework of Catholicism, individual practice and the strictness with which official Catholic rulings are observed differ a great deal in different countries. There are therefore major differences in practice and observance among Catholics in Britain, often influenced by the areas of origin of their families, as well as by factors such as personal experience and education. At the same time it is important to bear in mind that for each Roman Catholic her or his own decisions on adherence to official Catholic rulings are a matter of individual conscience and must be respected.

ROMAN CATHOLICISM – A BRIEF DESCRIPTION

The Roman Catholic Church states that it represents the authentic tradition of the church that Christ founded based on a direct line of succession from Saint Peter. The Pope, the head of the Roman Catholic Church, elected by the body of cardinals, lives in the Vatican City in Rome and is generally regarded as Saint Peter's direct successor and as having God-given spiritual authority. He speaks out and writes on moral and spiritual issues, setting out matters of faith and what the church requires of its members.

After the Second Vatican Council led by Pope John XXIII in the early 1960s there were major changes within the Catholic Church, including, at least within many local communities, greater lay involvement and more open discussion. These coincided with major changes in social values and behaviour in Britain. Although official Vatican teaching is now more traditional, there is a wide variety of beliefs, attitudes and practices on many key issues within the British Catholic community. While some people adhere strictly to traditional Catholic practices and beliefs, others feel that it is acceptable to make their own decisions provided they are based on Christian principles and ethics and on their own conscience. It is very important therefore not to make any assumptions but to find out from each woman what is important to her.

RELIGIOUS OBSERVANCE

Sunday Mass and Holy Communion   Sunday is traditionally regarded as a holy day for prayer and family pursuits. Catholics are required to go to Mass once a week on Sunday or on Saturday evening.

Mass is the most important Catholic religious service, at which the sacrifice of Jesus Christ on the cross is remembered and bread and wine are consecrated and blessed by the priest. The bread (and sometimes the wine) is distributed to those Catholic children and adults who have made their first Holy Communion. The blessing of the bread and wine during Mass are believed by Catholics to transform them into the actual body and blood of Jesus Christ. Holy Communion is therefore regarded as extremely sacred and as a very special gift from God.

Out of reverence for the sacrament, people should fast, that is, not eat or drink for at least an hour before taking Holy Communion, though this is not always strictly observed. Some people, in contrast, may fast for longer. People should not take Holy Communion if they have done anything seriously wrong. If a person has committed a serious sin or has not been to Holy Communion for a long time they may want to go to confession (see below) before receiving Holy Communion.

Although attendance at Mass is officially required once a week and failure to attend may be regarded as a serious sin, many Catholics in Britain do not go to Mass regularly. For some, however, it is very important to attend Mass if at all possible. A few very devout people go to Mass every day. Some women would like Holy Communion brought to them on the ward on Sundays and possibly on other days. This should be arranged with the Catholic chaplain.

Confession   Confession (also called the Sacrament of Penance or Reconciliation) is a sacrament at which people confess their sins privately to a priest, say that they are sorry and promise to try never to do wrong again. They agree to do whatever penance the priest requires (usually to say certain prayers), and receive counselling and forgiveness (absolution). The priest is believed to act as a representative of Jesus Christ in confession. Once sins have been forgiven in confession they are regarded as forgiven by God.

The practice of attending confession has almost died out in many Catholic communities but is currently reviving a little. For some women it may be important to make a confession before receiving Holy Communion or if they are seriously ill. This should be arranged with the Catholic chaplain.

Food restrictions   Catholics should not eat meat or drink alcohol on Good Friday (the day on which Christ's death on the cross is remembered) or on Ash Wednesday (the first day of Lent, the period of repentance leading up to Good Friday). Traditionally it was also forbidden to eat meat on all Fridays, again in memory of Christ's death and some people still adhere to this. Abstaining from meat is seen as a symbolic sacrifice.

FAMILIES AND RELATIONSHIPS

The Catholic church lays down clear guidelines relating to marriage and relationships. The family and marriage are regarded as extremely important especially in relation to bringing up children. Sexual intercourse is only permitted within marriage. Divorce is prohibited except in a few situations such as the non-consummation of a marriage when the Vatican may grant an annulment. Divorced people cannot remarry in the Catholic Church. Divorced Catholics who remarry outside the Church cannot officially receive Holy Communion (see above).

Many Catholics regard Mary, the mother of Jesus, as particularly holy and virtuous, since she dedicated her life selflessly and generously to fulfilling God's will. It is part of Roman Catholic doctrine that Mary remained a virgin all her life. Traditionally Mary is regarded as a role model for Catholic women. Nowadays, attitudes to the role and sexuality of women vary a good deal among Catholics but the official Church ruling is that women have a special role as mothers and should be supported and honoured in this role. Many Catholics regard Mary as having a special power to help get their prayers answered.

CHILDBEARING ISSUES

Antenatal screening Some Catholics may consider screening to detect fetal abnormalities unacceptable, particularly if they would not consider a termination (see below). However, others may prefer to know the true situation, even if they regard termination of pregnancy as prohibited. Catholics of African, African-Caribbean, Mediterranean, South Asian and Far Eastern descent may be at risk of haemoglobinopathies (see Chapter 25).

Baptism The Catholic church practises infant baptism, though there may be some variation in Catholic families of Middle Eastern heritage. Traditionally, babies were baptised in the first few days after birth, since it was believed that if an unbaptised baby died he or she could not go to heaven. However, beliefs have now changed and, provided the baby is not seriously ill, baptisms are now sometimes delayed for weeks or months, especially if parents wish close relatives from abroad to attend. At the baptism the baby is officially given his or her Christian name. (For emergency baptism see the general section on Christianity above.)

Contraception The Roman Catholic Church officially forbids all artificial contraception, including sterilisation, on the grounds that it interferes with God's natural law. Contraception using the safe period (or rhythm method) is, however, permitted. Although no figures are available it is believed that most Catholics in Britain use artificial methods of contraception, regarding this as an issue where it is acceptable for individual conscience and belief to override official religious rulings. A few devout Catholics, however, do not use artificial contraception. When discussing contraception with a Catholic woman or couple it is important to start by ascertaining their own views and to be aware that the Church's ruling may cause tensions for some people.

PREGNANCY LOSS

Infertility The Roman Catholic church officially forbids all forms of infertility investigation or treatment that involve masturbation because these dissociate the sexual act from the procreative act. The donation of sperm or eggs by another person and surrogate motherhood are forbidden. Some Catholics who accept certain methods of investigation and treatment may reject the destruction of 'unused' fertilised embryos and the 'selective reduction' of implanted embryos.

Although the Church recognises the suffering caused by infertility, it enjoins infertile couples for whom no acceptable treatment is effective to express their generosity through adoption or by performing services for other people. As with contraception, many Catholics feel that it is acceptable to obey their own consciences on this issue and to use any form of treatment or screening that is necessary. For those who follow the Church's ruling it may be important, where possible, to use methods of collecting sperm during intercourse between husband and wife.

Termination of pregnancy The Roman Catholic church strictly forbids all termination of pregnancy and regards termination as murder and a grievous or mortal sin. A baby is considered to have a soul and full human rights from the moment of conception.

Nevertheless, some Catholic women will consent to a termination, especially if the baby is known to have a serious congenital abnormality, if they are unmarried, or following rape. In discussing the possibility of termination with Catholic women it is important to be aware of the strength of the Catholic ruling on this issue and possible feelings of guilt at a later date if a woman has a termination. Strict confidentiality is also extremely important.

Miscarriage   There is no specific religious service for a baby that has miscarried. Some ministers will conduct a simple funeral service after a late miscarriage. Not all parents will be aware of this possibility and it may be helpful to suggest it.

Stillbirth and neonatal death   A funeral service is held for babies who are stillborn or die shortly after birth. It is not necessary for the baby to have been baptised. The prayers said at the funeral differ slightly depending on whether the baby was baptised. For some parents the fact that their baby was not baptised may add to their distress.

Seventh-Day Adventism

The information below will only apply to certain Seventh-day Adventist clients. Never assume. Always check everything with the person concerned.

INTRODUCTION

The Seventh-Day Adventist Church developed from Protestant Christian roots in Europe and the United States during the ninteenth century. There are now about 8 million Seventh-Day Adventists in 204 countries world-wide. In Britain there are approximately 17,000 Seventh-day Adventists, 11,000 of whom live in southern Britain. Approximately 85 per cent of British Seventh-Day Adventists are of African-Caribbean heritage.

RELIGIOUS BELIEFS AND PRACTICES

The Seventh-Day Adventist Church bases its beliefs wholly on the Old and New Testaments of the Bible and has developed twenty-seven fundamental beliefs. Amongst these are belief in the Trinity, consisting of God the Father, God the Son and God the Holy Spirit; in the Second Coming of Jesus Christ when the righteous dead will be resurrected; and in the importance of the Ten Commandments.

The Church teaches the importance of strengthening family relationships, of monogamy, of chastity before marriage, and of the equality of men and women. Divorce is viewed as a last resort. The Church offers education and guidance to its congregants and expects them to maintain high moral standards in all areas of life, while also emphasising personal responsibility and individual choice about observance and religious practice.

On the basis of the biblical statement that the body is the temple of the Holy Spirit, the Church places great emphasis on the importance of health and supports medical research. The Church runs 160 hospitals throughout the world. Many local churches run health education programmes for their communities. The Church also stresses the importance of education and runs primary and secondary schools and colleges in many countries. In the UK and Eire there are eight primary schools, two secondary schools and one Seventh-Day Adventist college.

Each community has a pastor who offers support and comfort as well as being a source of information and advice.

'Adventists as a whole have tremendous respect for the quality of life and this affects the decisions we make for ourselves and our families. We ask that you are sensitive to our needs and wishes.' Seventh-Day Adventist pastor

Prayer   Although there are no set times for prayer, many Seventh-Day Adventists pray, meditate and read the Bible every day. In hospital, it is important to respect and accommodate people's privacy and need for quiet at these times.

The Sabbath

'The Sabbath, Saturday, is our rest day. How we observe it is a profoundly personal choice. It is not imposed on us by the Church and we would like our individual needs and beliefs to be respected.' Health care assistant and mother of three

Seventh-Day Adventists observe Saturday as the Sabbath, the seventh day of the week, a day of rest and worship. The Sabbath starts on Friday night at sundown and ends at sundown on Saturday. Traditionally it is a day for prayer and meditation and for being with family and the community. Most Adventists, including infants and older children, regularly attend church and Bible study sessions on the Sabbath. Some women prepare food beforehand in order to cut down their work on the Sabbath, so Fridays may be particularly busy days and unsuitable for antenatal appointments. Many people do not watch television on the Sabbath and may be disturbed if there is a television on in their hospital ward.

Other festivals   Christmas and Easter are celebrated to varying degrees by different congregations. Seventh-Day Adventists recognise that the dates on which most Christians celebrate these festivals are not historically accurate.

Food restrictions   The religious dietary restrictions followed by Seventh-Day Adventists vary and are to some extent a matter of personal choice influenced by family traditions and cultural origins. Many Seventh-Day Adventists are vegetarians. Some are vegan and do not eat cheese, eggs or milk. Others avoid shellfish and certain meats such as pork and offal. Although these decisions are individual, they are firm and should be respected. It is important to find out from each woman what her dietary preferences are, to ensure that any advice on diet takes these into account, and to see that she is offered food that is acceptable to her while she is in hospital.

When Seventh-Day Adventists are baptised they promise to abstain from alcohol and recreational drugs including tobacco. Many Seventh-Day Adventists do not drink tea or coffee. There is, however, no restriction on the medical use of narcotics, for example, to control pain in labour or during and after surgery.

CHILDBEARING ISSUES

Antenatal screening   Since termination of pregnancy may be unacceptable to many Seventh-Day Adventists (see below), women should always be given clear explanations of the purpose of the various screening tests and the decisions which could arise as a result. Seventh-Day Adventists of African-Caribbean and other heritages may be at risk of haemoglobinopathies.

Welcoming the baby   There is no religious ceremony at birth. As soon as the parents feel ready, they bring the baby before the congregation for a service of dedication. During this they promise to care for the child spiritually and physically, and the congregation acknowledges and welcomes the child and accepts communal responsibility for him or her.

Baptism is not performed in infancy. Instead Believer's Baptism takes place later when the individual has gained sufficient understanding of scripture.

Contraception   The Church emphasises that both men and women should take responsibility for family planning and teaches that family planning is part of a Christian's responsibility in today's world. In general, Seventh-Day Adventists are likely to choose birth control methods that prevent conception rather than those that are effective after conception.

PREGNANCY LOSS

Infertility   Decisions about accepting investigations and treatment for infertility are matters of personal choice.

Termination of pregnancy   Although the Seventh-Day Adventist Church affirms the sanctity of all human life it also acknowledges the right of individual women to decide whether or not to terminate a pregnancy. A decision about termination is therefore ultimately a matter of personal choice and belief rather than a religious obligation. Termination is most likely to be acceptable in exceptional circumstances, for example when the pregnancy endangers the mother's life or is the result of rape, or when the baby is diagnosed as having a severe congenital defect. If a woman decides to terminate a pregnancy, the Church teaches that the congregation should offer her and her family 'gracious support'.

Miscarriage, stillbirth and neonatal death   There are no particular religious require-ments when a baby dies during pregnancy or around the time of birth. As always, bereaved parents will full need information about their choices, and support to decide what is best for them.

The Pentecostalist Churches

The information below will only apply to certain Pentecostalist clients. Never assume. Always check everything with the person concerned.

The Pentecostalist movement is historically rooted in Protestantism but came into prominence in the twentieth century. In Britain the main Pentecostalist churches include the Elim Pentecostalist Church, the Church of God, the Assemblies of God and Apostolic Church and include a number of black-majority churches, many of which have their roots in the Caribbean (Weller, 1993). The term Pentecostalist is derived from Pentecost, the fortieth day after the ascension of Jesus Christ into heaven, when the Holy Spirit descended to a gathering of his apostles and disciples. It refers to a group of churches, some of which are very small, and there is a great deal of variation in practice and custom within the overall framework of Pentecostalist belief.

The Pentecostalist churches stress the importance of each person's active and loving relationship with God through Jesus Christ, the Saviour of the world, and through the Holy Spirit. Faith in God, in His purpose and love for humankind and His power to intervene directly in people's lives are very important; although life can be very hard, God will help people get through the difficult times. Many members of Pentecostalist churches follow the literal meaning of the Old and New Testaments, and believe that everything that happens is the will of God.

RELIGIOUS OBSERVANCE

Prayer   There are no formal times for prayer but people may pray privately at any time of the day or night. It is considered very important to pray for other people. Sometimes visitors may wish to pray out loud or sing hymns with a woman in hospital. Privacy should be provided for this where possible. Many Pentecostalists believe in physical and emotional healing through the power of prayer to God. Some may practise the laying on of hands.

Sunday services   Sunday is traditionally regarded as a special day, set apart for congregational worship and private prayer. People often read the scriptures and spend time with their families. In some homes there is no television on a Sunday.

Congregational worship is very important and is often lively and enthusiastic. In some Pentecostalist churches there may be services of healing, and people may be moved to speak in tongues. Speaking in tongues – speaking in an 'ecstatic, unlearned language other than one's own which can then be interpreted by another worshipper' (Weller, 1993) – is recorded in the New Testament as a sign of the coming of the Holy Spirit and is generally regarded in Pentecostalist churches as a great gift.

Every month Pentecostalists celebrate the Lord's supper with bread and wine and ceremonial washing of feet. This is known as congregation (communion). If a woman is in hospital for any length of time a minister may come to celebrate congregation with her.

Christmas and Easter are celebrated and Good Friday is a solemn day.

The minister   In many churches the minister, and sometimes his family, are the focus of much community activity. One of his main duties is to preach the word of God based on biblical revelation. The minister also has important pastoral duties. A Pentecostalist minister may visit families in hospital to pray with them.

Fasting   Fasting is part of the Pentecostalist tradition though individual practices vary. There are no set times for fasting. Sometimes a church sets aside special days for fasting and communal prayer, sometimes people decide to make a fast themselves. Sometimes people fast and pray because the congregation or particular person is in special need of help. Communal fasts may also be held for someone who is sick so that they may be healed.

The length of the fast varies. Sometimes a fast lasts for several days during which people drink and eat very little.

FAMILIES AND COMMUNITIES

Most Pentecostalist churches stress the importance of traditional family values and sexual morality. They also stress social responsibility and practical and emotional support for other members of the congregation, especially those who are ill, lonely or troubled.

CHILDBEARING ISSUES

Antenatal care   Many women will want to dress modestly at all times and may be anxious about physical exposure during check-ups and labour (see Chapter 20). Most are prepared to be examined by a male doctor.

Antenatal screening   Some Pentecostalists may consider screening for fetal abnormalities unacceptable, particularly if they would not consider a termination (see below). Others may prefer to know the true situation, even if they would not consider a termination. Pentecostalists of African-Caribbean and other heritages may be at risk of haemoglobinopathies.

Termination of pregnancy   Termination of pregnancy is generally prohibited and is regarded as the taking of a life.

Baptism   Baptism is very important in most Pentecostalist churches and recalls the coming of the Holy Spirit on the disciples of Jesus Christ in the form of tongues of fire, and the gift of speaking in tongues. There is no infant baptism. Prayers may be offered in thanks for the baby's safe arrival and future well-being. If a baby is very ill or dying, the family and members of the congregation gather at the bedside to pray and sing hymns for the baby.

Most Pentecostalist churches carry out the sacrament of baptism (often by full immersion in water) at an age when the person can freely and knowingly choose to dedicate their life to Christ.

Welcoming the baby   When babies are about six to twelve weeks old they may be brought to church for a service of dedication. This is their welcome into the community. Prayers are offered in thanks for the baby's safe arrival and also for the well-being and protection of the baby and his or her family.

DEATH AND FUNERALS

When a person is seriously ill or dying the minister and the family pray and sing at the bedside. There is no ritual anointing. Burial is generally preferred to cremation.

The information below will only apply to certain Hindu clients. Never assume. Always check everything with the person concerned.

This chapter focuses particularly on those Hindu beliefs, practices and customs likely to be relevant to the majority of Hindus in Britain whose families originated in north-western India. The religious practices and customs of Hindus from other parts of the Indian subcontinent may differ to some extent.

Hindu communities in Britain

Most Hindu families settled in the UK in the 1950s and 1960s and emigrated from the north-western states of Gujarat and Punjab (see Figure 34.1). (For more about traditional South Asian culture and language see Chapter 34.) The families of most Hindus from East Africa also originated in Gujarat and Punjab, having emigrated to East Africa earlier during the twentieth century (see Figure 31.1). Most of them arrived in Britain in the late 1960s and 1970s, many as refugees (see Chapter 34). A small number of Hindu families have come from other parts of India, as well as from countries such as Fiji, Guyana and some Caribbean islands, to which their forebears emigrated in the nineteenth century. In addition there are a number of Tamil Hindu families from Sri Lanka, most of whom have arrived in Britain as refugees more recently.

It is estimated that there are about 400,000 Hindus in the UK and about 30,000 Jains (see Jainism below) (Weller, 1993). Most Hindu women now of childbearing age were born and brought up in Britain and are the children and grandchildren of the immigrant generation.

THE HINDU NAMING SYSTEM (See Chapter 14)

HINDUISM – A BRIEF DESCRIPTION

Hinduism is the religion of most of the people of India. It is however much more than many Western people would think of as a religion. It is a social system and a way of life as well as a set of beliefs, values and religious practices, and a way of understanding the world.

Hinduism has no one founder, no one holy book, no central authority or hierarchy. It has developed over thousands of years in India, in response to many different developments of thought and practice. As a result, there is a tremendous diversity within Hinduism, depending mainly on people's region of origin, caste and subcaste, and family. There are also many different Hindu sects whose members may observe different practices and customs. Although there is great variation within Hindu practice and belief, for each individual his or her own religious beliefs and duties are clear and very important.

There are certain fundamental truths and values which almost all Hindus acknowledge, including: the existence of a Supreme Spirit; the immortal soul that exists in all living things; reincarnation – the cycle of birth, death and rebirth through which everyone must go; release from reincarnation as the ultimate aim of life; karma, the natural cycle of reward and punishment for every act and thought; a clear code of dutiful and right behaviour; non-violence; and the supreme duty of seeking Truth.

Most Hindus worship God, the Supreme Spirit, through one or more symbols or manifestations, that is, through gods and goddesses. Each god or goddess has certain qualities and characters.

Jainism

Some people whose families originated in Gujarat are Jains. Jainism is a development of Hinduism which occurred around the sixth century BCE. Jains believe that all living things, including beings too small for the human eye to see, are part of the great cycle of birth and rebirth. Most Jains are very strict vegetarians (see below). In India some very devout Jains sweep the ground before them to avoid treading on any living thing.

RELIGIOUS OBSERVANCE

Prayer Many devout Hindus pray three times a day; at sunrise, around noon, and before sunset. It is important to wash and, if possible, to put on clean clothes before praying. Women do not pray formally when they are menstruating or for forty days after giving birth.

A Hindu woman who has been admitted to hospital antenatally may wish to pray in the morning before she eats and drinks. If she cannot get out of bed she may need a bowl of water and a cup so that, at the very least, she can pour water over her hands and can sprinkle it over her head to symbolise washing.

Some women may wish to sit cross-legged on the bed to pray, sometimes covering their head with a scarf or cloth. They may set up a small shrine in front of them with a picture or statue on it. Some people use a mala – a string of beads – to help their concentration while they pray. A mala, and any holy books, pictures or statues should always be treated with reverence and should only be touched with clean hands. People should not be disturbed while praying. Some may prefer to have their curtains drawn for privacy.

Some women may bring holy books into hospital with them, often wrapped in a cloth for protection. The most popular Hindu Holy Book is the Bhagavad Gita (often simply called the Gita). All holy books must be kept clean and safe. They should not be put on the floor or near the feet or near shoes or dirty clothes, and nothing should be put on top of them. People should wash before they touch a holy book.

At home Many Hindu homes contain a small shrine with statues and pictures of the Hindu gods where family members can worship. This may be in a separate room, or, if space is short, may be set up in a corner or a glass-fronted cabinet. Sometimes the shrine is in the kitchen, which is regarded as the purest and cleanest room in the house since food is prepared there.

If a family has a separate room for prayer this must be kept pure and should not be entered without an invitation. Anyone who enters must take off their shoes at the door. Women visitors may be asked to cover their heads. No one should touch anything on a shrine unless specifically invited to.

The pandit Almost every Hindu temple (mandir) in Britain has a resident priest, a pandit, whose main role is to perform ceremonies in the temple. The pandit does not traditionally have a pastoral role though this is changing in some communities in Britain. Such duties as visiting the sick, praying over the dying, and comforting the bereaved are usually undertaken by relatives and other members of the community. In certain cases the pandit may be called upon to give advice and guidance on religious matters.

Festivals   The three most important festivals among Hindus in Britain are Holi (in February or March), Navratri, the festival of the nine nights (in September or October), and Diwali, the Hindu New Year's Eve (in October or November). The dates of Hindu festivals vary slightly each year, depending on the date of the full moon. (For more on the dates of festivals see Walshe and Warrier, 1993.)

FAMILIES AND RELATIONSHIPS

The family is traditionally central to Hindu life and to Hindu communities, as to all communities from the Indian subcontinent. In many areas of India the family is still a large unit comprising several generations and including cousins of different degrees (see Chapter 34). Even when Hindu families no longer live in extended family units, their family responsibilities and commitments may remain strong. Extended families are less common in certain communities, for example, among Tamils in Sri Lanka.

Marriage   Hindus are expected to marry and have children, with both men and women taking an active part in bringing up the children. Parents remain responsible for their children all their lives. Children are expected to repay this by obedience, and by marrying and bringing up their own family well. Showing respect for and caring for one's elders are religious duties. Sexual morality is traditionally strict.

Within most traditional Hindu families, although men are considered to have ultimate public authority, men and women generally share decisions. Women are considered mainly responsible for the comfort and well-being of their families, the upbringing and spiritual and moral education of their families, and the atmosphere and conduct of the home. One of the traditional religious duties of a Hindu woman is to honour and obey her husband. In turn, it is the duty of a Hindu man to treat his wife with kindness and respect. Women are particularly honoured when they become mothers.

Divorce   Marriage is regarded by Hindus as a holy and indissoluble sacrament. Divorced people, particularly women, may be strongly disapproved of and even rejected in some communities.

The caste system

Hindu society is traditionally divided into four castes and many hundreds of interdependent subcastes, based on social and occupational status and on geography. Traditionally, the caste and subcaste into which a person was born have defined their social and spiritual status, occupation, social contacts, and social and religious duties. People in higher castes had more important religious duties and were expected to be more strict in their observances. A person's caste is believed to be determined by karma, the natural cycle of reward and punishment for every act and thought. It is linked to reincarnation and is regarded by many Hindus as divinely ordained and part of natural law.

There are also people who fall outside the four main caste groupings. They do the jobs that are considered particularly spiritually polluting, such as cleaning streets and lavatories and dealing with dead animals. They used to be known as Outcastes or Untouchables. Strictly speaking they had no social relationship with anyone in the caste system, lived apart from other people and did not mix with them. Mahatma Gandhi (1869–1948), a Gujarati who, like many Hindu reformers, fought against the caste system, was particularly concerned to raise the status of the Outcastes. He called them Harijans, Children of God, and made a point of mixing and eating with them. It is now illegal in India to discriminate on grounds of caste.

The caste system has existed for thousands of years, during which different subcastes have lived completely separately, mixing little except in certain defined roles, and intermarrying very rarely. Despite the pressures of the twentieth century, the caste system is therefore slow to change, and subcaste identity and feeling often remain even when people have moved away from their roots. The caste system also has clear benefits as well as disadvantages for most people. People in each subcaste see themselves as a community, more or less as cousins. The family, and its extension, the subcaste, are traditionally the two most important groups to which an individual belongs. Most people marry and mix socially within their own subcaste. People may look to other members of their subcaste for company and support as well as for financial help with, for example, a loan for a house or money for a good cause.

In Britain, caste awareness is particularly likely to remain among older people. Caste bonds were very important and necessary during the early years of migration and settlement and many subcaste organisations were set up to help members in need. As time passes in Britain, other caste differences to do with occupation and wealth are increasingly blurred and less significant. Caste is still, however, likely to be important when it comes to marriage. Many Hindu parents will try to encourage marriage within their subcaste, believing that such a marriage is, for social, religious and economic reasons, likely to be more successful and lasting.

HINDU FOOD RESTRICTIONS

Many Hindus in Britain follow dietary restrictions, though there is a good deal of variation. In general, women, people who are more devout, and older people, are more likely to be careful about what they eat. In addition, members of certain Hindu sects are particularly strict about following food prohibitions. Although food restrictions vary, they are not flexible. It is important to ask each woman what she can and cannot eat (see also Chapter 18).

Hindus whose families originated in Gujarat are particularly likely to eat a vegetarian diet. Some Gujarati Hindus whose families emigrated from East Africa may be less strict but this cannot be assumed. Hindus whose families originated in other areas of the Indian subcontinent may also be less strict, but again this depends on subcaste and sect, as well as on family tradition and personal choice. Hindus whose families originated in the south-west coast of India may, for example, include fish in their diet. Hindus whose families originated in Sri Lanka may eat meat but will probably not eat pork or beef.

A vegetarian diet   Hindus traditionally believe that all forms of life are interdependent, and that all living things are sacred. Many devout Hindus do not eat any food that involves the taking of life, including meat, fish, eggs or anything made from or containing them. A strict Hindu vegetarian who eats any of these, even unknowingly, is likely to feel revolted and also polluted.

The cow   The cow is a sacred animal in Hinduism. It is considered a symbol of the gentleness and unselfish love of a mother, and is generally revered and protected. The eating of beef is particularly strictly prohibited, and many Hindus who eat other meat will not eat beef. Some may also refuse pork since the pig is a scavenging animal in India and pig meat is generally regarded as dirty. Some Hindus do not eat cheese made with animal rennet. (Some people also dislike the taste of European cheese.)

Other restrictions   Some conservative Hindus, including members of the Swami Narayan sect, do not eat onions or garlic, which are hot foods and believed to be harmful stimulants. They may also avoid root vegetables. Some people also avoid tea and coffee as stimulants. Jains may avoid all root vegetables, including onions and garlic. Some may also avoid butter, cheese and honey.

Alcohol is regarded as prohibited by most conservative Hindus and by most Jains.

Fasting   Some Hindu women fast during certain festivals every year. Some may also make regular fasts on days of special significance, sometimes as often as once or twice a week. Fasting is believed to bring both physical and spiritual benefits, and may also be regarded as helping to ensure good fortune in the future. Some women may undertake a special fast for a particular intention, such as a successful pregnancy or the recovery of a relative. Some may fast in thanksgiving for, for example, an easy pregnancy or birth.

A Hindu fast does not usually involve abstaining from all food, though some people do make a complete fast. Jains, for example, may abstain from all food and liquid from sunrise to sunset. More usually, people who are fasting eat one meal a day, eating only foods that are considered pure, such as fruit or yoghurt, nuts or potatoes. Some people may refuse medication when they are fasting.

PHYSICAL CARE

Jewellery   Some Hindu women wear a special wedding necklace of gold and black beads. This, like a wedding ring, is never removed. Other wedding jewellery may include glass or gold bangles, rings (sometimes with precious stones), or nose jewels.

Some women may also wear other jewellery with a religious significance, often on a black string around the arm, neck or body. Sometimes this is put on specially to ensure a successful pregnancy or birth, or recovery from illness. In some families a woman in her first pregnancy is given a gold bangle by her sister-in-law to ensure a safe delivery. This should not be removed until after the baby is born. If an important item of jewellery must be removed, discuss it with the woman first to reach a mutually acceptable solution.

Make-up   Many Hindu women wear a small coloured spot (bindi or chandlo) on their forehead. Traditionally this indicates that they are married, though unmarried women increasingly also wear a bindi purely for decoration. Many married women traditionally wear a red streak of vermilion powder (sindur) in the parting of their hair, especially in the early years of their marriage or on special occasions. Some Hindu women in hospital will wish to apply their bindi and sindur fresh every morning.

Some widowed Hindu women may wear white, the traditional colour of mourning. Some do not wear any make-up. Others wear a bindi in a dark colour.

PREGNANCY ISSUES

Traditions during pregnancy   There are many Hindu customs and ceremonies associated with pregnancy and childbirth. These vary a good deal between families, communities and geographical areas of origin. For example, in some communities women hold a special celebration during the seventh month of the first pregnancy in which the new mother's sister-in-law gives her presents. Some women then do not wash their hair until after the birth. This ceremony does not take place if the woman has had a previous miscarriage or stillbirth.

Antenatal screening and care   See Chapters 19 and 25

POSTNATAL CARE

Immediately after the birth   Hindu customs and ceremonies differ. In some communities, soon after the birth, a member of the family writes 'OM', a mystical sound representing the Supreme Spirit, on the baby's tongue with honey or ghee (clarified butter). The person who does this may take on a role similar to that of a Christian godparent. In Britain this ceremony may be delayed until the mother and baby return home.

Some families may wish to wrap the baby in a special cloth with religious significance after the birth. It is also traditional in some families for a close married female relative to symbolically wash the mother's breasts before offering the baby a first feed. A mixture of cow's milk and water is used and prayers are said.

On the sixth day after the birth in some communities the women of the family gather to congratulate the mother, pray, give thanks and bring presents for the child. The father's sister or another close female relative may perform a special ceremony and give the baby a set of clothes. The sixth day is also the day on which the child's fate is traditionally written by the goddess of learning. Some parents may leave a symbolic blank sheet of paper and a pen near the baby's cot.

After five or six weeks the mother and baby may both have a ritual wash before going to the temple for a blessing. Women do not usually go to the temple while they are bleeding postnatally.

It may be important for some Hindu parents to know the exact time of the birth so that they can get an accurate horoscope worked out by the pandit at the temple. This may be referred to later in life, for example, when a marriage or some other important step is being considered. Astrological influences are often believed to have a strong effect on each person's character, personality and future.

Naming the baby   The first letter of the baby's name may be chosen by the person who makes out the baby's horoscope. The full name is then chosen, often by an older member of the family or by the baby's father's sister, and the baby may then be given his or her name by the priest at the temple, traditionally on the tenth day after the birth (see also Chapter 21).

Contraception   For most Hindus there is no specific religious ruling on birth control, though members of some sects may follow special rulings. Both Hindu and Asian tradition however, stress the value of the family, children as the purpose of marriage, and motherhood as a woman's chief joy and fulfilment. For a Hindu man it is traditionally most important to have a son who will light the funeral pyre at his cremation.

Contraceptive methods that cause spotting or irregular periods, or particularly long periods, may be unacceptable to a woman whose religious and household activities are restricted during menstruation (see below).

Menstruation   Hindu women are traditionally regarded as unclean during menstruation. Some women do not pray formally or touch holy things. A few women do not cook though this is not normally possible in the UK. At the end of this time a woman may take a special shower before returning to her normal routine.

CHILDBEARING LOSSES

Termination of pregnancy   Abortion is traditionally disapproved of but individual attitudes may differ a good deal. Many women will only consider a termination if their situation is desperate. Confidentiality and support are absolutely essential (see Chapter 22).

Miscarriage   According to traditional Hindu belief, the soul enters the body of the baby during the seventh month of pregnancy. If a baby miscarries before this time there are no special traditional religious requirements, though individual families may have their own wishes. After seven months the baby should normally be given a proper religious funeral.

Stillbirth and neonatal death   Stillborn babies, babies and young children are usually buried rather than cremated. Some families may prefer to wash and prepare the baby's body themselves. They may also wish for a religious ceremony to take place, possibly at the hospital, before the burial. Burial should take place as soon as possible. Traditionally, women do not attend funerals. All bereaved parents need full information about their choices, and support and time to decide what is best for them (see also Chapter 22).

In some Hindu families the stigma traditionally attached to pregnancy loss may still be important. A woman who has had one or more miscarriages, stillbirths or neonatal deaths may sometimes be regarded as carrying bad luck and may not be welcome at traditional women's events and ceremonies surrounding weddings, pregnancy and so on.

DEATH AND FUNERAL RITES

The information in this section applies mainly to adult deaths. Some or all of it may also apply to miscarriages, stillbirths and neonatal deaths although there may also be significant differences. It is important to check everything with the parents in every case.

Prayers   A devout Hindu who is very ill or dying may receive comfort from hymns and holy readings. Some families may call a pandit to perform holy rites. He may tie a thread around the neck or wrist of the dying person to bless them. He may also sprinkle blessed water from the Ganges over the dying person or place a sacred leaf or blessed water in the person's mouth. Staff should not remove any religious items before or after death.

Some people may very much wish to die at home for religious reasons. All possible steps should be taken to achieve this.

Last offices   Some Hindu families are extremely concerned about who touches the body after death. If a non-Hindu touches or washes the body this may sometimes cause real distress. Ask the family about this and about all other procedures. The family may wish to wash the body as part of the funeral rites.

Unless the family wishes otherwise, close the eyes and straighten the limbs. Non-Hindu staff should use disposable gloves if the body must not be touched. Do not remove jewellery or other religious objects. Wrap the body in a plain sheet without religious emblems.

The body may then be taken home or to a funeral director's and washed by the family. In the case of an adult death, the eldest son traditionally takes charge of the funeral arrangements. If the body is kept at the hospital members of the extended family and other people are likely to wish to come and pay their last respects. This is a binding duty for many Hindus.

Cremation   Adults and older children are usually cremated. It is normally important that the cremation should take place as soon as possible (see Chapter 22).

The family may hold a religious ceremony around the twelfth day after the death. This releases the soul which until this time is believed to have remained near the family. In some communities, special rice balls are symbolically cut to symbolise the separation and release of the soul. Another ceremony may be held on the fortieth day after the death. This often marks the end of the period of strict mourning, during which people often prefer to remain at home. Many bereaved families may continue to lead restricted lives for up to a year after the death, possibly staying away from festivals and family parties.

Post mortems   There is no specific Hindu prohibition against post mortems but many people find them abhorrent and disrespectful and may be distressed if the post mortem delays the funeral. Some families may be very concerned that all the organs should be returned to the body before cremation or burial.

37 Islam

The information below will only apply to certain Muslim clients. Never assume. Always check everything with the person concerned.

Islam is a major religion with more than 900 million adherents throughout the world (Zaidi, 1994). Although the basic beliefs and practices of Islam are the same everywhere, Islam contains several major sects and branches each of which has its own traditions and practices. Members of those Muslim sects which stress the literal meaning of the Quran, the Muslim holy book (see below) are generally more conservative and adhere more strictly to traditional practices and external observances. Members of other sects may place more emphasis on the internal aspects of religion and behaviour and may be less concerned about external practices.

The families of British Muslims originated in many different countries (see below) and so, within the overall framework of Islam, are likely to be influenced by different local and national cultures, traditions and history as well as by membership of different Islamic sects.

The Muslim communities in the UK

There has been a significant Muslim presence in the UK since the early nineteenth century when seamen and traders from the Middle East began to settle around the major ports such as South Shields, Liverpool and Cardiff. A number of Muslims from the Indian subcontinent settled in Britain after the First World War after having fought with the British army in Europe. The main period of Muslim immigration to Britain occurred in the two decades after the Second World War and was mostly of people from rural areas of the Indian subcontinent (see Figure 34.1). Some of these families had already been displaced at Partition in 1947, when they had to leave their homes in India and try to settle in the new state of Pakistan (Anwar, 1979). A smaller number of South Asian Muslims came to Britain from East Africa, during the 1970s, often as refugees (see also Chapter 34).

There are also Muslim communities whose families originated in other areas, including the Middle East, North Africa, Cyprus, Turkey, Malaysia, Indonesia and Sri Lanka. Certain other Muslim groups have come to Britain seeking asylum, including people from Somalia and Bosnia. In addition, there are people of white and black British origin who have converted to Islam. There are now approximately 1.5 million Muslims in Britain, about two-thirds of them of South Asian origin (Weller, 1993).

Although this chapter deals with Islam in general, some of the cultural details it contains are likely to apply particularly to Muslims whose families originated in rural areas of the Indian subcontinent, since they form the largest group in Britain (see also Chapter 34). It is important to be aware of the many differences in outlook and practice among Muslim clients and not to assume uniformity of culture, adherence or practice.

ISLAM – A BRIEF DESCRIPTION

Islam means submission and peace. A Muslim is someone who obeys God's will and so is at peace with Him and with other people. To become a Muslim, a person must make the following statement of faith sincerely and with true belief in front of two witnesses: 'I bear witness that there is no god but God and that Muhammad is the messenger of God.' The Arabic word for God, used by most Muslims, is Allah.

Islam was founded in the seventh century CE by the Prophet Muhammad through revelations from God. As a sign of respect, most Muslims normally follow the name of Muhammad with the phrase 'Peace be upon him'. The power of Islam was such that in the first hundred years after the Prophet Muhammad's death, its message spread all over the Middle East, North Africa and into Spain, much of Central Asia, and into and beyond the Indian Subcontinent.

Muslims believe that Muhammad was the last of a long line of human prophets and that he completed everything that had gone before. Abraham, Moses, David, Job, John the Baptist and Jesus, among others, are regarded by Muslims as forerunners of Muhammad. Their messages were, however, distorted by those who heard them. Jesus is particularly revered in the Quran, though the idea of his divinity is regarded as heresy. Much of the teaching of the Old Testament is shared by Muslims, Jews and Christians (Henley, 1982).

Being a Muslim involves following a complete way of life. There is no division between the religious and the secular. Most Muslims follow five main duties or pillars of Islam: faith, prayer at five set times every day, giving alms, fasting during the month of Ramadan, and making a pilgrimage to the sacred city of Makka (Mecca) in Saudi Arabia. (Members of some sects may have a number of additional duties.) Islam also contains other very clear practical rules which cover most aspects of personal, family and community life. Muslims are expected to follow these and also to accept the truths and the laws and code of behaviour laid down in the Quran, the Muslim holy Book, and as recorded in the deeds and sayings of the Prophet Muhammad. Muslim law has evolved over time and continues to evolve, based always on the original revelations in the Quran.

Muslims should try to live perfectly as God's servants, following all His commands. Personal difficulties and tragedies are an inevitable part of life and are part of God's plan that each person should develop their inner strength and their capacity to cope. Most Muslims believe that God never puts a greater burden on a person than she or he has the capacity to bear (Anionwu, 1993). People should try to bear difficulties and sorrow with patience and acceptance, knowing that God will support them and will reward them both in this life and after their death. For many Muslims, their faith is a vital source of support, comfort and strength.

Many Muslims in Britain continue to live by the detailed code of Islam and reject those aspects of modern Western culture and lifestyle that they see as conflicting with their religious beliefs and practices. For example, the free mixing of the sexes, aspects of the dress of Western women, Western attitudes towards sex and marriage, gambling and alcohol may all be seen as unIslamic, especially by conservative sects and communities. Many observant Muslims feel that to adopt Western ways would require them to go directly against important beliefs and practices of their faith and would damage them both physically and spiritually. At the same time, there are also clear differences in practice and observance between the different Muslim communities in Britain, depending largely on which branch of Islam the community belongs to and on practice and observance in the countries from which families originally emigrated.

RELIGIOUS OBSERVANCE

Prayer Most adult practising Muslims say formal prayers (salat) five times a day; after dawn, around noon, in the mid-afternoon, in the early evening after sunset, and at night. Before praying people always wash using running water. The private parts, the hands, face, ears, forearms and feet must be washed three times, and the nose and mouth rinsed out three times with water. If a person is bed-bound, they may make a symbolic wash using a small quantity of water.

Prayers are recited in Arabic standing on a clean surface – a prayer mat or a towel is often used – and facing the Ka'bah, the sacred shrine in Makka (Mecca) in Saudi Arabia. Makka is the holy city of Islam and is south-east of Britain. The person should be fully dressed with everything but their face and hands covered. The head should also be covered and the shoes removed. While praying people go through a set series of physical movements including standing, kneeling, bowing, and touching the ground with their forehead. People who cannot get out of bed can pray sitting. Many devout Muslim women at home pray for a good part of the day, especially during Ramadan (see below) when there are extra prayers to be said after sunset.

Women do not usually say formal prayers up to forty days after giving birth or while menstruating. They need not say formal prayers after 36 weeks of pregnancy because of the physical movements required, though some will wish to do so. Women in hospital should be asked if they wish to pray and, wherever possible, offered a clean, quiet room where they will not be disturbed. It has been suggested that the direction of the Ka'bah could be marked by a discrete golden arrow on the ceilings of side wards, chapels, quiet rooms and other rooms in which people might pray (McIntosh and Andrews, 1992).

Where no private room is available for prayer, women should be asked if they would like their curtains drawn while they pray. Women confined to bed should be asked if they wish to wash before praying and, if so, given a bowl of water and a glass or cup to wash with. Men visiting their wives in hospital or accompanying them in labour may also need a quiet room in which to pray. It is important not to interrupt or walk in front of a person who is praying except in an emergency (Gatrad, 1994a).

The Quran   The Muslim holy book, the Quran, is regarded as the direct word of God and is sacred. It must always be treated with great care. Nothing may be placed on top of it, and it should never be placed on the floor or near, for example, dirty clothes or shoes. No one should eat, speak or smoke while the Quran is being read. It should only be touched by people who have performed the ritual wash.

The imam   In Britain there is usually an imam in charge of each mosque who performs religious functions and teaches the children. Such tasks as visiting the sick, praying with the dying and supporting those in trouble are usually performed by ordinary Muslims within the community, women for women and men for men. In most countries, therefore, the imam does not traditionally have a pastoral role though in many communities in Britain his role is becoming extended. Although every Muslim makes their own decisions about religious observance, people may also turn to imams for information and guidance.

In general, because of differences in tradition, language and heritage, different Muslim communities in Britain worship separately, though there is a strong sense of unity among many Muslims.

Festivals   The Muslim holy day is Friday, when men, and in some communities, women, are expected to attend the mosque at noon to say a special additional Friday prayer. In some Muslim countries Friday is also the official day of rest.

The two most important Muslim festivals are Eed-ul-Fitr (which marks the end of the holy month of Ramadan), and Eed-ul-Adha (which commemorates the willingness of the Prophet Abraham to sacrifice his son at God's command). Eed means anniversary. (The Turkish word is bayram.) Each of the eeds begins with prayers. The rest of the day is usually spent visiting friends and relatives and exchanging sweets and gifts.

The precise date of the eeds depends on the sighting of the new moon (the eed is the following day) and so can only be roughly predicted in advance. Women's family responsibilities usually keep them at home over the eeds and they may, for example, miss antenatal appointments. (For more on the dates of Muslim festivals see Walshe and Warrier, 1993.)

FAMILIES AND RELATIONSHIPS

Men and women   The treatment of women in Arabia at the time of the Prophet Muhammad was appalling. Women were bought, sold and inherited as possessions. Unwanted daughters were buried alive. Islam abolished this and gave women legal status with special emphasis on their economic rights. Under Islamic law women can control and dispose of their own money and property without reference to husbands or fathers. (Women in England and Wales only received these rights in the nineteenth century; until then they had no more status in law than children.) They can run their own businesses and are not required to contribute to family expenses. A marriage contract is only valid if the husband has covenanted a sum of money to be given to the wife if he dies or divorces her (Dearden, 1983).

At the same time, many Muslims believe that the equality of role demanded by many Western women is against the fundamental nature of men and women as ordained by God. They consider that although women and men are spiritually and morally equal, they have clearly differentiated and complementary roles and responsibilities. In most Muslim societies, men are traditionally responsible for all matters outside the home and all contact with non-family members, and for the financial support of their families. Women are traditionally responsible for the comfort of the family, the upbringing and moral education of the children, and the atmosphere and conduct of the home. In conservative families women are expected to spend most of their time at home, though again this has more to do with social and cultural traditions than with Islam.

In matters outside the home, a Muslim woman may be under the guardianship and protection of a man: her father, her husband, or her sons if she is a widow. This may be important, for example, when consent is being sought for surgery or other procedures. In many conservative families almost all non-domestic decisions are made by men. A strict code of public behaviour is observed between Muslim men and women in many communities.

Marriage   Marriage is a civil contract in Islam, not a religious sacrament. It involves mutual consent and clear mutual responsibilities. Conducting a responsible marriage and raising children well are religious duties and are considered fundamental to a good life. The Quran stresses the importance of the family and of family responsibilities.

Sexual morality is strict, to protect the family and society. Sex is only permitted within marriage, in which men have specific and clear responsibilities to protect and provide for women and children. Deep shame for the whole family usually follows the discovery of illicit sexual liaisons.

Sexual relationships outside marriage, in which a man need take little or no responsibility for a woman and any children, are strictly forbidden. At the time of Muhammad the local men often had large numbers of wives as well as extramarital relationships. As a result of tribal warfare there were also many widows, most living unprotected and in poverty. Limited polygamy was intended to protect women and to restrain male excesses (Dearden, 1983). Under certain clearly defined conditions, therefore, a Muslim man can have up to four wives: The husband must be sure that he can treat all his wives exactly the same and must have the means to support them all equally at a suitable level. Each wife also has the right to a separate home. Economic realities and human nature mean that most Muslim men nowadays have only one wife (see also Chapter 17).

In many Muslim countries, polygamy is forbidden unless permission is obtained from a special court. This is normally only granted if the wife is permanently infirm or in cases of infertility.

Divorce   Divorce is permitted in Islam but is usually severely disapproved of. Before a divorce can be granted, at least three attempts must be made by three different parties over several months to reconcile the couple. There are different Islamic divorce procedures for men and women, and practices differ somewhat within different branches and sects.

Divorced men and women are generally encouraged to remarry. Muslim couples living in Britain who want a divorce must also go through the British courts.

Under Islamic law the children of divorced parents may be raised by the mother while they are young; boys up to seven years, girls up to eleven. Their father remains responsible for supporting and educating them.

Cousin marriage   Marriage between first and second cousins is common in certain Muslim communities and is highly regarded as promoting family well-being and stability. In some communities a cousin is the first choice as a partner for a son or daughter. In an extended family (see Chapter 34) cousin marriage also reduces the potential strains; the bride moves into a family with whom she already has a good relationship. For farming families cousin marriage helps prevent the break-up of property over the generations. Cousin marriage may be regarded as having a religious sanction since the Prophet Muhammad himself married a cousin.

In Britain, cousin marriage is most common among families originating from Pakistan. A study in Birmingham found that 69 per cent of marriages within the Pakistani Muslim community were consanguineous. This compares with 46 per cent within the Arab community, 44 per cent within the Indian Muslim community (mainly families from East Africa), and 14 per cent among the Bangladeshi Muslim community. In about half these families there was also a history of earlier consanguineous marriages (Bundey et al., 1990). The rate of consanguineous marriage within the Pakistani Muslim community in Britain appears at present to be higher than in Pakistan, possibly because of the social and cultural isolation of the community and of British immigration policies. It has been alleged that immigration officials seem more ready to consider a planned marriage with a spouse from overseas to be genuine, and therefore to permit the spouse to enter the country, if he or she is a close relative (*Lancet*, 1991).

Genetic issues   Marriage between people who are closely related is now known to increase the risk of transmitting a number of serious or fatal recessive genetic disorders. Babies born to consanguineous parents of Pakistani origin in Britain have a significantly higher rate of serious or lethal congenital malformations than babies born to other minority ethnic groups where consanguineous marriages are not the norm. Studies in Pakistan have also shown that perinatal mortality and childhood deaths are increased in the offspring of consanguineous marriages (Shami et al., 1989, quoted in Bundey et al., 1990).

The rate of serious disease or malformation in the offspring of a first cousin marriage from a family with no previous consanguinity is about one in twenty. The rate in a non-consanguineous marriage in the general population is about one in forty. In a family with one or more previous consanguineous marriages, the rate for the children of a first cousin marriage is thought to be about one in eleven (Parsons et al., 1993).

The picture is, however, not simple and there is a lot still to be learnt about genetics and consanguinity. Only about half the lethal malformations identified in the Birmingham study could be attributed to recessive diseases (Bundey and Alam, 1993). There was also an increased frequency of cardiac malformations among Pakistani and Bangladeshi Muslim children which was not associated with parental consanguinity (Bundey et al., 1990). The Birmingham study also found that the children of non-consanguineous marriages in families with previous consanguineous marriages had a lower rate of lethal or serious malformations than the general population (Bundey et al., 1990). In areas of South India where close consanguineous marriages have occurred for about 100 generations, there is little if any evidence of high rates of lethal or serious malformations, possibly because certain recessive genes have been redistributed or bred out through repeated consanguineous marriages in earlier generations. Consanguineous marriages have only occurred in the Indian subcontinent since the introduction of Islam in the sixteenth century (Bundey *et al.*, 1990).

Certain congenital problems, in particular some heart conditions and limb malformations and many metabolic conditions, can be clearly traced to genetic factors (Parsons *et al.*, 1993). However, there are many other well-researched factors that are known to have an adverse effect on birth outcome and which affect the majority of Muslim communities in Britain. These include, for example, poverty, poor housing, overcrowding, poor nutrition, exposure to teratogens and poor access to health care services (Ahmad, 1994; Proctor and Smith, 1992). Muslim parents also tend to have a larger number of children and to have babies when they are older than the average in the general population.

Since the range of potential genetic disorders is wide, it is not feasible to offer **genetic counselling and screening** to the whole population. Where possible, however, genetic counselling and screening should be publicised and made available to all couples who are planning a consanguineous marriage. Family histories can then be taken to detect potential disorders and the couple advised accordingly. Related couples who have not received counselling and screening before conception should be offered them during pregnancy or after the birth.

Attitudes to and understanding of genetic counselling and screening vary a good deal within the Muslim communities. Some people may accept screening because it offers them the opportunity to make an informed choice in the light of medical expertise. Some may regard all termination as unacceptable and so refuse screening. Others may wish to know the outcome of tests and then make their decision (see also Chapter 19). It is very important that parents should have all the information they need about screening methods, risks and possible consequences.

Discussing the issues Some Muslim families are reluctant to discuss cousin marriages with British health professionals since they are aware that cousin marriage is generally thought to be irresponsible and bizarre in Western European culture. Some may feel that any enquiry about their family structure or relationships is loaded. They also know, from their own experience, that most couples who are cousins have healthy children. It is therefore vital to approach the subject, where necessary, objectively, with tact and understanding and with clear respect for the traditions, views and decisions of the people involved.

General advice from health professionals to avoid cousin marriage is also likely to be ineffective. The strong tradition of cousin marriage has been in existence and has had proven personal and social benefits for several centuries. Although the proportion of genetic disorders is high compared to the proportion in a population that does not have cousin marriage, most children of parents who are closely related are perfectly healthy. The problem tends to be relatively isolated and to affect a few couples very severely.

Avoiding cousin marriages cannot ensure that children will not inherit recessive disorders, especially if there is a high proportion of carriers within the community, nor that children will not be born with other problems.

Although cousin marriages are known to increase the risk of transmitting recessive disorders, it is important to keep the issue in proportion and, in particular, not to ascribe all health problems experienced by Muslim families to cousin marriage. Ahmad (1993), for example, relates meeting several consultants – a paediatrician, a haematologist, and an oncologist and an ophthalmologist – who all linked consanguinity to significant aspects of their work with South Asian patients. He writes:

> 'It has been argued that the medical scientific community has failed to maintain high standards in research on black people and has favoured interpretations which locate problems of health care in black people's cultures and genetics . . . Consanguinity is fast becoming the 'cause' of all the health problems of the Pakistani and Muslim minorities. (From Ahmad, 1993, by permission)

Telling people to change such a fundamental and in many ways positive aspect of their culture is as likely to be successful as outsiders telling English families that they must all start making arranged marriages from now on in order to increase the likely success of

318 Culture, Religion and Childbearing in a Multiracial Society

marriage. Change, if it is to occur at all, must be led and motivated from within a community and must be based on a sensitive and thorough understanding of all the factors involved and of the social costs and benefits of such a major change.

'If we don't start with respect we won't change attitudes. We have to work with the community, and have clear communication and understanding.' Genetic counsellor

MUSLIM FOOD RESTRICTIONS

Muslim food restrictions are laid down in the Quran and so are regarded as the direct command of God. They are based on the belief that the health of the body and the soul are connected. Most practising Muslims follow them.

Muslims may not eat pork, anything made from pork (e.g. sausage, ham, bacon), or anything made with pork products (e.g. food fried in bacon fat, food containing lard). All fish is permitted provided it has fins and scales.

Muslims can eat all other meat and meat products provided they are **halal** (which means permitted), that is, killed according to Islamic law. Because they only eat halal meat and meat products many Muslims eat a vegetarian diet in hospital, and may avoid processed and other foods that may contain non-halal animal products (e.g. rennet in cheese, gelatine in jelly). Many Muslims will also avoid any food whose ingredients they are not sure of (see also Chapter 18).

Practising Muslims may also try to avoid prohibited substances in medication, for example, capsules with gelatine coatings or additives derived from animal fat. Nevertheless, in an emergency or where there is no alternative, the use of medication containing animal products is allowed.

Alcohol is forbidden in the Quran and Muslims in most communities do not drink. Alcohol is permitted as a constituent of essential medication if there is no alternative.

Fasting All healthy Muslims over the age of 12 should fast during the month of Ramadan, the ninth month of the Muslim year (pronounced Ramzaan by most South Asian Muslims). The dates of Ramadan, and of other Muslim festivals vary each year, as they are based on the lunar year (see above).

Fasting is regarded as one of the most valuable forms of worship, enabling people to come closer to God, to practise self-discipline and to share and understand the suffering of poor and hungry people all over the world. The shared deprivation and sacrifice of fasting, and the celebrations that follow the end of the fast, also bring families and communities together. Many people are keen to participate and to observe the fast properly.

Fasting for Muslims means taking no liquid or food at all between dawn (about one and a half hours before the sun rises) and when darkness falls. Timetables are printed and distributed by local mosques to help people keep the fast correctly (Gatrad, 1994a). When Ramadan occurs during the summer months in Britain, it can mean many hours without any liquid or food. Even the use of toothpaste is forbidden during fasting hours. Some people may also try to avoid swallowing any saliva.

Exemptions from fasting Certain people are exempt from fasting. However, people who miss any of the Ramadan fast must normally make up the days lost as soon as possible.

Women who are pregnant or breast feeding need not fast. However, pregnancy provides many Muslim women with a rare opportunity to make the full four-week fast since they do not menstruate. (Menstruating women are not allowed to fast.) Some women are very keen to fast both for its spiritual benefits, and in order to participate fully with their families in the festival. Some may also feel that fasting will help ensure a successful pregnancy. Making up the full month's fast at a later date can be very difficult and unpleasant when women are cooking for the rest of the family.

Current research (Cross *et al.*, 1990; Rashed, 1992) shows no effect on babies' birth weights of maternal fasting during Ramadan at any stage of pregnancy. Provided, therefore, that the pregnancy is going well and the woman is generally healthy, and eats and drinks properly at night (simply reversing her usual eating pattern), there is normally no reason to get alarmed or to intervene. Unnecessary pressure from staff not to fast, including, as has sometimes happened, quoting from the Quran by non-Muslims, may offend and alienate women and lead them to avoid important appointments. However, if fasting is causing genuine problems for the woman's own health or that of her baby, it is important that the medical issues are carefully explained to her so that she can make an informed decision.

People who are ill need not fast. However, this is an individual decision and many people may still choose to fast. People with chronic illnesses, such as insulin-dependent diabetes, or who must take medication regularly throughout the day, are also not bound to fast but many wish to for spiritual reasons. If this causes problems, discuss the situation with the woman and where necessary with her family so that she can make an informed decision.

The restriction on taking food or liquid also covers all forms of medication. Medicines for fasting Muslim women should, if possible, be prescribed taking the fast into account. For example, it may be possible to prescribe tablets to be taken twice a day, or at sunset, midnight and before dawn. It may also be necessary to consider the effects of medication on an empty stomach (Gatrad, 1994a). Discuss this with the woman, stressing, if appropriate, the importance of taking the medication at the prescribed times even if she feels well.

Routines during Ramadan   During Ramadan, people usually get up an hour or two before dawn and eat before the fast begins. When darkness falls they end the fast with a date or a little salt followed by a light meal and plenty of fluid. Relatives and friends are often invited to share the breaking of the fast. Children are usually encouraged to begin fasting with their parents for a few days from the age of about seven.

The routines of many Muslim households change drastically during Ramadan (depending partly in Britain on the time of year in which it falls). Women, in particular, who may have to get up early to prepare the first meal and stay up late to clear up the last one, may spend much of the day in bed. They may become very tired as Ramadan progresses. It may also be necessary to adjust the times of morning home visits so as not to disturb sleeping families. Most people who are fasting also feel the cold (Gatrad, 1994a).

Ask Muslim women in hospital if they intend to fast and what they will need at what times. This will include suitable food when it is dark before dawn and after sunset, and a glass of water with which to rinse out their mouths before praying during the day and a bowl for spitting the water into. Women who are fasting may prefer to go and sit in a day room at mealtimes, away from people who are eating. Many women do not like to have blood taken during Ramadan, possibly because they fear it may further exhaust them. Sexual intercourse is also forbidden during the hours of fasting; some women may refuse vaginal examinations (Gatrad, 1994a).

PHYSICAL CARE

Clothes   Traditionally, Muslims should wear clothes that are both modest and allow the freedom of movement that is needed for prayer. Although the traditional style of dress varies in different counties, many conservative Muslim women prefer to cover themselves from head to foot whenever they go out, possibly showing only their hands and faces. Some women always wear a scarf or shawl over their head in public. Some conservative South Asian women wear a full length dress called a burqah and some very conservative Turkish women wear a similar garment called a charshaf. For many, this form of dress provides complete privacy and freedom outside the home as well as often being a positive statement of their Muslim identity. Muslim women in some communities wear Western clothes.

Some conservative Muslim men may keep their heads covered at all times.

Jewellery Some women may wear religious jewellery to protect them while they are pregnant and when they come into hospital. Practice in different communities varies but some women may wear, for example, a medallion or a small amulet made of cloth, leather or metal containing words from the Quran, often worn on a black string around the waist, arm or neck. Religious jewellery should be treated with respect and never removed without consent.

PREGNANCY ISSUES

Modesty Modesty is an important religious obligation and is laid down in the Quran. Many Muslims regard physical contact between a man and a woman who are not husband and wife or close family as strictly forbidden. Many conservative Muslim women feel that the Islamic requirement that they should not be touched by any other man, even a doctor, should only be over-ruled in an emergency. All possible steps should be taken to respect and accommodate women's needs in relation to modesty during pregnancy, labour and postnatally (see also Chapters 19, 20 and 21).

Antenatal screening Some Muslim couples may not want screening to detect fetal abnormalities, particularly if they would not consider a termination. Others may prefer to find out about possible problems during the pregnancy, even if they regard termination as prohibited. For some couples very early screening may be more acceptable (Anionwu, 1993).

Muslims of African, African-Caribbean, South Asian, Far Eastern and Mediterranean heritages may be at risk of haemoglobinopathies (see Chapter 25). (See also Cousin Marriage above.)

LABOUR AND BIRTH

Labour Some Muslim women regard prayer during labour as very important. A woman in labour may continue to say the formal daily prayers until she starts to bleed after the birth. Some women may also say a special prayer known as the 'Shahadah' or Witnessing. If he is present, the husband may, for example, read the Quran to his wife, and may recite the chapter which tells the story of the birth of Jesus, whom Muslims regard as a major prophet. Some men may wish to pray as normal if they are with their wives during labour. Where possible they should be given privacy for this (see above).

A few Muslim women may be reluctant to use narcotic methods of pain relief on religious grounds, as narcotics are forbidden in the Quran except in cases of overriding medical need. For these women, personal support and encouragement during labour may be particularly important (Zaidi, 1994). Most women feel that labour qualifies as overriding medical need and feel able to accept analgesia if they need it. For reasons of modesty, some women may be unwilling to expose their backs to male anaesthetists to have an epidural inserted. (See also Chapter 20.)

Immediately after the birth Many Muslim parents consider it very important that a baby should be washed immediately after the birth to get rid of any impurity. Some may be distressed if the baby is given to them unwashed and may not want to hold or feed the baby until he or she has been cleaned properly. It is important in such cases not to make any assumptions about the mother's or the father's attitude towards their baby (Zaidi, 1994). Parents' wishes on this and other issues should be discussed and recorded antenatally.

The mother may then take the baby and hand it to the father who whispers the Muslim call to prayer (Adhan) into the child's ears. For many parents it is important that these should be the first words that the child hears since they are its introduction to the Muslim faith. Families should be given privacy to do this if they request it. In some cases a family may wish to bring a male relative or a learned member of the community into the delivery suite to do this (Zaidi, 1994).

POSTNATAL CARE

Feeding the baby   The Quran enjoins a woman to breast feed her baby as soon as possible after the birth, and to continue for two years, though few women nowadays find this practically possible. A mother's milk is seen as a gift from God to that particular baby. Attitudes towards breast feeding are also likely to be influenced by the traditions of the woman's own community and by her personal experience (see Chapter 21).

Naming the baby   Traditions vary in different Muslim communities. Some families may prefer not to choose a name before the birth. In some communities the name is traditionally chosen by the baby's parents. Among South Asian and Turkish Muslims, it may be chosen by an older relative who has been given the honour of choosing the names of all the children in the extended family. The name may be given on the day the baby's hair is shaved. (For more about South Asian Muslim and Somali names see Chapter 14.)

Circumcision   All Muslim boys should be circumcised before they reach puberty. In most communities this is carried out in the first few days after the birth. In some communities, for example, the Bangladeshi and Turkish communities, circumcision may sometimes be done when the boy is about eight years old.

There is no religious ceremony attached to circumcision, but in some communities it is an occasion for celebration and a party may be held for relatives and friends.

Shaving the baby's head   In some communities the baby's head is shaved to symbolise removing the uncleanness of birth and also to help the hair grow thickly, often on the sixth or seventh day after the birth but sometimes later. In some communities oil and saffron are rubbed onto the baby's head.

Postnatal bleeding and menstruation   Women do not usually say formal prayers, fast, or have sexual intercourse for forty days after giving birth or while menstruating. At the end of this period some women take a special bath and remove their pubic and underarm hair before resuming their normal routines. Some women shave their pubic and underarm hair as part of their normal cleansing routine before going into hospital to give birth.

Contraception   Beliefs and practices with regard to contraception vary a good deal among Muslims. There is no Islamic ruling against contraception, though much is written on the value of the family and of children (see Chapter 21). Some conservative Muslims may consider it forbidden to decide never to have another child, even if parents are concerned about their ability to provide for their family (Bignall, 1993). Irreversible contraception is not permitted.

Some Muslims consider that all artificial contraception is wrong, since it interferes with God's plan. They may regard the arrival of any child as the gift of God which should be accepted, and may only use contraception if there is a good medical reason to delay another pregnancy. Some Muslims regard all forms of contraception as permitted, and believe that parents should only have as many children as the husband or family can support. Barrier methods or withdrawal may sometimes be more acceptable than the pill or the coil which are often perceived as interfering with normal physiological processes. Some women may reject the pill if it causes breakthrough bleeding (see above). Sterilisation may only be acceptable if the mother's life would be endangered by another pregnancy.

In some conservative couples, the final decision about contraception may be made by the man. Many Muslims find discussion of contraception and other sexual matters with a member of the opposite sex shameful and embarrassing. In such cases, women should discuss such issues with women and men with men.

CHILDBEARING LOSSES

Infertility   Treatment that may help a couple conceive, including artificial insemination with the husband's sperm, is normally acceptable. Artificial insemination by donor is not generally acceptable (Bignall, 1993).

The overwhelming importance of children in some cultures, and often especially of sons, can have serious implications for couples who have fertility problems. Tradition and culture, not religion, may lead to infertility being regarded as the woman's fault. Infertility may sometimes be grounds for divorce or for the husband to take a second wife (see Chapter 22).

According to the Quran, Muslims may foster a child, but may not legally adopt since a child always belongs to its biological parents. In communities where the extended family is the norm, however, it is traditional for a childless couple to bring up one or more children of a relative. In Britain, such informal arrangements may be difficult because of legal restrictions and processes.

Termination of pregnancy   Infanticide and abortion were prevalent in Arabia at the time of Muhammad and are specifically forbidden in the Quran. However, individual attitudes may vary. Some couples will consent to a termination if the mother's life is at risk or if the baby has died in utero. Others may consent to a termination before 120 days' gestation if the baby is known to have a serious congenital abnormality (Bignall, 1993). Others will consider a termination at any gestation if the baby is severely handicapped or in other very difficult situations. As always, the option of termination should be offered sensitively and in complete confidence.

Miscarriage   The remains of the baby should not be incinerated or cremated. Some parents may wish to take them home for burial. No formal religious ceremony is required. Parents whose baby miscarries at a later gestation may wish to follow the practices set out below.

Stillbirth and neonatal death   For every parent, whatever their religious beliefs, the decisions to be made after a baby has died or miscarried are difficult and unfamiliar (see Chapter 22). According to Muslim tradition, a baby who dies at or after birth must be given a name (Gatrad, 1994b). The body must be buried in its entirety and nothing, including hair, should be removed.

Most Muslim parents find it acceptable to have photographs taken, but it is important to check since some may regard photography as unacceptable. Figures and statues of the human form are traditionally forbidden in Islam (Gatrad, 1994a). It takes tact and sensitivity to distinguish between those parents who initially find the idea of a photograph bizarre and unattractive but may later be grateful and those who are refusing on religious grounds. All parents are likely to need patient and sensitive support to help them decide what is right for them.

A stillborn baby does not need to be ritually washed before burial. A formal religious ceremony is not required under Islamic law.

A baby who dies at any time after birth should be ritually washed in the normal way as part of the normal funeral rites. Provided the family wishes, hospital staff should prepare the body as set out below.

In most Muslim communities, women do not attend the actual funeral (see below). They may go into an anteroom to wash and wrap the baby.

DEATH AND FUNERAL RITES

The information here applies mainly to adult deaths. Some or all of it may also apply to miscarriages, stillbirths and neonatal deaths although there may be significant differences. It is important to check everything with the parents in every case.

Death   Most Muslims prefer to die in their own homes (Gatrad, 1994b). The presence of a religious leader is not necessary. Members of the family recite verses from the Quran and perform religious ceremonies and rites themselves. It is an important religious for all Muslims to visit the sick; a very ill or dying person may have a large number of visitors. The dying person should if possible lie or sit facing the Ka'bah (south-east in Britain) (see above).

Last offices   The human body is regarded as sacred and must always be treated with respect. For many families it is preferable that the body is not touched by non-Muslims after death. Nursing staff and others should check with the family before carrying out any procedures and should wear disposable gloves. Some families prefer to do everything that is necessary themselves.

Provided the family wishes, the following should be done: close the eyes and mouth, straighten the limbs, and, if possible, turn the head towards the right shoulder so that the body can be buried with the face towards the Ka'bah (see above). If this is not possible, the whole body will be turned towards the Ka'bah during burial. The body should be wrapped in a plain unstitched sheet without emblems. The body should not be washed; this is part of the funeral rites to be carried out by the family or other members of the community later. The hair and nails should not be cut.

Funeral preparations are often carried out at home rather than at the mosque. The body is washed according to special Muslim procedures. Women usually wash a female body and men a male body. In some communities women who are menstruating or bleeding postnatally do not go near the dead body. Many families in Britain prefer not to use a funeral director. They may, for example, arrange all transport themselves and keep the body at home or at the mosque until the funeral. Often members of a local Muslim funeral committee collect death certificates and arrange funerals in order to take the immediate pressure off the family (Gatrad, 1994b).

Burial   Muslims should be buried, not cremated. After the ritual washing, the body is wrapped in a simple white shroud. Passages from the Quran are recited and the family prays. The men normally take the body to the mosque or to the graveside for prayers before the burial. Heads are covered as a mark of respect. The most qualified person present usually officiates. Women may go to the mosque but under Islamic law do not go to the graveside in case they become too distressed. This restriction applies even in the case of the death of a baby or of a female relative. Some women may go to the graveside at other times, though, strictly speaking, this is frowned upon (Gatrad, 1994b). Flowers are not traditional at Muslim funerals but may be sent in Britain.

According to Islamic law and practice the burial must take place as soon as possible, normally within 24 hours. Delay can cause great distress. Families may worry that the body of the person they loved will decay. (Embalming is prohibited.) Many families do not eat until after the burial as a sign of respect. In Britain, where most Muslim communities are very closely knit, a large number of relatives and community members may come to stay or to spend their days at the family's home from the moment they hear of the death until the burial has taken place. A delayed burial can therefore put a great burden on the family (Gatrad, 1994b).

The initial period of mourning after a death lasts for three days, during which prayers are recited continuously (Gatrad, 1994b). The full period of mourning lasts several weeks or months. It is very important to visit and sit with bereaved family members.

Muslims would not normally be buried in a coffin. According to Islamic law the area above the grave should be slightly raised and the grave should be aligned so that the face of the dead person faces the Ka'bah. Some sects do not mark the grave. Some local authorities provide special areas for Muslim burials.

Post mortems   In Islam, the body of a Muslim is considered to belong to God. No part of a dead body should normally be cut out or harmed. Post mortem examinations are therefore forbidden and most families will refuse. If a post mortem is legally required, the reasons must be clearly explained to the family and all efforts must be made to return the body for burial as soon as possible. All the organs should be returned to the body before burial.

Jehovah's Witnesses in Britain

There are Jehovah's Witnesses in approximately 230 countries throughout the world. In the UK there are around 117,000 baptised and committed adult Jehovah's Witnesses with an additional number of children and associates (Green, 1992).

The families of Jehovah's Witnesses in Britain originated in many parts of the world, including the UK, the West Indies, the Indian subcontinent, Greece, Italy and Spain. Individuals may be influenced by their family's cultural heritage as well as by their religious faith.

The information below will only apply to certain Jehovah's Witness clients. Never assume. Always check everything with the person concerned.

RELIGIOUS BELIEFS AND PRACTICES

Jehovah's Witnesses accept the whole of the Bible, both the Old and the New Testament, and try to live their lives by God's commands. Their highest priority is faithfulness to God and this transcends earthly considerations. Jehovah's Witnesses believe in the immortality of the soul and that, after death, there is a period of rest until the resurrection when the Kingdom of God will be restored on earth. Jehovah's Witnesses regard Jesus Christ as the Son of God. They have a strong commitment to spreading their faith.

Jehovah's Witnesses are baptised when they have reached 'the age of understanding'. Each Jehovah's Witness must make their own baptismal commitment, it cannot be made on their behalf. The conscience of the individual is very important: Everyone makes their own decisions in life while taking official Jehovah's Witness rulings and biblical teachings into account.

There are no salaried ministers, but each community has lay elders who have pastoral responsibilities. The meeting place of the congregation is called the Kingdom Hall.

Jehovah's Witnesses regard the cross as a pagan symbol and shun its use.

Religious festivals   Once a year Jehovah's Witnesses celebrate an important ceremony, the Memorial, at which some people take bread and wine, representing Christ's body and blood. Jehovah's Witnesses do not observe Sunday as a holy day and do not celebrate Christmas or Easter. A woman who is in hospital during these festivals may not want to participate actively in celebrations.

FAMILIES AND RELATIONSHIPS

Jehovah's Witnesses observe traditional family values. The local Jehovah's Witness community is often regarded as an extension of the family.

FOOD RESTRICTIONS

Jehovah's Witnesses are forbidden to eat blood or blood products. Foods such as black pudding are therefore unacceptable. Since animals are bled after slaughter, meat is normally acceptable. Some Jehovah's Witnesses are vegetarian.

BLOOD TRANSFUSIONS

'We are totally ordinary, normal people who value medical treatment providing it doesn't include blood transfusions. We want to be treated like everyone else and appreciate health professionals who are patient and understanding about our religious prohibition about receiving blood products.'   Church elder

'Other people besides Jehovah's Witnesses refuse blood transfusions, but it seems that we are pre-judged and treated with greater intolerance, more prejudice and less understanding.'   Mother of three

Jehovah's Witnesses seek alternatives to blood transfusions because of their deeply held religious belief that a human must not sustain his or her life with another creature's blood (Acts 15: 20, 28–29). Jehovah's Witnesses believe that if they knowingly allow transfusion of blood they risk losing eternal life and will not experience the Kingdom of God on earth (see above). A practising Jehovah's Witness is therefore likely to refuse a blood transfusion for him or herself or for a child whatever the possible consequences (Butler Sloss, 1992). Most Jehovah's Witnesses carry a small personal card which directs medical staff not to use blood or blood products as a means of treatment and releases them from responsibility in this regard. Hospitals should have a standard form for refusal of blood which a Witness will sign when necessary. A parent will sign in the case of a child (Green, 1992).

Jehovah's Witnesses are able to receive all medical treatment and care providing that this does not include receiving blood. The prohibition includes whole blood, red cells, white cells, platelets and plasma. Blood fractions such as Factor 8, anti-D and globulins are considered to be substantially different from whole blood and from the constituents that nourish and sustain the body. These are therefore not strictly prohibited and it is up to individual Witnesses to decide whether to accept these products. Jehovah's Witnesses with haemophilia, for example, may accept Factor 8. People with hereditary conditions affecting the blood, such as sickle cell disease and thalassaemia (see Chapter 25), need special consideration.

Auto-transfusion   Auto-transfusion (where the patient's own blood is infused), which may sometimes be a suitable medical course of action, is acceptable to some Jehovah's Witnesses provided that the blood is not stored and that it is returned immediately to the patient through a continuous circuit constantly linked to the patient. This can be seen as an extension of the patient's own circulation. Haemodialysis and heart bypass surgery are acceptable to many Jehovah's Witnesses provided that no blood prime is used.

Blood is generally seen to represent life itself and should always be handled with respect. It should not be stored or re-used. Blood samples may be taken for testing, provided any unused blood is disposed of and not re-used (Green, 1992).

Care of a premature or sick baby   Jehovah's Witnesses accept and appreciate that health professionals have a responsibility to do the best for each patient and are prepared to accept all forms of treatment for their child that do not involve the transfusion of blood. Most parents will refuse a blood transfusion whatever the immediate consequences for their baby. Parents who are likely to be already anxious and stressed need sensitive and understanding care and should not be pressurised, either overtly or covertly, into consenting to blood transfusion.

Since blood transfusion is prohibited it is particularly important to ensure that the management of pre-term infants does not precipitate anaemia. One way of reducing the need for red blood cell transfusion is by holding the new-born infant 20 centimetres below the introitus for 30 seconds before the cord is clamped (Kinmond *et al.*, 1993). Another is to ensure that the minimum amount of blood is taken from the baby for testing and that blood samples are used efficiently. Specialists who have devised special techniques for taking samples from babies of Jehovah's Witnesses may be contacted through the Hospital Liaison Committees or through the Hospital Information Desk (see Useful Addresses below).

Alternatives to transfusion should be sought whenever possible. The nearest Hospital Liaison Committee can provide information about these and may have the names of paediatricians with experience of managing similar situations without blood transfusions.

In extreme cases, the parents' wishes may be over-ruled by a court order. In such a case it is important that the parents, whose sincerely held beliefs and concerns must be respected, should be represented in court, so that justice can be seen to be done (Times Law Report, 1993). Contrary to common belief, Jehovah's Witnesses will not normally reject their baby because he or she has received blood against their will.

Help and advice   Local elders are often very well informed about medical issues and especially about alternatives to blood transfusion. There is also a country-wide network of thirty-six Jehovah's Witness Hospital Liaison Committees. The members of these committees are extremely well informed about medical and surgical procedures. They have detailed information about alternatives to blood transfusion and some are in regular contact with physicians and surgeons who are experienced in giving medical and surgical treatment without the use of blood.

The Hospital Information Desk at International Bible Students Association House (see below) can provide information about local Hospital Liaison Committees.

CHILDBEARING ISSUES

Antenatal screening   There is no religious prohibition on taking blood for tests and most Jehovah's Witnesses will accept all antenatal screening. It is, however, very important that women understand the purpose and potential consequences of each test as some may decide to refuse tests that could lead to a decision to terminate the pregnancy.

Depending on their family origins some Jehovah's Witnesses may be affected by particular hereditary conditions such as haemoglobinopathies (see Chapter 25).

Labour and birth   There is no restriction on pharmacological methods of pain relief. Most Jehovah's Witnesses will refuse a blood transfusion even if they are severely anaemic or have a life-threatening haemorrhage (see above). It is, however, acceptable to use volume expanders such as Ringer's lactate, normal saline and Dextran.

Baptism   Babies are not baptised, even if they are very ill. It is believed that babies and children are spiritually protected by the dedication of their parents (Green, 1992).

Contraception   Contraception is generally a matter for personal choice. The morning-after pill, however, is unacceptable since it acts after fertilization and is therefore viewed as an abortifacient. For the same reason some Jehovah's Witnesses might not wish to use an IUD.

CHILDBEARING LOSSES

Infertility   Infertility treatment using donated sperm or eggs is likely to be unacceptable. Other forms of treatment, including IVF using the couple's own eggs and sperm, are a matter for personal decision.

Termination of pregnancy   Termination of pregnancy is prohibited since it involves the taking of life. For the same reason Jehovah's Witnesses are conscientious objectors and do not do military service.

Miscarriage, stillbirth and neonatal death   There are no particular formal religious requirements if a baby is miscarried, stillborn or dies shortly after death. Parents should receive the normal support and care and be given patient and sensitive support to help them decide what is right for them. Many Jehovah's Witnesses find comfort and support in their religious community.

DEATH AND FUNERALS

There is no formal ritual to be used when a person is dying. Congregational support is normally important. Jehovah's Witnesses may be buried or cremated.

Post mortems   There is no religious prohibition against post mortems.

USEFUL ADDRESSES

Hospital Information Desk (8 am–9 pm)
International Bible Students Association House
The Ridgeway
London NW7 1RN
Tel.: 0181-906-2211

The information below will only apply to some Jewish people. Never assume. Always check everything with the person concerned.

Jewish communities in Britain

There has been a long-standing Jewish presence in Britain, where, as in the rest of Europe, Jewish communities suffered frequent persecution and expulsions until the eighteenth century. The families of most British Jews originated in Eastern European countries such as Russia, Poland and Germany (sometimes known as Ashkenazi Jews). A smaller number originated from Spain and Portugal mainly in the seventeenth and eighteenth centuries (sometimes known as Sephardi Jews). The main periods of modern Jewish immigration into Britain occurred between 1880 and 1914, during anti-Jewish pogroms in Russia and Poland, and in the 1930s and 1940s when Hitler's Third Reich in Germany systematically attempted to murder all European Jews (Weller, 1993). There are also a number of Israelis who have made their homes here.

Most Jews of childbearing age in the UK were born here. Although English is their main language, some traditional Ashkenazi families speak Yiddish at home and with friends. Yiddish is an old language derived mainly from Old German, Polish and Hebrew. Israeli families speak modern Hebrew (Ivrit).

The term Jewish can mean many different things and is an ethnic and cultural as well as a religious label. According to Orthodox Jewish tradition, a Jew is someone whose mother is Jewish or someone who has converted to Judaism according to Orthodox law. However, within the British Jewish community there are many different groups, degrees of religious observance and a wide spectrum of belief. There are, for example, Orthodox, Reform and Liberal Jews, each group attending their own synagogues and following their own traditions. Some Jews are secular and have no religious beliefs or requirements; for other Jews their religion influences most aspects of their daily life. There may also be differences in certain customs and traditions depending on the family's area of origin. **It is important to identify the needs and wishes of each individual woman and her family.**

'Because we speak English, health professionals assume we are part of the indigenous population and that we have the same needs and attitudes as everyone else. But this is not true. We may sound the same and maybe look the same but we have specific needs and wishes that are different.' Orthodox Jewish mother

Most of the practices described below apply mainly to people who are strict Orthodox or ultra-Orthodox Jews. Reform, Liberal and secular Jews may not have the same customs or expectations.

JUDAISM – A BRIEF DESCRIPTION

Religious Jews believe in one God who is merciful and just, and that humankind's purpose on earth is to worship and serve God, to live justly and do good deeds, and to study. Jews believe that the human soul is immortal but that it is more important to concentrate their religious efforts on creating an ideal world for the living on this earth than to focus on the life hereafter.

The written and oral law   For Jews, the holy books are what Christians call the Old Testament of the Bible, the most important being the first five books called the Pentateuch or Torah. These are known as the Written Law. There is also the Oral Law which consists of detailed comment by distinguished rabbis over many centuries on legal and ethical issues and on the Written Law and how it should be applied to everyday living. The Oral Law was eventually written down and is called the Talmud. Orthodox Jews are likely to stick strictly to the letter of the Law as it is written down.

RELIGIOUS OBSERVANCE

Prayer   Religious Jews pray each morning and evening. Women who wish to pray while in hospital may draw their bed curtains. Their privacy should be respected.

The rabbi   A Jewish religious leader is called a rabbi (teacher). Traditionally the rabbi has religious authority and teaches and advises on religious issues. Rabbis do not traditionally have a pastoral role. Since Judaism places great emphasis on health, many rabbis are very well informed about medical issues.

The Sabbath   Shabbat (pronounced 'shabbat' or 'shabbos') or the Sabbath starts at sundown on Friday and ends after nightfall on Saturday. It is a major festival and a day of rest when Orthodox Jews do not work and may avoid all kinds of activities such as carrying anything outside the confines of the home, any activity that involves turning electrical or gas appliances on or off, driving, being driven, using a telephone or a lift, or writing. Any necessary activity is however permitted if life or health are threatened. For example, an expectant father can telephone for an ambulance if his wife is in labour and will travel with her, but may walk home from the hospital afterwards. Some Orthodox Jews may be unwilling to sign non-urgent papers or consent forms on Shabbat. An Orthodox Jewish mother whose baby is in a neonatal unit on a different floor may not want to use the lift on Shabbat.

Strictly observant Jews also avoid tearing paper on Shabbat, and may prefer to use interleaved lavatory paper. They may be unwilling to open paper packages or to remove the paper covering from the sticky tabs of disposable nappies. Some people also avoid altering the shape of anything (other than food) and may prefer to use liquid soap rather than a bar of soap, tooth powder rather than toothpaste and to avoid using any creams or ointments on Shabbat.

Shabbat begins with the ritual lighting of two candles which are left to burn down and with a festive family meal at which a blessing is recited over wine and bread. In hospital, Orthodox Jewish women may wish to light candles. If this is forbidden for safety reasons, a woman may want to keep her bedside light on throughout Shabbat. It is important to check with her as she may also have left the light on simply because she cannot switch it off. She may also not want to use the bell to call a midwife except in a real emergency.

Other religious festivals   There are numerous festivals during the year. The most important are Rosh Hashanah and Yom Kippur. The dates vary to some extent because they are based on the lunar calendar. Some people observe all the festivals strictly, others only observe some and may be less strict. Jewish women in hospital during religious festivals should be asked if they have any special needs or requirements. (For more on the dates of festivals see Walshe and Warrier, 1993.)

Jewish festivals start an hour before sunset on the eve of a festival, and last until the nightfall the next day. The main festivals are (stressed syllables underlined):

Rosh Hashana (rosh ha<u>shana</u>) the Jewish New Year occurs in September or early October. It lasts for two days though some people observe only one day. It is a solemn festival, a time for reflection rather than celebration. Like Shabbat, it is also a day of rest and the same restrictions may be observed.

The New Year is announced by blowing the shofar (a ram's horn) which proclaims the need for spiritual revival. Since it is important for Orthodox Jews to hear the Shofar every New Year, a rabbi may bring one in and blow it for a woman in hospital.

Yom Kippur (yom kip<u>oor</u>), the Day of Atonement, falls ten days after Rosh Hashana. It is a day of repentance and is the most solemn festival in the Jewish year. Observant Jews fast strictly from before sundown the previous day (see Fasting below). As on Shabbat, no work is allowed and many activities are avoided.

Pesach (<u>pays</u>ah) or Passover is celebrated in the spring at the end of March or the beginning of April. It lasts eight days and commemorates the escape of the Jews from Egypt under the leadership of Moses.

Pesach starts with a ritual meal, the Seder (<u>sayder</u>). During the following eight days observant Jews eat no leavened bread or foods containing wheat flour. Instead they eat unleavened bread (matzo or matzah), and specially prepared cakes and biscuits baked without wheat flour. Fermented foods, or foods containing brewed or fermented ingredients such as vinegar or ketchup are also forbidden. Some people avoid rice and pulses. Orthodox Jews may be unwilling to take medication during the Passover week unless they can be sure that it contains no wheat, wheat derivatives or other prohibited ingredients.

Before Pesach, observant Jews spring clean their homes to ensure that no breadcrumbs remain. They also use a completely different set of cutlery and china during the festival. A woman who is in hospital just before the festival may want her locker cleaned out before Pesach begins. Preparations for Pesach involve a great deal of cooking, baking and cleaning and can be a very tiring time for pregnant and newly delivered women.

On the first two and last two days of Pesach observant Jews do no work as on Shabbat. Some people do no work only on the first and last days. It is permitted to take a bath or shower during the intermediary days of Pesach. On the second day of Pesach, a second Seder is often held.

Chanukah (<u>Hann</u>ooka), the feast of lights, is celebrated in December and lasts eight days. Each night Jews light candles on an eight-branched candlestick called a Chanukiah. Normal daily life and work continue.

Purim (<u>Purim</u>) is a joyful festival celebrated in February or March. Children dress up and the story of Purim, as told in the Book of Esther, is read. It is important for Orthodox Jews to hear the story every year, so an Orthodox woman in hospital may be visited by someone who will read it to her. Normal daily work and life continue during this festival.

FAMILIES AND RELATIONSHIPS

Family structures and relationships vary in different communities and from family to family. Broadly speaking, marriage and the family are the centre of traditional Jewish life and it is the duty of a married couple to create a peaceful home. Sexual morality is central to traditional Jewish values. In most Orthodox families, male and female roles are clearly delineated with the mother taking primary responsibility for the home and the children, though she may also work outside the home. Fathers take particular responsibility for the religious education of the children. Mutual respect between husband and wife are very important.

Marriage   In some very observant Jewish communities marriages are arranged or guided. Families may consult a marriage broker who will suggest potentially suitable partners who may then be introduced to each other with a view to marriage. The final decision about marriage is made by the couple themselves. Enquiries about suitability often include a check to ensure that two people who are both Tay–Sachs carriers (see Chapter 29) are not introduced. In some Orthodox communities young people normally marry in their late teens.

Divorce, though considered very undesirable, is permitted if a marriage is very unhappy and cannot be rescued.

JEWISH FOOD RESTRICTIONS

Food is very important in Jewish life and culture and many people feel strongly that it is important to eat properly especially at times of stress and vulnerability. Families may bring special delicacies into hospital. Chicken soup is often regarded as very nourishing and sustaining.

Kosher food   Orthodox Jews eat only kosher food. Kosher means ritually correct or fit:

- All meat must be slaughtered and prepared according to ritual Jewish law.
- Pork and shellfish or anything made from or containing them are forbidden.
- Milk or milk derivatives cannot be eaten at the same meal with meat and meat derivatives.
- Orthodox Jews will not eat any food prepared outside the home unless it has been produced under the supervision of the Rabbinate using special cooking utensils.

In order to keep milk and meat completely separate, many people leave a gap of several hours after eating meat foods and before eating dairy foods. At home many people keep a kosher kitchen with two complete sets of cutlery, china and cooking utensils, one for meat foods and one for dairy foods. These are always washed and stored separately. In an Orthodox Jewish family home, it is important to find out before using the kitchen if the family keeps a kosher kitchen and, if so, which equipment is kept for dairy foods and which for meat foods.

The level of dietary observance varies from family to family, so when an observant Jewish woman is booked for a birth in hospital it is important to ask her what her dietary needs will be. Some women only follow certain dietary laws and may be able to select carefully from hospital menus (see also Chapter 18). Others will need specially prepared and packaged kosher food ordered for them. Kosher meat is usually salted to remove excess blood in accordance with Jewish law. Women with pre-eclampsia or raised blood pressure may be advised not to salt their meat or to stick to non-meat sources of protein such as fish, eggs, pulses and cheese.

Some women may bring in their own milk, packaged under the supervision of the Rabbinate. They may also prefer to use disposable plates, cups and cutlery for breakfast and tea when kosher meals are not usually supplied to the wards. Space should be made available in the ward fridge to store kosher milk. Since it is forbidden to turn electrical appliances on or off, some Orthodox women may ask for the milk to be brought to them on the Sabbath and on Jewish festivals if the fridge has an internal light. Alternatively the internal light bulb can be removed, or a piece of tape put over the switch to prevent the light being turned on.

Fasting   There are two major religious fasts each year during which all food and drink, including water, are forbidden from before sundown on the eve of the fast until after sundown the next day. The dates of these fasts vary from year to year depending on the moon. In September or October there is a 25 hour fast on Yom Kippur, the Day of

Atonement and in July, a 25 hour fast on the Ninth Day of Av, which commemorates the destruction of the Temple built in Jerusalem by King Solomon. Many observant women will wish to continue to observe these important fasts during pregnancy and while breast feeding, though if this might endanger her health or that of her baby, she can get a dispensation from the Rabbi. A woman who misses a fast does not have to make it up later. If a woman is on essential medication it is important to discuss with her the necessity of continuing to take it during a fast.

There are several minor fasts during the year which some women may also observe. These start just before sunrise and end after dark. They are not considered as important as the two major fasts and most women will feel able not to fast if necessary.

PHYSICAL CARE

Modesty   Modesty is very important in traditional Judaism. Strictly observant Jewish women always keep their arms covered to the elbow and legs to below the knee. Married women cover their hair outside the home with a head scarf or a sheitel (wig). Most conservative women will find it important to observe these rules of modesty as far as possible during antenatal checks and during labour. Since they are likely to find hospital gowns inadequate they should be encouraged to wear clothing of their choice in labour. Care should be taken to maintain women's modesty and to avoid any unnecessary exposure during labour or at any other time.

In Orthodox Judaism, touch between a woman and a man is forbidden unless they are married. This prohibition does not include touch when it is part of a medical examination or part of medical care. Nevertheless, for reasons of modesty, some strictly observant women prefer to be examined by a female doctor. Some women may not wish to be examined with their husbands present.

Orthodox Jewish men may wish to keep their heads covered at all times. Out of modesty, some men may prefer not to discuss intimate matters with female health professionals.

Professionals   It is important to dress modestly when caring for Orthodox Jewish clients or visiting them at home. Women should keep their arms and legs covered and should normally wear a skirt. Some Orthodox men avoid all contact with unrelated women and may not shake hands. A few Orthodox men avoid eye contact or looking at an unrelated woman.

Washing   If a meal contains bread, Orthodox Jews may wish to wash their hands and say a blessing before eating.

Some Orthodox Jews do not bath or shower during Shabbat or the other major festivals since running hot water activates the heating system. Some women may be happy to take a bath or shower provided that the water is turned on and off for them. Orthodox Jewish women who give birth on the Sabbath or during a religious festival should be asked about their wishes concerning washing. Washing in warm water after childbirth is usually considered part of essential health care and is therefore acceptable.

PREGNANCY AND ANTENATAL CARE

Pregnancy   In some Orthodox communities, women lead a very sheltered existence and marry young. For first-time mothers, antenatal contact with the health service may be the first time they have stepped out of their own close-knit community. Some may never have spoken to anyone outside their community and so may be shy and anxious. Their behaviour is sometimes misinterpreted and wrongly labelled as withdrawn or odd. Some, especially very young women, may be accompanied by their mothers. Most Orthodox Jewish couples expect to have several children.

Antenatal screening   Attitudes to antenatal screening vary. Some Orthodox Jews may refuse all screening since they are likely to find termination of pregnancy unacceptable. (For Tay–Sachs disease see Chapter 29.)

Antenatal education   Most observant women will attend antenatal classes though some may prefer to attend women-only classes run within their own community. Strictly observant women will be concerned about modesty and may not want to discuss intimate physical details or watch videos showing labour or birth, especially with men present. Since touch is forbidden during established labour (see below), Orthodox couples may not want to practice massage or positions that involve the husband supporting the woman. Orthodox men may also wish to leave the room during exercises, so as not to watch other men's wives. Some people may not want to sit on the floor as this traditionally indicates mourning.

LABOUR AND BIRTH

Expectations and traditions   In some communities, Orthodox women expect to have large families. Eight to ten children are not uncommon. Birth is usually considered a normal process. Although there are no religious objections to any medical procedures or interventions, Orthodox couples may want clearly explained reasons for anything that is suggested, such as induction, before they can accept it. Many Orthodox women will be anxious to avoid a caesarean which might make subsequent births more difficult and potentially restrict the number of babies they might have.

> 'We have large families and it can be embarrassing to say "I have three children under 4 years old and I am expecting my fourth". A woman having her fifth or sixth baby is often more experienced than the people who are caring for her.'   Orthodox Jewish mother of three

If a planned induction or elective caesarean is necessary, parents may prefer to avoid the Sabbath. A few may ask if the procedure can be carried out on a Tuesday since they may consider this an especially auspicious day.

Some women may wear a red cord around the wrist during pregnancy and labour to ward off the evil eye. This should not be removed unless it is essential and only with the woman's consent. Some women have a special card, called a Shir Hamaalot, containing verses from the Psalms. They will want to keep this near them throughout labour and place it in the baby's cot after the birth.

Where there are serious problems and a choice has to be made between the life of the mother or the life of the baby during pregnancy or labour, the mother's life takes precedence under Jewish law.

Labour   Strict Orthodox couples are prohibited from any physical contact once there has been a show or any blood loss. Although a husband can stay with his wife during labour and actively support and encourage her verbally, he cannot touch her or hand her anything directly. Some Orthodox couples may decide that the man should only participate spiritually; in this case he will normally sit in the corner of the room and recite psalms (Bash, 1980). Staff who do not understand the prohibition on touch may become unnecessarily anxious or make incorrect assumptions about the couple's relationship. The prohibition lasts until the woman has had seven clear days without blood loss and has been to the mikvah (see below). It can, however, be disregarded if the husband's help is needed, for example, to move the woman in an emergency when life is threatened.

For reasons of modesty, some Orthodox men prefer to leave the room during internal examinations. They may also leave for the birth, or may position themselves so that they are facing the head of the bed rather than the foot.

Immediately after the birth   Some mothers and fathers may want the baby to be washed before they hold the baby. Some may not hand the baby directly to each other, in case they accidentally touch. Instead, they will put the baby down or give the baby to the midwife as an intermediary.

Very occasionally, a couple may want to take the placenta home to bury it.

The sex of the baby   From a religious viewpoint, Orthodox Jews are enjoined to have two sons or a son and a daughter. As in many other cultures, some traditional Jewish families may place extra value on boys, and may be particularly pleased if their first child is a son. However it is important not to make assumptions and to realise that many parents will be equally delighted by the birth of a daughter.

POSTNATAL CARE

Feeding the baby   Attitudes to infant feeding depend on each woman's upbringing and expectations. Some women strongly prefer to breast feed because it is natural. Conservative women will not breast feed in the presence of others and some not in the presence of their husband. In hospital, women's needs for privacy while breast feeding should be respected.

Some women with large families to care for may find bottle feeding more practical. Some artificial baby milks are not acceptable to Orthodox Jews since they contain non-kosher animal products.

Naming the baby   A male baby is traditionally named on the eighth day at his circumcision (see below). The name of a baby daughter is traditionally announced by her father in the synagogue at the first Torah (Bible) reading after the birth. Ashkenazi Jews may honour a deceased relative by naming the baby after them. Sephardi Jews may honour a living relative by naming the baby after them. In some communities it is considered important not to tell anyone the baby's name before the official naming ceremony. Traditionally this was considered to protect the child.

Circumcision   Male infants are traditionally given their name and circumcised on or after the eighth day at a ceremony called Brit Milah. Circumcision is performed by a mohel (or circumciser) who decides whether the baby is well enough for the circumcision to be performed. If the baby is jaundiced or if there is any concern about his health or progress, the ceremony is postponed. Brit Milah takes place between sunrise and sunset, usually in the morning and is normally held in the presence of a quorum of ten men (a minyan). The mohel gives precise instructions about the care of the baby after circumcision.

Mohels are especially trained and those in the Orthodox community belong to the Initiation Society. Members of the Initiation Society only perform Brit Milah when the baby's identity as a Jew is certain. Since in the Orthodox community Jewish status is dependent on having a Jewish mother, distress can be caused for parents when the father is Jewish but the mother's Jewish status is uncertain. The Association of Reform and Liberal Mohelim (see Useful Addresses) will always help in such cases.

Many women are anxious about the physical process of circumcision for their baby and may need extra support and understanding at this time. Circumcision is an important part of Jewish culture as well as being fundamental in religious terms. Even Jews who do not regard themselves as in any way religious may therefore decide to have their sons circumcised. For some parents the decision on whether to circumcise is only reached after much heart-searching.

Many mohels are willing to perform a non-religious circumcision for non-Jews who want their sons to be circumcised.

The first-born son   After the birth of a first-born son a religious ceremony, known as 'Pidyon Ha'ben' or the redemption of the first-born, is held on the thirtieth day. Boys who were delivered by caesarean section or whose mothers have had a previous miscarriage or stillbirth do not have a Pidyon Ha'ben. Women who are adjusting to motherhood can find the prospect of preparing for this ceremony stressful since it often involves a gathering of large numbers of family and friends.

Menstruation   Jewish law states that while a woman has any vaginal blood loss and for seven days after the loss ends, touch between her and her husband is forbidden. Strict Orthodox couples sleep in separate beds during menstruation and afterwards, and avoid any touch. After seven clear days without bleeding observant women go to the mikvah, a special bath house for women attached to the synagogue, to take a ritual cleansing bath. The couple can then resume physical contact.

In some Orthodox households women who have recently given birth may sleep in a separate bed until they have stopped bleeding postnatally.

Contraception   Sex within marriage is regarded as joyful and positive and a husband has a duty to satisfy his wife sexually. Contraception is not encouraged within the Orthodox community, but can be used if a woman's life or well-being would be jeopardised by pregnancy. An Orthodox couple would normally discuss the situation with their rabbi who would take the woman's health and her family circumstances into consideration. The most acceptable form of contraception is likely to be the contraceptive pill. The diaphragm or the coil may also be acceptable. Condoms are unlikely to be acceptable because of the biblical prohibition against the spilling of seed. Any contraceptive method that precipitates irregular bleeding or spotting is likely to be unacceptable (see above).

Some women may regard breast feeding as a way of spacing their pregnancies and may need information about the likely effectiveness of this.

CHILDBEARING LOSSES

Infertility   The Torah (the first five books of the Old Testament) exhorts couples to 'be fruitful and multiply'. Strictly speaking a couple should have either two sons or a son and a daughter. In some Jewish communities, large families are expected. A woman's aim and purpose is traditionally to be a good wife and a good mother and much of the life of a religious Jew revolves around the family. These factors can increase the anguish felt by all infertile couples.

Jewish women who ovulate early in their cycle and who observe the prohibition against sexual intercourse during the first seven days after a period may have difficulty in conceiving. Some Orthodox couples in this situation may seek artificial insemination with the husband's sperm rather than break the religious prohibition. However it may be important, where possible, to use methods of collecting sperm during intercourse between husband and wife since masturbation is forbidden in Jewish law. Artificial insemination by donor may be unacceptable since it raises serious issues about the child's legitimacy and may be considered akin to adultery. Similarly, IVF using the couple's own eggs and sperm may be acceptable while using donated eggs or sperm may not.

Termination of pregnancy   In Jewish law an unborn fetus is regarded as part of the mother's body and is not considered a separate being until labour has begun. Nevertheless, Judaism holds that all human life is of infinite value. Orthodox Jews are unlikely to accept termination of pregnancy at any stage in cases of fetal abnormality. However, since in Judaism the health of the mother takes precedence over that of the fetus, termination may be considered if the mother's physical or mental health is endangered, or if the pregnancy is the result of rape.

Miscarriage   In Jewish law, life does not begin at conception; the embryo is regarded as 'mere water' for the first forty days of pregnancy. Thus in Jewish law, a miscarriage during the first six weeks of pregnancy is not officially viewed as the loss of a baby and the products of the pregnancy may be disposed of in the usual way.

From 40 days' gestation and until the birth, the fetus is recognised in Jewish law but is not considered to be a full life. Whatever the gestation, following the miscarriage of a recognisable baby, parents should be asked how they would like the baby's body to be prepared.

Stillbirth and neonatal death   All parents should be offered the opportunity of seeing and holding their baby. Some parents may not want to, possibly because it is traditionally considered wrong to see or handle a dead body unless essential. Men of certain Orthodox Jewish families, descended from the priesthood, are not allowed to be near a dead body and may have to leave abruptly if a baby is stillborn or dies.

When a baby is stillborn or dies after birth, the parents should be asked if they want their community's Burial Society to be called (see below). In this case, staff should put on gloves before wrapping the baby in a sheet to await their arrival. If the parents prefer the staff to prepare the baby's body, ask whether they would prefer non-Jewish staff to wear gloves. The baby should be laid out with the arms beside the body and should be wrapped in a plain sheet with no religious emblems.

A baby is considered in Jewish law to have full human rights immediately after birth. However, a baby who has not lived for thirty days is not legally considered to be a fully viable human being and so the full traditional mourning rituals (see below) are not followed. As a result, although a baby who is miscarried, stillborn or dies within thirty days of birth is buried in the normal way, his or her parents do not have all the other usual rituals and traditions surrounding death to support them. Some parents may be distressed by this. Others may accept it and be supported through it by their religious faith. For some parents the requirement to bury the baby as soon as possible may cause difficulties (see Chapter 22).

It may be helpful to encourage parents to give the baby a name and to attend the funeral, both of which are acceptable in Jewish law.

DEATH AND BURIAL

The information in this section applies mainly to adult deaths. Some or all of it may also apply to miscarriages, stillbirths and neonatal deaths although there may also be significant differences. It is important to check everything with the parents in every case.

Last rites   There are no official last rites in Judaism. Prayers are said by the family and a rabbi is not needed unless the person who is dying or the relatives want one to be called.

Last offices   Traditionally, when a religious Jew dies, the eyes and mouth are closed and ritual purification of the body is carried out by members of the community's Burial Society, the Chevra Kaddishah (<u>h</u>evra ka<u>d</u>eesha). After the body has been washed and dressed in a special shroud, the arms and hands are placed along the body which is then put on the floor with the feet towards the door. A lighted candle is placed at the head and any mirrors are covered. The body is never left alone. Watchers sit with it night and day until the burial reciting psalms. Women attend to the bodies of women and children, while men attend to the bodies of men. Members of the Chevra Kaddishah perform their duties voluntarily and anonymously so that the bereaved family does not feel under any obligation to them.

When an Orthodox Jew dies in hospital, the relatives should be asked about their wishes. If they wish, the Burial Society of their synagogue should be contacted. In preparation, provided the relatives consent, staff should close the eyes, straighten the limbs and remove any tubes and equipment. The body should then be covered and left unwashed. It may be taken to the mortuary to await the arrival of members of the Burial Society. Non-Jewish staff should wear gloves while handling the body.

If the family does not wish the Burial Society to be called, they should be asked about their wishes concerning last offices.

Burial   Burial should normally follow as soon as possible after the death, usually within 24 or 48 hours. If the death occurs on or just before Shabbat, burial must be delayed till afterwards. Cremation is not acceptable to Orthodox Jews, but may be to Reform and Liberal Jews.

Mourning rituals   During the seven days following the burial, Orthodox families 'sit Shiva' (seven in Hebrew). Formal mourning is suspended on Shabbat. During the seven days the dead person's immediate family stay at home to be visited and comforted by family, friends and acquaintances. In some communities visitors may support the bereaved by bringing food. Close relatives may tear their clothing as a sign of mourning and men may not shave. Male relatives recite Kaddish, the prayer for the dead, in the synagogue. Each year after the death the anniversary or 'Yarzeit' (yartzite) will be commemorated by the family lighting a candle which burns for 24 hours. Within the first year of the death, a ceremony is held at the graveside at which a tombstone is erected. These mourning rituals are not followed in the case of a baby who is miscarried, stillborn or dies within thirty days of birth.

Certification   Because burial must take place very quickly after a death it is important to issue a Cause of Death Certificate as soon as possible. In areas where there is an Orthodox Jewish community, Registrars of Births, Marriages and Deaths may make special arrangements to issue death certificates out of normal office hours.

Post mortems   Orthodox Jews are unlikely to consent to a post mortem unless it is required by law since it is considered a desecration of the body. Many believe that when the Messiah comes, the dead will be revived and therefore bodies must be buried complete and intact.

Orthodox Jews are likely to be distressed if a post mortem is legally required, both because they fear that the body will be desecrated and because this is likely to delay the burial. In such a case, relatives must be treated with respect and sensitivity and special care should be taken to ensure that the body is complete after the post mortem. Where appropriate a partial post mortem should be performed.

USEFUL ADDRESSES

Association of Reform and Liberal Mohelim
80 East End Road
London   N3 2SY

The Secretary,
Initiation Society,
15 Sunny Hill Court,
Sunningfields Crescent,
London
NW4 4RB

The information below will only apply to certain Rastafarian clients. Never assume. Always check everything with the person concerned.

The Rastafarian movement began in the Caribbean and most Rastafarians are of African-Caribbean heritage. It is primarily a spiritual movement but has important political aspects. Rastafarians may also be influenced to some extent by other aspects of traditional African-Caribbean culture (see Chapter 30).

RASTAFARISM – A BRIEF DESCRIPTION

Rastafarism is a personal and private religion and does not place great emphasis on formal theology. All adherents have a deep love of God and believe that God, known as 'Jah', is incarnate within each individual. All members are equal, nobody has any special position or power, and everyone can speak directly to Jah.

Many Rastafarians derive strength and support from the Bible. They do not regard themselves as Christians but believe that Christ's spirit has been reborn in Ras Tafari, the Emperor of Ethiopia (Haile Selassie I). Ras (Prince) Tafari is considered to be a divine being, the Messiah, who will ultimately lead all black people to freedom. Rastafarians claim that there is a direct link between the biblical King David and Ras Tafari who also bore the biblical titles 'King of Kings' and 'Lion of Judah'. Rastafarians believe that they are the true Jews who will eventually be redeemed by return to Africa, their true home and heaven on earth. Many Rastas see Western society as the biblical Babylon, the place of exile and slavery, in which black people will never have a chance of equality and freedom.

Rastafarians hold meetings called 'reasoning sessions' which provide forums for people to discuss and debate any topic as well as for mutual support. These are usually held in people's homes. People may also gather at 'groundations' to sing and praise Jah. Some Rastafarians take part in formal religious services, called temple worship, at which a Rastafarian priest reads liturgies. Rastafarians may belong to the Coptic Church, the Ethiopian Orthodox Church, of which Haile Selassie is the head, or the Church of Haile Selassie I.

Spiritual values are central to Rastafarism, but some Rastafarians are also very politically aware. The Rastafarian movement began in the West Indies in the 1930s, mainly in Jamaica, and spread rapidly throughout the Caribbean. It was inspired by Marcus Garvey (1887–1940) who advocated pride in black consciousness and greater self-respect. He stressed the importance of black people becoming aware of world-wide white economic and cultural domination and of their own mental enslavement which taught them to view themselves as less able and deserving and to accept the role of second-class citizens. He encouraged them to cast aside notions of inferiority and to develop their own independent potential. The Rastafarian movement also highlighted and rejected many aspects of colonial and white influence prevalent in Jamaica. Most Rastafarians are, therefore, particularly conscious of white racism and its effects, and of the tendency of white people to regard themselves and their culture as superior. They also feel strongly that many white people downgrade Rastafarism and accord it little respect or status.

LANGUAGE

Many Rastafarians speak to each other in a language based on Jamaican patois (see Chapter 30) but with additional features including the phrase 'I and I' instead of 'I and you'. This indicates the oneness of two persons and the belief that God is in all people.

FAMILIES AND RELATIONSHIPS

Traditionally women are mainly responsible for child care though many fathers are also involved. Economic changes have meant that more women go out to work and may be the main breadwinners. Both men and women are encouraged to develop their own potential and in many relationships there is equality, with decisions being taken jointly after discussion.

RELIGIOUS ASPECTS OF FOOD

Rastafarism regards the body as a Temple of God which should be protected from contamination, especially from chemicals. Food is regarded as having a major influence on the health of the body and of the soul.

Most Rastafarians prefer to eat food that is as natural, fresh and pure as possible, known as I-TAL food, though individuals vary in what they find acceptable. The needs of each woman should be accepted and respected. Some Rastafarians are vegans; some are vegetarians; some follow a raw food diet, eating only a minimal amount of cooked food. Some Rastafarians eat meat, but do not eat pork or pork products. Rastafarians may also avoid salt or foods to which salt has been added. Tinned or processed food and foods that contain additives are likely to be unacceptable. Tobacco and alcohol are not usually used and some people may not eat grapes. Some Rastafarians use ganga (marijuana) (see Chapter 28).

Women are likely to pay particular attention to their diet during pregnancy and when they are breast feeding to ensure that their food is especially pure and wholesome. Advice about diet should only be given if there are clinical reasons for concern, and should always respect the woman's knowledge and the care she takes about the food she eats.

PHYSICAL CARE

Modesty   Modesty in dress is important. Women may wish to keep themselves covered at all times and may prefer to wear their own clothes in hospital as hospital gowns are often inadequate. If internal examination is necessary, most women would prefer it to be done by a woman.

Hair   For some Rastafarians, uncut locks are a sign of their covenant with God. They are often known as dreadlocks. This reflects religious awe and wonder, rather than fear. Some devout Rastafarians wear their hair long, others wear it short. Most keep their hair covered at all times with a hat or scarf. Not everyone with locks is religious.

CHILDBEARING ISSUES

Attitudes to medical care and screening   Since the body is the Temple of God, Rastafarians considers it essential to avoid anything which might be contaminating or harmful. Many will therefore want detailed information about the risks and benefits of routine or special tests, investigations, screening and treatments before giving their consent. Some may question the need for internal examinations. Some Rastafarians may prefer to avoid any medication, and, if medication is necessary, may wish to know what it contains. Some Rastafarians, because of negative experiences with health services, may also be sceptical about the motives of the medical establishment. It is important to ensure that people's concerns are respected and listened to and that questions are answered fully.

> *'When I was expecting my fourth baby I said I didn't want an internal as there seemed to be no real purpose. The doctor was very rude to me and wrote 'un co-operative' in my notes. This upset me a lot. I was frightened that as a consequence I would not get the sort of care given to everyone else.'*   Rastafarian mother of four

Some Rastafarians prefer to use complementary therapies such as herbalism or acupuncture.

Labour   Some women may prefer to labour without using pharmacological pain relief. Many Rastafarian women prefer another woman to accompany them. However, fathers are also increasingly choosing to attend and some women will want to have two supporters.

Blood transfusions   Because it is important to avoid anything that might contaminate the body, some people may find blood transfusion unacceptable. This is a matter of personal choice and should be discussed antenatally.

Welcoming the baby   There is normally no ceremony to welcome the baby at birth. The baby is named by the parents. When the baby is 3 or 4 months old a religious ceremony may be held at which the spiritual name is given.

Postnatal care   Rest and a good diet are considered to be important and breast feeding is the norm. Women who need to bottle feed their babies are likely to want information about the content of baby milks. They may want to avoid those that contain animal products.

Contraception   Decisions about contraception are a matter for personal choice. However many Rastafarians follow the Old Testament teaching 'be fruitful and multiply'. Children are regarded as a blessing and are seen as a continuation of life so the use of contraception may be unacceptable. Community awareness of higher infant mortality and morbidity rates in black babies is another reason why people might choose not to use contraception (see also Chapter 21).

CHILDBEARING LOSSES

Infertility   Infertility investigations and treatments are a matter of personal choice. Some people may be reluctant to accept them because of their invasive nature.

Termination of pregnancy   This is a matter for personal choice. However many Rastafarians will not want to terminate a pregnancy.

Miscarriage   Parents are unlikely to have any special requirements if a baby miscarries before 24 weeks, and may rely on the hospital to make the necessary arrangements. Some may choose not to give the baby a name. However parents should always receive information about the choices available to them so that they can decide what is best for them.

Stillbirth and neonatal death   Some Rastafarians may not wish to see or hold a baby who is stillborn or who has died, or to have photographs taken or to have a lock of hair cut. In some cases this may be because the body is felt not to be important (see below). Parents should be asked about their wishes and have an opportunity to decide what is right for them. Some parents may wish to arrange the funeral themselves, others may want this to be done for them.

DEATH AND FUNERAL RITES

Attitudes to death vary. Many Rastafarians regard death as something to be accepted. Some believe that because God is eternal, people live forever, and that it is more important to focus on the living than the dead. For some the body of the person who has died is therefore irrelevant. Some Rastafarians may not attend funerals. Others feel that it is important to acknowledge the departure of a soul and to support each other through their grief.

Last offices   Some Rastafarians carry out ceremonies at the bedsides of people who are very sick or dying. After death, there are no particular requirements and, with the relatives' consent, the body can be prepared in the usual way with the arms placed at the sides.

Funerals   Most Rastafarians prefer burial to cremation but this is a matter of personal choice. Funerals are generally plain and simple (unlike the elaborate funerals often held in African-Caribbean tradition). Usually only close family and friends attend.

Post mortems   Post mortems are likely to be unacceptable to many Rastafarians.

The information below will only apply to some Sikhs. Never assume. Always check everything with the person concerned.

Sikh communities in Britain

The Sikh community has a long-standing military tradition and more recently a tradition of emigration and settlement, mainly in parts of the British Empire such as Singapore, Hong Kong, East Africa, and Canada. There have been small Sikh communities in Britain since the First World War, when a number of Sikh servicemen who had fought in the trenches in Europe settled here after being demobbed. Between the wars Sikh traders settled in the ports. After the Second World War, a number of Sikh ex-servicemen again stayed in Britain. Many others were recruited to come and work in Britain by private industrial companies whose staff had fought beside Sikh servicemen in the Second World War (Henley, 1983; Weller, 1993).

It is estimated that there are about four hundred thousand Sikhs in the UK (Weller, 1993). The families of most Sikhs in Britain originated in Punjab in northern India (see Figure 34.1). Most of these families arrived in Britain in the 1950s and 60s. A few Sikh families came to Britain from East Africa (to which their forebears had emigrated from Punjab) (see Figure 31.1). They came mainly in the 1970s, often as refugees.

The very different backgrounds and experiences of these two groups may mean that, at least among older people, there is a tendency to live, worship and socialise separately, and to see themselves to some extent as separate communities. Almost all Sikh women now of childbearing age were born and brought up in Britain and are the children and grandchildren of the immigrant generation.

LANGUAGE

The first language of many Sikhs in Britain is Punjabi (see also Chapters 34 and 13).

THE SIKH NAMING SYSTEM (See Chapter 14)

SIKHISM – A BRIEF DESCRIPTION

The Sikh religion was founded as an offshoot of Hinduism in the sixteenth century in Punjab in northern India. Almost all Sikhs are Punjabi in origin, and Sikhism has remained essentially a Punjabi religion (see also Chapter 34).

Sikhs believe in one personal God who is the eternal creator and the source of all being. Sikhs stress the need for each person to develop their own individual relationship with God, seeking truth and leading a virtuous life. Prayer and meditation, family duties and community involvement are all important in Sikhism. Most Sikhs, like Hindus, believe in reincarnation: each soul must go through many cycles of birth and rebirth in the world. The ultimate aim of each soul is to reach perfection and so to become united with God and avoid reincarnation into this world. Reincarnation is linked to belief in karma, the cycle of reward and punishment for all thoughts and deeds. Sikhs believe that a person's karma can be changed and improved through the grace of God.

Sikhism was founded by Guru Nanak (1469–1539 CE). Guru Nanak was born into a Hindu family and wanted to get away from the caste system, and from the excessive ritual and priestly domination of the Hinduism of his time. Sikhism stresses community and equality between all people, whatever their caste, class or occupation. Men and women are considered equal, though they may have different traditional roles. Sikhism has no ordained priesthood or official priestly hierarchy, and all the members of each community play a part in worship and in running their own temple (gurdwara).

Guru Gobind Singh   The tenth and last of the great living Sikh gurus, Guru Gobind Singh (1666–1708 CE) wanted to make the Sikhs into a visible community and to strengthen them as a fighting force against the Mughal emperors who were attacking them at the time. He gave them five symbols which all initiated Sikh men and women should wear: uncut and unshaven hair and (for men) beard, a special comb to fix the hair, a steel bangle, a dagger, and special underwear (see below). Guru Gobind Singh also wore a turban, and a turban has become the best-known mark of a Sikh man.

In order finally to eradicate caste-consciousness from the Sikh community, Guru Gobind Singh also required Sikhs to stop using their family names, which indicated their position in the Hindu caste system. Instead all Sikh men were to use the last name Singh (Lion), and all women the last name Kaur (Princess) (see also Chapter 14). Nevertheless, caste awareness and divisions, which were as deeply rooted in society as class awareness and divisions in Britain, proved difficult to destroy completely. Awareness of caste status still influences many Sikhs, particularly with regard to social life and obligations and marriage. Different Sikh caste and subcaste groups in Britain tend to remain separate; some are more traditional and orthodox in their religious practices than others.

Guru Gobind Singh stated that he would have no human successor. After his death spiritual authority among the Sikhs would pass partly to the Guru Granth Sahib (the Sikh Holy Book), and partly to the Sikh community itself. Many Sikhs have pictures of the gurus, who are highly revered, in their homes and by their beds.

RELIGIOUS OBSERVANCE

At home   The time before sunrise is considered a good time to pray without distraction and many devout Sikhs wake up very early to pray. People also pray in the evenings. It is important to be physically clean when praying and Sikhs normally wash or shower beforehand. Privacy during prayer (for example, with bed-curtains drawn in hospital) is appreciated. If a woman cannot wash properly, she may wish to make a symbolic wash by sprinkling a little water over herself. If she is bed-bound she may need water and a towel.

Some Sikhs may bring holy books, prayer books, pictures and prayer beads into hospital. These should only be touched with clean hands, if at all, and nothing should be put on top of them. They should not be put near dirty clothes or shoes, nor on the foot of the bed near the woman's feet. They should never be allowed to fall on the floor.

The gurdwara   Sikhism is a community-based religion. Communal worship and social activities at the gurdwara (the Sikh temple) are very important. Most gurdwaras contain a room for prayer in which the Guru Granth Sahib, the Sikh holy book, is kept on a dais, a kitchen and a communal dining area where meals may be served for the whole congregation after services and on special occasions, and facilities for washing. Non-Sikhs are welcome providing they behave with respect.

Before entering into the gurdwara both men and women must remove their shoes and cover their heads. Some people wash their hands and feet. By tradition men and women normally sit separately. Everyone sits with the soles of their feet pointing away from the Guru Granth Sahib as a matter of courtesy.

Although there is no fixed day for Sikh worship, Sikhs in Britain generally hold their main services on Sundays. At the end of a service everyone is given a small portion of karah parshad (a specially prepared and blessed sweet dish). The sharing of karah parshad emphasises the equality and fellowship of all Sikhs. Sikh families may bring a portion of karah parshad to relatives in hospital. They may also sometimes bring amrit (a blessed mixture of water and sugar).

The granti   Most Sikh communities in Britain employ a granti, an elected caretaker or leader, to lead services and look after the gurdwara. The granti does not traditionally have a pastoral role.

Festivals   The two main festivals celebrated by Sikhs in Britain are Diwali, the festival of light, in October or November (also a Hindu festival), and Baisakhi, the Spring festival, in April. The precise dates vary each year depending on the date of the full moon. (For more on the dates of festivals see Walshe and Warrier, 1993.)

THE FIVE SIGNS OF SIKHISM

Each of the five signs of Sikhism – the kara, kesh, kangha, kirpan and kaccha – also known as the five Ks, has a symbolic meaning. Sikhs in Britain differ a good deal in how far they adhere to the five Ks; for example, many Sikh men have cut their hair and no longer keep it in place with a special comb. Most men and women still wear a kara and many wear a symbolic kirpan. A few Sikhs no longer wear any of the five Ks, though some are now re-adopting them as a sign of increased confidence and pride in their identity and religion. Some devout Sikhs wear all five Ks all the time and never remove them completely, even when they are ill, in bed or washing.

Some adult Sikhs devote themselves more closely to their religion and undergo a special kind of initiation or confirmation known as taking amrit. In some ways this has a similar significance to Christian communion and confirmation. A Sikh man or woman who has taken amrit is likely to be particularly careful never to remove any of the five Ks.

Kara (bangle)   Most Sikhs, even those who may not consider themselves religious, wear a steel (or sometimes gold) bangle on their right wrist. Left-handed people wear it on their left wrist. Most people never remove their kara. It should normally be taped before an operation. If this is not possible, explain the reasons and find a mutually acceptable solution.

Sikh children usually wear a kara from a very early age, and relatives may give a tiny kara, often gold or silver, to a new born Sikh baby. Again, this should not normally be removed without permission.

Kesh (uncut hair and beard)   In South Asian tradition the head is regarded as the most sacred part of the body. Many devout Sikh men and women never cut their hair, and men never shave or trim their beards, though this may be less important for younger people. The hair and beard must always be kept clean and tidy. Some devout Sikh women may be distressed if the hair on any part of their body is cut or shaved. If this is really unavoidable it must be discussed and an acceptable solution found.

The prohibition on cutting or shaving hair specifically bans the use of razors and scissors. If it is essential to remove body hair and the woman is reluctant, it may sometimes be more acceptable to use a depilatory cream. Discuss this with her.

The hair of a Sikh baby should be treated with the same respect and should not be cut or shaved, for example to attach a scalp clip, without the parents' permission.

Sikh men with uncut hair wear a turban. A very few extremely devout Sikh women also wear turbans.

Kangha (comb)   Men and women with uncut hair usually fix it on their head in a bun kept in place by a kangha, a small wooden or plastic semi-circular comb. Many people never remove this and may keep it in a pocket, for example, when their hair is loose. A Sikh woman who has cut her hair may carry a kangha in a pocket or wear a miniature one on a chain around her neck. Again, some women will wish to keep this with them at all times.

Kirpan (symbolic dagger)   The kirpan symbolises the Sikh's traditional readiness to fight in self-defence and to protect the oppressed and needy. A few very devout Sikh women wear a full-sized kirpan under their clothes in a cloth sheath slung over one shoulder and round the body. Most people wear a kirpan-shaped brooch or pendant instead.

Devout Sikhs may not wish to remove the kirpan even when showering or bathing. It must always be kept clean and dry. The sheath may, for example, be wound round the neck when showering. In the past, health professionals have sometimes caused distress by removing kirpans, thinking they were dangerous weapons. A woman who wishes to wear her kirpan should be able to do so throughout labour. If it would be safer for medical reasons to remove it, it is important to obtain her consent.

Kaccha (underwear)   Kaccha are to remind Sikhs of the duties of modesty and sexual morality. Traditionally they were knee-length but now most devout Sikhs in the UK wear conventional underwear as kaccha.

A few devout Sikh men and women never remove their kaccha completely. They keep them on while showering and then put on a dry pair. When changing, people often put one foot in the new pair before completely removing the old pair. A few devout Sikh women may prefer to leave at least one leg or ankle in the kaccha all the time and tuck them to one side, even during antenatal examinations and during childbirth. This is common practice in Punjab and causes no inconvenience.

FAMILIES AND RELATIONSHIPS

Guru Nanak stressed that men and women could come closer to God by being active members of their families. Providing for the family (traditionally and, in many cases still, the extended family) and caring for all its members' spiritual and emotional well-being are religious duties for Sikhs (see also Chapter 34). Involvement in the community is also important.

One of Guru Nanak's explicit aims was to raise the status of women. Sikh women are traditionally educated equally with men. Socially and within the family they usually have a good deal of freedom and authority, though in practice, as in most communities, Sikh women are not always given equal rights, and most major decisions are made by men. In the early days in Britain, Sikh women were often the first South Asian women to go out to work.

Traditional female virtues, such as decorum and modesty, are important to many Sikh women and are not generally seen as conflicting with the equality of the sexes. There is also a system of etiquette which influences behaviour between the sexes in public.

Marriage   Sikhs are expected to marry, and both men and women are expected to take an active part in bringing up children (see also Chapter 34). Many believe that Sikhs should marry within their own community to avoid future conflict and difficulty. Marriages between Hindus and Sikhs do occur, depending on caste and subcaste position. Marriages between Sikhs and Muslims are very rare.

Divorce   Sikhs traditionally regard marriage as in indissoluble sacrament. Divorce is generally regarded as shameful and occurs only when the marital situation is desperate. There is a strong stigma attached to divorced people, especially women.

FOOD RESTRICTIONS

Religious restrictions   The only explicit Sikh prohibition regarding food is against eating halal meat, that is, meat killed according to Muslim regulations. Most Sikhs do not follow other food restrictions though a few devout Sikhs, particularly women, are vegetarians. Like Hindu vegetarians (see Chapter 36), Sikh vegetarians do not eat meat, fish, eggs or anything made with them. Some non-vegetarian Sikhs do not eat beef. Some do not eat pork since the pig is a scavenging animal in India and pig meat is generally regarded as dirty.

Although, as a group, Sikhs are generally less strict than, for example, Hindus and Muslims in following dietary restrictions, the dietary practices of each individual woman are still binding and must be respected (see also Chapter 18). A few devout Sikh women fast on certain days. Sometimes this involves eating only a few foods such as fruit, yoghurt or nuts.

Alcohol and tobacco   Alcohol and tobacco are traditionally forbidden, though many less devout and younger Sikhs both drink and smoke. Some devout Sikhs feel strongly about not being exposed to tobacco smoke.

PHYSICAL CARE   (see also The Five Signs of Sikhism above)

Jewellery   A few Sikh women wear special religious jewellery apart from the kara and kangha (see above) to protect them while they are pregnant and when they come into hospital.

When a Sikh woman marries she usually receives a number of glass or gold wedding bangles, equivalent in significance to a British wedding ring. Some women may be very reluctant to remove their wedding bangles and it may be impossible to do so without breaking them. Religious and other jewellery should always be treated with respect and never removed without consent.

Make-up   A few Sikh women may wear a bindi, a small dot on the forehead. This has religious connotations among Hindus but for Sikhs is usually purely decorative.

CHILDBEARING ISSUES

After the birth   There is usually no religious ceremony at the birth of a Sikh baby. On the thirteenth day some families hold a religious ceremony at which prayers are said and the baby blessed. Both mother and baby may be given blessed sweetened water (amrit).

When a baby is about forty days old there may be another larger celebration when the parents take the baby to the gurdwara to pray and give thanks.

It is traditional to choose a name by opening the Guru Granth Sahib (the Sikh Holy Book) at random and choosing a name that begins with the first letter of the first word of the first complete paragraph on the left hand side of the page. Until the formal naming ceremony, often on either the thirteenth or the fortieth day after the birth, the baby may be known by a pet name.

Contraception   There is no religious prohibition against contraception.

CHILDBEARING LOSSES

Infertility   Fertility treatment is generally acceptable but some Sikhs may be reluctant to use donor eggs or sperm.

Termination of pregnancy   Abortion is traditionally disapproved of but individual attitudes vary.

Miscarriage, stillbirth and neonatal death   Stillborn babies and very young infants are usually buried rather than cremated. The parents may want to wash the baby's body themselves. All bereaved parents need full information about their choices, and support and time to decide what is best for them (see also Chapter 22).

DEATH AND FUNERAL RITES

The information in this section applies mainly to adult deaths. Some or all of it may also apply to miscarriages, stillbirths and neonatal deaths although there may also be significant differences. It is important to check everything with the parents in every case.

Death   A devout Sikh who is very ill or dying may receive comfort from hymns from the Guru Granth Sahib. Family members may also read or pray with the dying person. There are no specific religious ceremonies at the death of a Sikh.

Last offices   Most Sikhs are not concerned about non-Sikhs touching the body. Staff may therefore perform the normal last offices providing the family has no special wishes. However, in South Asian tradition the family is responsible for all ceremonies and rites connected with death, and some Sikh families may prefer to wash and lay out the body themselves.

If the family wishes to wash the body, only do the following. Close the eyes, straighten the limbs, and wrap the body in a plain sheet without religious emblems. The body may then be taken home or to the funeral director's and washed and dressed by the family. Every Sikh is cremated wearing the five signs of Sikhism.

Cremation   Adult Sikhs are cremated, not buried. The cremation should normally take place as soon as possible, normally within 24 hours of death. The ashes are normally thrown into the sea or a river, or buried.

Post mortems   There is no religious prohibition against post-mortem examinations but it may be important to the family that burial or cremation take place as soon as possible.

References and further reading

GENERAL (references referred to in several chapters in this section)

Green, J. (1991) *Death with Dignity, Vol. I*, Nursing Times, London
Green, J. (1992) *Death with Dignity, Vol. II*, Nursing Times, London
Hill, Sara E. (ed.) (1990) *More than Rice and Peas: Guidelines to Improve Food Provision for Black and Ethnic Minorities in Britain*, The Food Commission, London
Mares, P., Henley, A. and Baxter, C. (1985) *Health Care in Multiracial Britain*, National Extension College, Cambridge
OPCS (1993) *1991 Census: Ethnic Group and Country of Birth – Great Britain (CEN 91 TM EGCB)*, Office of Population Censuses and Surveys, London
Walshe, J. G. and Warrier S. (1993) *Dates and Meanings of Religious and Other Festivals*, Foulsham Educational Press, London
Weller, P. (ed.) (1993) *Religions in the UK: a Multi-faith Directory*, University of Derby/Interfaith Network for the UK

30 TRADITIONAL AFRICAN-CARIBBEAN CULTURE

Coombe, V. (1986) African-Caribbean families in Britain. In *Race and Social Work: a Guide to Training*, V. Coombe and A. Little (eds), Tavistock, London
Hiro, Dilip (1973) *Black British, White British*, Penguin, London
Larbie, J. (1985) *Black Women and the Maternity Services*, National Extension College, Cambridge (out of print)
Larbie, J., Mares, P. and Baxter, C. (1987) *Trainer's Handbook for Multiracial Health Care*, National Extension College, Cambridge
Peach, C. (1968) *West Indian Migration to Britain*, Oxford University Press, Oxford
Sutcliffe, D. (1982) *British Black English*, Basil Blackwell, Oxford

32 TRADITIONAL CHINESE CULTURE

Au, Wing K. L. and Au, Kerrie P. K. Lin (1992) *Working with Chinese Carers*, Health Education Council/King's Fund Centre, London
Bloomsbury Health Authority (1984) *The Health Care Needs of Chinese People in Bloomsbury Health District: the Report of a Survey*, Bloomsbury Health Authority, London
Fong, L. C. and Watt, I. (1994) Chinese health behaviour: breaking barriers to better understanding. *Health Trends*, **26**(1), 14–15
Goodburn, P., Falshaw, M. and Hughes, H. (1987) Chinese food and diet. In *Food and Diet in a Multiracial Society*, National Extension College, Cambridge

Home Affairs Commitee (1985) *The Chinese Community in Britain* (HC 102–1), HMSO, London

Li, Pui-Ling (1992) Health needs of the Chinese population. In *The Politics of 'Race' and Health* (ed. W. I. U. Ahmad), Race Relations Research Unit, University of Bradford

Mares, Penny (1982) *The Vietnamese in Britain: a Handbook for Health Workers*, National Extension College, Cambridge

Neile, E. (1995) The maternity needs of the Chinese community. *Midwifery*, **91**(1), 34–5

Runnymede Trust (1986) *The Chinese Community in Britain: the Home Affairs Committee Report in Context*, Runnymede Trust, London

Shang, Anthony (1986) 'Seeds of Chinatown: the Chinese in Britain. In *Race and Social Work: a Guide to Training*, V. Coombe and A. Little (eds), Tavistock, London

33   TRADITIONAL SOMALI CULTURE

Home Office (1992) *Control of Immigration Statistics, United Kingdom 1992*, HMSO, London

Karmi, G. (ed.) (undated) *The Ethnic Fact File*, North West/North East Regional Health Authorities, London

Lem, I. M. (1994) Physical and social geography. In *Africa South of the Sahara 1994*, 23rd edn, Europa Publications, London

Northwick Park and St Marks NHS Trust (1994) *Somali Foods and Dietary Habits*, Department of Nutrition and Dietetics, Northwick Park Hospital, Harrow, Middlesex

Refugee Council (1994) *Somali Refugees in the UK/Somalia*, Factfile 5, Refugee Council, London

34   TRADITIONAL SOUTH ASIAN CULTURE

Ahmed, G. (1990) Family planning – religion and culture. *Maternity Action*, **43**, Jan./Feb., 8–9 (Maternity Alliance, London)

Ahmed, G. and Watt, S. (1986) Understanding Asian women in pregnancy and confinement. *Midwives Chronicle and Nursing Notes*, May, 98–101

Ahmet, L. (1990) A model for midwives – support for ethnic breast-feeding mothers. *Midwives Chronicle and Nursing Notes*, January, 5–7

Aitchison, C. (1994) By prior arrangement. *Independent*, 12 Feb, 47

Alibhai, Y. (1986) Can't they see I'm me? *Nursing Times*, 1 Jan, 56

Anwar, M. (1979) *The Myth of Return: Pakistanis in Great Britain*, Heinemann, London

Atherton, D. J. (1994) Towards the safer use of traditional remedies. *British Medical Journal*, **308**, 673–4

Attenburrow, A. A., Campbell, S., Logan, R. W. and Goel, K. M. (1980) Surma and blood levels in Asian children in Glasgow. *Lancet*, **1**, 323

Bahl, V. (1986) Breastfeeding and Asian mothers. *New Generation*, **5**(2), 34 (National Childbirth Trust)

Blanchet, T. (no date) *Women, Pollution and Marginality: Meanings and Rituals of Birth in Bangladesh*, University Press Ltd, Dhaka, Bangladesh

Boore, J. R. P. (1978) *Prescription for Recovery*, Royal College of Nursing, London

Bowler, I. (1993) Stereotypes of women of Asian descent in midwifery: some evidence. *Midwifery*, **9**, 7–16

Brown, C. (1984) *Black and White Britain: The Third PSI Survey*, Heinemann, London

CRE (1993) *The Sorrow in my Heart: Sixteen Asian Women Speak about Depression*, Commission for Racial Equality, London

D'Alessio, A. (1993) Culture clash. *Nursing Times*, **89**(38), 16–17

Gordon, P. and Klug, F. (1985) *British Immigration Control: a Brief Guide*, Runnymede Trust, London

Hayward, J. (1975) *Information – a Prescription Against Pain*, Royal College of Nursing, London

Healy, M. A. and Aslam, M. (1989) *The Asian Community – Medicines and Traditions*, Silver Link Publishing, UK

Mamdani, M. (1972) *The Myth of Population Control*, Monthly Review Press, USA

Moore, R. (1975) *Racism and Black Resistance in Britain*, Pluto Press, London

Narang, I. and Murphy, S. (1994) Assessment of the antenatal care for Asian women. *British Journal of Midwifery*, **2**(4), 169–73

Niven, C. (1992) *Psychological Care for Families Before, During and After Birth*, Butterworth-Heinemann, Oxford

Rose, E. J. B. (1969) *Colour and Citizenship*, Oxford University Press, Oxford

Sen, D. (1989) Asian culture and communications in midwifery. *Midwife, Health Visitor and Community Nurse*, **25**, 16–18

Tandon, Y. and Raphael, A. (1978) *The New Position of East African Asians: Problems of a Displaced Minority*, Minority Rights Group, London

Vadgama, K. (1982) *Indians in Britain*, Maddison Press

Woollett, A. and Dosanjh-Matwala, N. (1990) Postnatal care: the attitudes and experiences of Asian women in East London. *Midwifery*, **6**, 178–84

35 CHRISTIANITY

Catechism of the Catholic Church (1994) Geoffrey Chapman, London

Hornsby-Smith, M. P. (1991) *Roman Catholic Beliefs in England: Customary Catholicism and Transformations of Religious Authority*, Cambridge University Press, Cambridge

Keeley, R., English, D., Fackre, G. *et al.* (1982) *The Lion Handbook of Christian Belief*, Lion Publishing, Tring

The Ministerial Association General Conference of Seventh-Day Adventists (1988) *Seventh-Day Adventists Believe . . . A Biblical Exposition of Fundamental Doctrines*, MAGCSA, Washington

36 HINDUISM

Ahmed, G., and Watt, S. (1986) Understanding Asian women in pregnancy and confinement. *Midwives Chronicle and Nursing Notes*, May, 98–101

Henley, Alix (1983) *Caring for Hindus and their Families*, National Extension College, Cambridge

Jones, Meg (1991) A valued tradition. *Nursery World*, 19 December, 18–19

37 ISLAM

Ahmad, W. I. U. (1993) Making black people sick: 'race', ideology and health research. In *'Race' and Health in Contemporary Britain* (ed. W. I. U. Ahmad), Open University Press, Buckingham

Ahmad, W. I. U., (1994) Reflections on the consanguinity and birth outcome debate. *Journal of Public Health Medicine*, **16**(4), 423–8

Andrews, I. and McIntosh, V. (1992) *Respect for Religious and Cultural Beliefs*, Mount Vernon Hospital NHS Trust, Rickmansworth Road, Northwood, Middlesex

Anionwu, E. (1993) Sickle cell and thalassaemia: community experiences and official response, in *'Race' and Health in Contemporary Britain* (ed. W. I. U. Ahmad), Open University Press, Buckingham

Anwar, M. (1979) *The Myth of Return: Pakistanis in Great Britain*, Heinemann, London

Bignall, J. (1993) Family planning in Islam (letter). *Lancet*, **341**, 687

Bundey, S. and Alam, H. (1993) A five-year prospective study of the health of children of different ethnic groups, with particular reference to the effect of inbreeding. *European Journal of Human Genetics*, **1**, 206–19

Bundey, S., Alam, H., Kaur, A. *et al.* (1990) Race, consanguinity and social features in Birmingham babies: a basis for a prospective study. *Journal of Epidemiology and Community Health*, **44**(2), 130–5

Cross, J. H., Eminson, J. and Wharton, B. A. (1990) Ramadan and birth weight at full term in Asian Moslem pregnant women in Birmingham. *Archives of Disease in Childhood*, **65**, 1053–6

Dearden, A. (1983) *Arab women*, rev. edn, Minority Rights Group, London

Gatrad, A. R. (1994a) Medical implications of Islam for women and children. *Maternal and Child Health*, July, 225–7

Gatrad, A. R. (1994b) Muslim customs surrounding death, bereavement, postmortem examinations, and organ transplants. *British Medical Journal*, **309**, 521–3

Henley, Alix (1982) *Caring for Muslims and Their Families*, National Extension College, Cambridge

Islamic World League (undated) *Funeral Regulations in Islam*, Dar Al-kitab Al Masri, Cairo

Lancet (1991) Consanguinity and health (Editorial). *Lancet*, **338**, 85–6

McIntosh, V. and Andrews, I. (1992) *Patient's Charter Standard: Respect for Religious and Cultural Beliefs*, Mount Vernon Hospital, Rickmansworth Road, Northwood, Middlesex

Parsons, L., Macfarlane, A. and Golding, J. (1993) Pregnancy, birth and maternity care. In *'Race' and Health in Contemporary Britain* (ed. W. I. U. Ahmad), Open University Press, Buckingham

Proctor, S. R. and Smith, I. J. (1992) A reconsideration of the factors affecting birth outcome in Pakistani Muslim families in Britain. *Midwifery*, **8**, 76–81

Rashed, A. D. (1992) The fast of Ramadan. *British Medical Journal*, **304**, 521

Shami, S.A., Schmitt, L. H. and Bittles, A. H. (1989) Consanguinity-related prenatal and postnatal mortality of the populations of seven Pakistani Punjab cities. *Journal of Medical Genetics* **26**, 267–71

Townsend, P. and Davidson, N. (eds) (1988) The Black Report. In *Inequalities in Health*, Pelican, Harmondsworth

Zaidi, F. (1994) The maternity care of Muslim women. *Modern Midwife*, March, 8–10

38   JEHOVAH'S WITNESSES

Butler Sloss, Lord Justice (1992) Re T. *All England Law Reports*, **4**, 665

Kinmond S., Aitchison T. C., Holland B. M. *et al.* (1993) Umbilical cord clamping in preterm infants: A randomised trial. *British Medical Journal*, **306**, 172

Times Law Report (1993) *The Times*, 19 March

39   JUDAISM

Bash, D. M. (1980) Jewish religious practices related to childbearing. *Journal of Nurse-midwifery*, **25**(5), 39–42

Berkovits, D. (1992) *A Guide to Jewish Practice for Nurses and Medical Staff*, The Federation of Synagogues, 65 Watford Way, London

Feldman, D. M. (1968) *Birth Control in Jewish Law*, New York University Press, New York

Gold, M. (n.d.) *And Hannah Wept: Infertility and Adoption and the Jewish Couple*, Jewish Publication Society, Philadelphia, USA

Jakobovits, I. (1975) *Jewish Medical Ethics* Bloch Publishing, USA

Neuberger, J. (1987) *Caring for Dying People of Different Faiths*, Austen Cornish, London

Office of the Chief Rabbi (n.d.) *Stillbirth and Neonatal Death: a Guide for the Jewish Parent*, Office of the Chief Rabbi, Adler House, Tavistock Square, London

Pearl, C. and Brookes, R. (1975) *A Guide to Jewish Knowledge*, Jewish Chronicle Publications, London

Rosner, F. (1986) *Modern Medicine and Jewish Ethics*, Yeshiva University Press, New York

40   RASTAFARISM

Cashmore, E. (1979) *The Rastafarian Movement in England*, Allen and Unwin, London

Cashmore, E. (1984) *The Rastafarians*, Minority Rights Group, London

Coombe, V. (1986) Afro-Caribbean families in Britain (Appendix). In Coombe, V. and Little, A. (eds), *Race and Social Work: a Guide to Training*, Tavistock, London

41   SIKHISM

Henley, Alix (1983) *Caring for Sikhs and Their Families*, National Extension College, Cambridge

Singh, T., Singh, B.J., Singh, K. *et al.* (trans.) (1960) *Selections from the Sacred Writings of the Sikhs*, Allen and Unwin, London

Appendix I The population of Great Britain

The 1991 Census

The 1991 Census was the first British census to record ethnic group as opposed to country of birth. People were asked to classify themselves and were then placed in one of the following groups: White, Black Caribbean, Black African, Black Other, Indian, Pakistani, Bangladeshi, Chinese, Other Asian, and Other (Non-Asian). White includes people of Irish and other European descent. Black Other includes people of mixed race, and black people from areas other than the Caribbean and Africa. Other Asian includes Asian people of other than Chinese, Indian, Pakistani, Bangladeshi and Sri Lankan origin.

Black and minority ethnic groups in Great Britain

The 1991 Census showed that out of a population of almost 55 million people, just over 3 million people belong to minority ethnic groups (OPCS, 1993). This is 5.5 per cent of the total population of Great Britain (see Table A1). OPCS defines minority ethnic groups as all ethnic groups other than White. Northern Ireland is excluded because it runs separate censuses. Note that ethnic origin is not the same as birthplace.

Table A.1   The population of Great Britain by ethnic group

Ethnicity	*Number ('000)*	*% total population*
Black communities	891	1.6
African	212	0.4
African Caribbean	678	1.2
South Asian communities	1 480	2.7
Bangladeshi	163	0.3
Indian	840	1.5
Pakistani	477	0.9
Other minority groups		
Chinese	157	0.3
Asian	198	0.4
Various	290	0.5
All minorities	3 015	5.5
Majority communities	51 874	94.5

Source: *Multi-ethnic Britain: Facts and Trends*, Runnymede Trust, 1994, by permission.

The largest single minority ethnic group in Great Britain is Indian, making up 1.5 per cent of the total population. Taken together, the three groups identified by OPCS as Black (Black Caribbean, Black African and Black Other) make up 1.6 per cent of the total population.

In general, the minority ethnic population is concentrated in metropolitan and industrial areas, reflecting the fact that most immigration (excluding refugees) after the Second World War was of people coming to fill vacancies in the less attractive areas of British industry. Over a quarter of the population in nine London boroughs, in Slough and in Leicester belongs to minority ethnic groups.

Age ranges

In general, the minority ethnic population is younger than the white population. According to the Census, a third of the minority ethnic population is under 16, compared with a fifth of the white population. Only 3 per cent of the minority ethnic population is over 65, compared with 17 per cent of the white population. This reflects the large-scale immigration of young adults and their families for work in the 1950s and 1960s (OPCS, 1993).

Where people were born

Ninety-three per cent of the total population was born in the UK. This includes 96 per cent of the white group and 47 per cent of all minority ethnic groups.

The proportion of people born outside the UK varies between age groups. For example, almost one in ten people in the age group 30–44 was born outside the UK, reflecting large-scale immigration in the 1950s and early 1960s. Younger people are less likely to be immigrants. Only one out of every 30 people aged under 16 was born outside the UK.

People born overseas

Seven per cent of people now in the UK were born overseas. Of these:
- 45 per cent were born in the New Commonwealth (mainly in India, Pakistan, Bangladesh, the West Indies and Hong Kong).
- 16 per cent were born in the Irish Republic.
- 13 per cent were born in other countries of the European Community. (At the time of the 1991 Census, the European Community consisted of Belgium, Denmark, France, Germany, Greece, the Irish Republic, Italy, Luxembourg, the Netherlands, Spain, Portugal and the UK.)
- 5 per cent were born in the Old Commonwealth (Australia, New Zealand and Canada).

Age ranges of people born overseas

The proportion of different minority ethnic groups born overseas varies according to age:

- 70 per cent of Black Caribbean people aged between 30 and 44 were born overseas, but only 9 per cent of Black Caribbean people aged between 16 and 29.
- 95 per cent of Indian people aged between 30 and 44 were born overseas, but only 48 per cent of people aged between 16 and 29.
- In contrast, among the Bangladeshi group a higher proportion of all age groups were born overseas; 96 per cent of people aged between 30 and 44, 82 per cent of people aged between 16 and 29, and 44 per cent of children aged between 5 and 15. This reflects the much slower rate of family reunion in the Bangladeshi community.

• The Chinese and Black African groups also have a relatively high proportion of younger people born overseas. In the 16–29 age group 74 per cent of Chinese people and 60 per cent of Black Africans were born overseas. In the case of the Chinese group this probably reflects a high proportion of ethnic Chinese refugees from Vietnam.

REFERENCES AND FURTHER READING

OPCS (1993) *1991 Census: Ethnic Group and Country of Birth – Great Britain (CEN 91 TM EGCB)*, Office of Population Censuses and Surveys, London
Runnymede Trust (1994) *Multi-Ethnic Britain: Facts and Trends*, Runnymede Trust, London

Index

In order to avoid encouraging generalisations and stereotyping, this index refers mainly to Parts One to Four of the book. It is essential to understand the broad principles of providing care in a multiracial society before considering specific factors which may be relevant to some individuals of different cultural and religious groups. We have not given detailed individual references to Part Five, since it is important to read each of these chapters as a whole, not to pick out and use one or two 'facts' in isolation.

CRANFIELD
BATH